D1728683

Progress in Drug Research
Fortschritte der Arzneimittelforschung
Progrès des recherches pharmaceutiques
Vol. 37

Progress in Drug Research
Fortschritte der Arzneimittelforschung
Progrès des recherches pharmaceutiques
Vol. 37

Edited by / Herausgegeben von / Rédigé par
Ernst Jucker, Basel

Authors / Autoren / Auteurs
John A. Salmon and Lawrence G. Garland · Brian D. Hoyle and J. William
Costerton · Nikolaus Seiler · David Raeburn and Jan-Anders Karlsson
A. Polak and P. G. Hartman · Michel Rohmer, Philippe Bisseret and
Bertrand Sutter · Alfred Burger

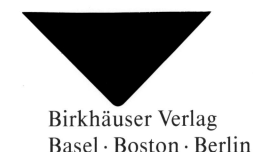

1991   Birkhäuser Verlag
Basel · Boston · Berlin

© 1991 Birkhäuser Verlag Basel
   P.O. Box 133
   4010 Basel
   Switzerland

Printed in Germany on acid-free paper

ISBN 3-7643-2626-3
ISBN 0-8176-2626-3

Contents · Inhalt · Sommaire

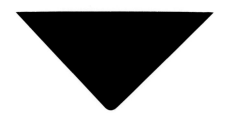

Foreword

Volume 37 of "Progress in Drug Research" contains seven articles and the various indexes which facilitate its use and establish the connection with the previous volumes. While all articles deal with some of the topical aspects of drug research, the contribution by Alfred Burger on "Isosterism and bioisosterism in drug design" is of great value to those researchers who are engaged in drug design and wish to include isosteric considerations in establishing a working hypothesis.

The remaining six reviews provide an overview of the work involved in the search for new and better medicines. All these articles contain surveys of the latest findings in the respective domain.

In the 31 years this series has existed, the Editor has enjoyed the help and advise of many colleagues. Readers, the authors of the individual reviews and, last but not least, the reviewers have all contributed greatly to the success of PDR. Although many comments received have been favorable, it is nevertheless also necessary to analyze and to reconsider the current position and the direction of such a series.

So far, it has been the Editor's intention to help spread information on the vast domain of drug research, and to provide the reader with a tool helping him or her to keep abreast of the latest developments and trends. The reviews in PDR are useful to the non-specialists who can obtain an overview of a particular field of research in a relatively short time. The specialist readers of PDR will appreciate the reviews' comprehensive bibliographies. Moreover, they may even get fresh impulses for their own studies. Finally, all readers interested in drug research can use the 37 volumes of PDR as an encyclopedic source of information.

It gives me great pleasure to present this new volume to our readers. At the same time, I would like to express my gratitude to Birkhäuser Verlag and, in particular, to Mrs. L. Koechlin and Mssrs. H.-P. Thür and A. Gomm. Without their personal commitment and assistance, editing PDR would be a nearly impossible task.

Basel, October 1991   Dr. E. JUCKER

Vorwort

Der vorliegende 37. Band der «Fortschritte der Arzneimittelforschung» enthält sieben Artikel sowie die verschiedenen Register, welche das Arbeiten mit dieser Reihe erleichtern.

Alle sieben Referate behandeln aktuelle Gebiete der pharmazeutischen Forschung und die umfangreiche Bibliographie vermittelt den Zugang zur Originalliteratur.

Besonders zu erwähnen ist der umfassende Artikel von Alfred Burger über die Rolle des Isosterismus in der Planung von Projekten der Arzneimittelforschung.

Seit der Gründung der Reihe sind 31 Jahre vergangen; in dieser langen Zeitspanne konnte der Herausgeber immer auf den Rat der Fachkollegen, der Leser und der Autoren zählen. Ihnen allen möchte ich meinen Dank abstatten. In diesem Dank sind auch die Rezensenten eingeschlossen, denn sie haben mit ihrer Kritik und mit ihren Vorschlägen wesentlich zum guten Gedeihen der Reihe beigetragen. Viele Kommentare und Besprechungen waren positiv und lobend. Trotzdem ist es angebracht, die Frage nach dem Sinn und Zweck der «Fortschritte» zu stellen und zu überprüfen.

Nach wie vor ist es unser Ziel, neueste Forschungsergebnisse in Form von Übersichten darzustellen und dem Leser auf diese Weise zu ermöglichen, sich verhältnismässig rasch und mühelos über bestimmte Gebiete und Richtungen zu informieren. Es wird ihm somit die Möglichkeit gegeben, sich im komplexen Gebiet der Arzneimittelforschung auf dem laufenden zu halten und den Kontakt zur aktuellen Forschung aufrecht zu erhalten.

Die Übersichten der «Fortschritte» bieten dem Spezialisten eine wertvolle Quelle der Originalliteratur dar, erlauben ihm nützliche Vergleichsmöglichkeiten und sie können u. U. seine eigene Forschung befruchten oder deren Richtung dem neuesten Stand anpassen.

Für alle Leser der «Fortschritte» stellt diese Reihe eine nicht zu vernachlässigende Quelle von enzyclopaedischem Wissen dar, so dass das gesamte Werk auch als Nachschlagewerk dienen kann.

Zum Gelingen dieses Werkes haben nicht zuletzt auch die Mitarbeiter des Birkhäuser Verlages, vor allem Frau L. Koechlin und die Herren H.-P. Thür und A. Gomm, wesentlich beigetragen; auch ihnen möchte ich an dieser Stelle meinen Dank aussprechen.

Basel, Oktober 1991 Dr. E. JUCKER

Leukotriene antagonists and inhibitors of leukotriene biosynthesis as potential therapeutic agents

By John A. Salmon and Lawrence G. Garland

The Wellcome Foundation, Langley Court, Beckenham, Kent BR3 3BS, England

1   **Introduction**

Arachidonic acid is converted by mammalian enzymes to a variety of oxygenated metabolites which include prostaglandins, thromboxanes and leukotrienes (collectively called *eicosanoids*). Many of these naturally occurring compounds have potent biological activities which suggest that they could be involved in mediating symptoms associated with various diseases (eg. allergic and inflammatory conditions). Thus, compounds which limit the effect of these mediators have therapeutic potential.

None of the eicosanoids are stored in tissues but are biosynthesized from the fatty acid upon appropriate stimulation of the cell (see Section 2). This implies that inhibitors of synthesis, as well as end organ antagonists, will decrease the magnitude of the biological responses mediated by eicosanoids. In this review, we will focus on the contribution of leukotrienes to disease processes and we shall describe the development of both leukotriene antagonists and inhibitors of leukotriene biosynthesis as potential new medicines. These new agents will also be invaluable experimental tools for establishing the pathophysiological roles of the leukotrienes.

2   **Biosynthesis of eicosanoids**
2.1   General metabolic pathways

The most important classes of prostaglandins and leukotrienes are formed from arachidonic acid. The amount of free fatty acid within cells is very low but there is a comparatively large amount esterified in phospholipids and glycerides. Therefore, the initial and rate limiting step in the biosynthesis of most eicosanoids is the enzymic liberation of free arachidonic acid from the ester pools. Arachidonic acid is located predominantly at the 2-acyl position of phospholipids, and its release occurs by hydrolysis which is catalysed either by phospholipase A_2 (PLA_2) or the combined action of phospholipase C (PLC) and a diglyceride lipase on phosphatidylinositol [1.2.3].

Until recently, research on arachidonic acid metabolism had mainly focussed on the prostaglandins and the closely related compounds, prostacyclin and thromboxanes. The initial reaction in the formation of all of these compounds from arachidonic acid involves a specific oxidation controlled by the fatty acid *cyclo-oxygenase* (or *prostaglan-*

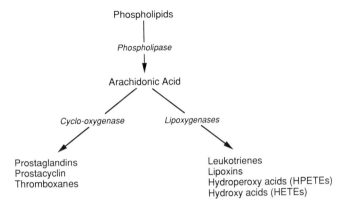

Figure 1
General pathways of arachidonic acid metabolism.

din synthase). The cyclo-oxygenase (CO) enzyme is inhibited by aspirin and other non-steroid anti-inflammatory drugs (NSAIDs), and this is believed to be the mechanism of the anti-inflammatory activity of this class of therapeutic agent [4,5]. Also, some side effects, such as the tendency for the formation of gastric ulcers, are probably related to the inhibition of the CO.

Other biologically active compounds are formed from arachidonic acid under the influence of different enzymes (see Fig. 1): the roles of lipoxygenases, and, in particular the 5-lipoxygenase (5-LO), are important. Arachidonic acid is converted into hydroperoxy derivatives (hydroperoxy-eicosatetraenoic acids; HPETEs) which are readily reduced to the corresponding hydroxy acids (HETEs) by glutathione peroxidase. There are several lipoxygenases in both the animal and plant kingdoms which catalyse the oxidation by molecular oxygen of *cis,cis-1,4*-pentadiene systems. Thus, arachidonic acid can be metabolized by these enzymes to several HPETE regio-isomers. Unlike the CO which acts comparatively specifically on arachidonic acid [6], lipoxygenases can efficiently catalyse oxidation of some other fatty acid substrates (e.g. eicosatrienoic and eicosapentaenoic acids) [7, 8]. The first lipoxygenation of arachidonic acid in mammalian tissues to be described was that occurring in blood platelets which resulted in the formation of 12-HPETE [8, 9]. However, another hydroperoxy derivative, 5-HPETE, is of more interest since it can be converted to a novel series of biologically active compounds known as leukotrienes (see Section 2.2). The leukotrienes (LT) were so named because they were described initially as products of arachidonic acid metabolism in leucocytes and they contain a conjugated triene system in their structure. As with the prostaglandins and thromboxanes, the leukotrienes are divided into groups (A–F) according to major structural differences and into sub-groups according to the number of double bonds in the side chains.

The first report of 5-LO activity was in polymorphonuclear leucocytes PMN [10]. Whereas the CO is widely distributed in mammalian cells, the 5 LO is restricted mainly to neutrophils, eosinophils, monocytes, macrophages and mast cells. These cells originate in the bone marrow and probably derive from the same stem cell. Also, these classes of cell are considered to be "inflammatory cells" and this suggests that products of the 5-LO could be involved in inflammatory responses (see Section 3.1).

Another difference between the CO and 5-LO is that the latter enzyme has to be activated selectively by a mechanism which involves calcium (eg. the calcium ionophore calcimycin [A 23 187] potently and selectively stimulates the synthesis of 5-LO products). However, the CO appears to be active constitutively and only requires free acid substrate for the reaction to occur. Also, unlike CO, 5-LO can use arachidonic acid directly from phospholipid pools [11,12]. The properties and activity of 5-LO are considered in more detail in Section 2.3.

2.2   Biosynthesis and metabolism of leukotrienes

The initial enzymic reaction in the conversion of 5-HPETE to leukotrienes is the loss of water to form the unstable 5,6-epoxide leukotriene A_4 (LTA$_4$; Fig. 2) [13]. As with the endoperoxides in the synthesis of prostaglandins, LTA$_4$ is pivotal in the formation of other leukotrienes. It is hydrolysed to 5(S),12(R)-dihydroxy-6,14-cis-8,10-$trans$-eicosatetraenoic acid (LTB$_4$; see Fig. 2) [14] under the influence of LTA$_4$-hydrolase which has been purified partially [15,16]. Also, LTA$_4$ can be hydrolysed non-enzymically to other 5,12- and 5,6-dihydroxy acids [13]. Additionally, glutathione can react with LTA$_4$ under the influence of a specific glutathione-S-transferase to form the 5-hydroxy-6-glutathionyl derivative (LTC$_4$; [17]) which can be metabolized successively by γ-glutamyl-transpeptidase and cysteinyl-glycine dipeptidase to LTD$_4$ [18,19] and LTE$_4$, respectively (see Fig. 2). Another leukotriene, LTF$_4$, has been identified as having cysteine-glutamate at C-6

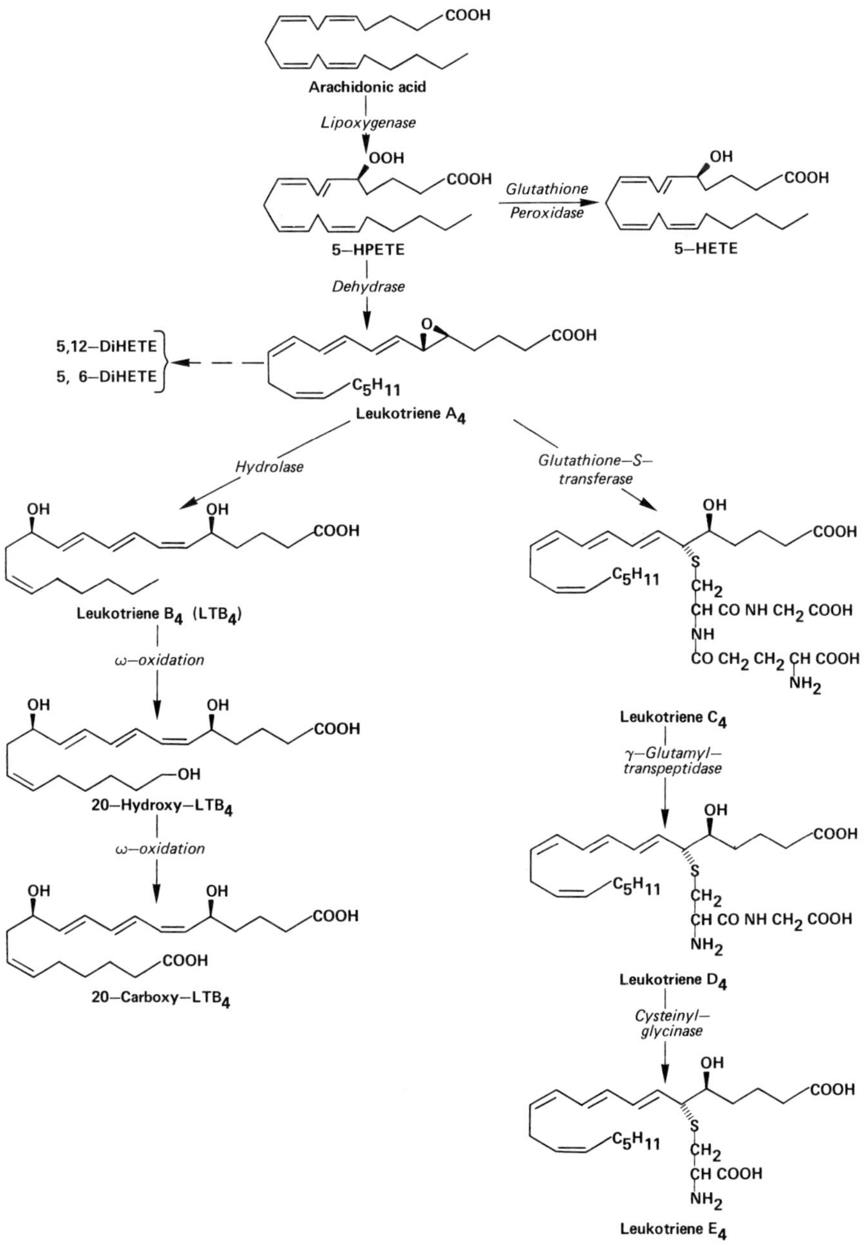

Figure 2
Metabolism of arachidonic acid by 5-lipoxygenase and the subsequent reactions to produce leukotrienes.

[20,21]. These peptido-lipid leukotrienes are now known to be the major constituents of a putative mediator which was referred to by pharmacologists as the "slow reacting substance of anaphylaxis" (SRS-A; [22]; see Section 3.2).

As with the prostaglandins, different leukotrienes are formed in specific cell-types. Thus, human eosinophils and neutrophils synthesize predominantly LTC_4 and LTB_4, respectively [23]; reports of the synthesis of either product by the other cell type probably reflects an impure preparation of cells. Monocytes and macrophages are able to synthesize both LTB_4 and the peptido-lipid leukotrienes [24].

As mentioned above, LTC_4 can be metabolized to LTD_4 and LTE_4 by the same cell in which it is formed; LTC_4 and the other peptido-lipid leukotrienes can also be transformed into 6-*trans*-LTB_4 by hypochlorous acid which is generated during the stimulated respiratory burst in leucocytes [25,26].

After intravenous administration, [³H]-LTC_4 is eliminated rapidly. In rats more than 50% of the radioactivity is excreted in the bile suggesting that there is an effective uptake mechanism in the liver [27,28]. However, negligible amounts of unchanged [³H]LTC_4 were recovered in bile; major metabolites were LTD_4, LTE_4, N-acetyl-11-*trans*-LTE_4, and N-acetyl-LTE_4 [27,29–32]. More polar metabolites were later identified as 20-carboxy-N-acetyl LTE_4, 18-carboxy-N-acetyl LTE_4 and 16-carboxy 14,15-dihydro-N-acetyl LTE_4 [33–35]. These metabolites are also formed during incubations of LTE_4 with rat hepatocytes and hepatic microsomes [36–38]. However, in species other than the rat, N-acetylation is not a major route of metabolism of the peptido-lipid leukotrienes: the major metabolite excreted by man is LTE_4 [39]. As will be discussed later (Section 6.1.4), the excretion of LTE_4 in the urine offers the opportunity of monitoring leukotriene synthesis non-invasively in human subjects during asthmatic attacks.

Leukotriene B_4 is also metabolized further by the cells in which it is biosynthesized; a unique membrane-bound cytochrome P_{450} enzyme converts it to 20-hydroxy-LTB_4 [40–43] and this can be further oxidised by a different, soluble enzyme to 20-carboxy-LTB_4 [40]. There is also evidence for a reductase/dehydrogenase in PMN which appears to be fairly specific for LTB_4 [44].

Thus, several enzymes are involved in the biosynthesis of leukotrienes and could be considered as targets for the design of novel therapeutic agents to reduce the formation of leukotrienes. However, as the 5-LO is the initial enzyme in the metabolic cascade its inhibition will cause a reduction in the generation of all leukotrienes. It is not, therefore, surprising that most effort has been directed to the design and development of 5-LO inhibitors. Consequently the properties and activity of 5-LO are considered in more detail below (Section 2.3).

For further information about the biosynthesis and metabolism of leukotrienes readers are referred to other reviews [45–48].

2.3   Properties of the 5-lipoxygenase enzyme

The 5-LO (*arachidonate: oxygen 5-oxidoreductase*, EC1.13.11.34) is an unstable and complex enzyme, and, therefore its complete characterisation has presented many biochemical challenges. It is believed to be a soluble enzyme but its precise intracellular location is uncertain. It was first purified from potatoes [49] but, importantly, it has now been isolated from mammalian sources. It was purified to homogeneity from the 20 000 × g supernatant of sonicated rat basophilic leukaemia (RBL-1) cells [50,51] primarily through the use of anion-exchange HPLC. Purification of the enzyme from human and porcine PMN and from mouse mastocytoma cells has also been accomplished [52–54]. The purified enzyme has a molecular weight of 73–76 kDa. When incubated with arachidonic acid the only enzymatic product formed under the conditions described by Goetze *et al.* [50] was 5-HPETE; this reaction exhibited a lag phase and premature cessation, which is also a characteristic property of the transformation using crude homogenates of cells as source of enzyme. The enzyme isolated by Hogaboom *et al.* [51] converted arachidonic acid to di-HETEs in addition to 5-HPETE. These di-HETEs were the non-enzymatic hydrolysis products of LTA_4 (ie 6-*trans*-LTB_4 and 12-epi-6-*trans*-LTB_4). The enzyme was also able to convert 5-HPETE to the same di-HETEs. Thus, these data provided evidence that 5-LO and LTA_4-synthase activities reside on a single monomeric protein.

The activity of the enzyme is dependent on the presence of both Ca^{2+} and ATP [51,55,56]. Full activation of 5-LO requires a Ca^{2+}-dependent translocation of the enzyme from the cytosol to a membrane-bound site [57,58]. Other studies have also shown that for maximum activity the human enzyme requires the presence of at least three non-dialysable factors – two cytosolic and one membrane associated (see below).

cDNA clones for human arachidonate 5-LO have been isolated [59,60]. Also, the cDNA clone for the rat enzyme was obtained [61]. A direct comparison of rat and human protein sequences shows that the 5-LO is remarkably well conserved between species: the two homologues show 93% identity.

As mentioned above, non-dialysable factors are required for optimal activity of the 5-LO. One such factor has been isolated recently from rat and human leucocytes and has been termed 'five-lipoxygenase-activating protein' (FLAP) [62,63]. The presence of FLAP was first proposed to explain the activity of a unique class of leukotriene inhibitor exemplified by MK-886 (see Section 6.2.4). MK-886 inhibits cellular leukotriene biosynthesis but fails to reduce soluble 5-LO activity. Evidence was obtained which indicated that MK-886 interacts with FLAP. It is uncertain how exactly FLAP contributes to 5-LO activity but it was postulated that it could play an essential part in the transfer of arachidonic acid to 5-LO [62]. Although 5-LO does not require free arachidonic acid as a substrate it is conceivable that lipase activity is needed to facilitate the biotransformation to 5-HPETE. However, it appears that FLAP is not a lipase (see [62]). Because translocation of 5-LO from the cell cytosol to the membrane is required for activity it was also suggested that FLAP could be a membrane anchor for activated 5-LO.

The experiments described by Miller et al. [62] and Dixon et al. [63] clearly demonstrate that the expression of FLAP, together with 5-LO, is essential for cellular leukotriene synthesis. Thus, FLAP, and possibly similar key proteins, offers a target for the design of specific inhibitors of lipoxygenases (see Section 6.2.4).

There are similarities between the enzymic reactions controlled by the CO and LO; each reaction is initiated by abstraction of hydrogen followed by the introduction of molecular oxygen. Thus, some anti-oxidants do inhibit both reactions (eg. BW755C, phenidone; see Section 6.2.2). However, there are important differences between the enzymes which suggests that it will be possible to develop specific inhibitors of each of the enzymes. Thus, the CO, which is present in the "microsomal" fraction of most cells, is a homodimer of molecular weight 70 kDa. The mammalian LOs are present in the cell cytosol and are monomers of molecular weight 75–100 kDa. A key difference between the two classes of enzyme is that the CO contains haem (one mole per sub-unit) but although the mammalian LOs are believed to

contain iron it is not present as haem; it has been difficult to demonstrate the presence of iron in the enzyme because it is believed to be tightly bound and this provides an explanation for why simple iron chelators do not inhibit enzymic activity. Investigation of the 5-LO protein has revealed a sequence which is reminiscent of the cysteine- or histidine-rich putative metal binding domains found in many proteins. Although metal binding has not been established for 5–LO it has been demonstrated in the 15-LO of rabbit reticulocytes (see [64]).
The recent advances made on the structure of the enzyme, its regulation and mechanism of action (see [65–67] for reviews) may provide the basis for the design of specific inhibitors of 5-LO. However, the current range of inhibitors have been obtained by a more pragmatic approach (see Section 6).

2.4 Other lipoxygenases

The major pathway of arachidonic acid metabolism in blood platelets is via 12-LO but the biological role(s) of 12-HPETE and its reduced derivative 12-HETE is uncertain. There are suggestions that 12-LO products maybe involved in pathological conditions (see 3.3) and, therefore, inhibition of this pathway could be a future therapeutic target. Molecular cloning, primary structure and expression of the human platelet, erythroleukaemia and porcine leucocyte 12-LO have been described [68,69]. Apparently, the enzyme has no cofactor requirement. Two types of 12-LO were found in mammalian tissues: one in platelets and the other in leucocytes [68].
The 12-LO in platelets produces 12(S)-HPETE/HETE. However, Woollard [70] found that the 12-HETE extracted from human psoriatic scale was in fact the 12(R)-enantiomer. Importantly, it was demonstrated that 12(R)-HETE was more potent biologically than the S-enantiomer; for example, it was much more active as a chemotactic agent for human PMN [71] and as an aggregating agent for rat leucocytes [72]. As LTB$_4$ contains a 12(R)-hydroxy group it was proposed that 12(R)-HETE acted on the LTB$_4$ receptor and indeed it has been shown that 12(R)-HETE competitively displaces [^{3}H]-LTB$_4$ bound to human leucocyte membranes [72]. Thus, the formation of 12(R)-HETE in psoriasis may be important in the pathogenesis of the disease. Consequently, inhibition of 12(R)-HETE could be useful therapeutically. However, the mechanism of the formation of

12(R)-HETE is unclear. As Humes and Opas [73] suggested it could be formed via (i) a 12-LO which is different to that producing 12(S)-HETE (ii) cytochrome P_{450} catalysed oxygenations (iii) coupled oxidation and reduction (iv) isomerization and (v) auto/photo oxidation of arachidonic acid. 12(R)-HETE can be formed by P_{450} dependent enzymes [74–77] but there is evidence that this mechanism is not responsible for the 12 (R)-HETE formed in the skin [73,78]. A possible explanation is that arachidonic acid could be auto-oxidised in the presence of molecular oxygen and ultraviolet radiation to racemic 12-HETE and the 12(S)-enantiomer is esterified preferentially into cellular phospholipids and triglycerides.

The exact roles of 15-HPETE and 15-HETE also have not been defined although there is some evidence that they could be involved in mediating some symptoms of the asthmatic response; the 15-LO pathway is the predominant route of arachidonic metabolism in human lung homogenates [79,80]. The products of 15-LO activity may be further metabolized to the lipoxins which may have other pathophysiological roles (see Section 2.6). The human 15-LO has been purified to homogeneity from eosinophil-enriched leucocytes [81]. There appears to be a high degree of homology between 15-LO and 12-LO; for example, porcine 12-LO exhibited 86% homology to human reticulocyte 15-LO [81] and it is known that the catalytic properties of the two enzymes are very similar.

2.5   Other enzymes involved in leukotriene biosynthesis

As noted earlier the 5-LO is capable of converting arachidonic acid not only to 5-HPETE but also to the unstable epoxide LTA_4. LTA_4-hydrolase, which controls the specific hydrolysis of LTA_4 to LTB_4, has been purified from leucocytes and erythrocytes [15,82], from lung [83] and liver tissue [84]. Interestingly the cDNA sequence for LTA_4-hydrolase shows no significant homology with the sequences for any other enzyme including those of rabbit and rat liver microsomal epoxide hydrolases [85]. As is the case with several of the enzymic reactions involved in the biosynthesis of leukotrienes, the conversion of LTA_4 to LTB_4 exhibits a "suicide-type" inactivation of the enzyme [82,83].

LTC_4-synthase, which conjugates LTA_4 with reduced glutathione to form LTC_4, has been purified from sensitized guinea-pig lung tissue [86]. Specific elution of the enzyme from an affinity column yielded a preparation showing two bands each of molecular weight of 17 kDa; it is uncertain if these products represent two sub-units of the same enzyme, isozymes of LTC_4-synthase or two unrelated proteins. There is evidence that LTC_4-synthase is a novel member of the family of microsomal GSH-S-transferases. Within the leucocytes, LTC_4-synthase was found predominantly in eosinophils, to a far lesser extent in monocytes and was not present in PMN [87].

2.6   Biosynthesis of other eicosanoids

Metabolites of arachidonic acid, in addition to those described above, have been reported. Bioactive compounds are formed by the combined action of two lipoxygenase enzymes and hence the term *lipoxin* (lipoxygenase interaction product) was introduced. Two main lipoxins are formed from arachidonic acid, and these are referred to as lipoxin A (LXA_4) and lipoxin B (LXB_4), both contain a conjugated tetraene in their structure [88,89]. These compounds exhibit a variety of biological activities (see [90–94]). There is evidence that LXA_4 competes for LTD_4 binding and antagonises the actions of LTD_4 on glomeruli [95] which suggests potential counter-regulatory interaction between leukotrienes and lipoxins. However, since there is no convincing evidence, as yet, that lipoxins are mediators of pathophysiological events they will not be considered further in this review.
Isomeric trihydroxyeicosatetraenoic acids (THETAs) and epoxy-hydroxyeicosatetraenoic acis (EPHETAs) can also be formed. Usually these metabolites are derived from a LO reaction and non-enzymic degradation of the initial hydroperoxy product (eg. [96]) or via a cytochrome P_{450} enzyme [97,98] (see [99] for review) to THETA and EPHETA. Pace-Asciak [100] introduced the term hepoxilins to describe a group of biologically active but short-lived hydroxyepoxides (e. g. hepoxilin A_3 and hepoxilin B_3). Since the formation of these metabolites has not been demonstrated *in vivo* it is unclear if they are pathophysiologically important.

3   **Lipoxygenase products in disease**
3.1   Role of lipoxygenase products in inflammation

Inflammation is a complex response involving several cell-types (e. g. polymorphonuclear leucocytes [PMNs], macrophages, lymphocytes and mast cells) and the participation of many putative mediators and modulators have been implicated (e.g. histamine, 5-hydroxytryptamine, kinins, chemotactic peptides, interleukins, interferons, prostaglandins, thromboxanes and leukotrienes). These mediators act in concert to amplify the inflammatory response which is characterised by erythema, oedema, hyperthemia, hyperalgesia, cell influx and loss of function. For example, (i) the pain induced by bradykinin is increased by prostaglandins [101] (see [102] for review), and (ii) oedema is potentiated if a chemotactic principle (e.g. the complement fragment C_{5a} or LTB_4) is present together with a vasodilator substance [103]. Since there is probably "mediator redundancy", it may seem unlikely that either inhibition of synthesis or antagonism of the response of one group of mediators could provide significant benefit. However, there is persuasive evidence that inhibition of arachidonic acid metabolism can give important anti-inflammatory effects. The evidence that CO products are important mediators of some cardinal signs of inflammation (e.g. erythema, oedema, hyperalgesia and hyperthermia) is substantial; prostaglandins have been detected in inflammatory exudate at biologically active concentrations [5,102,104], and the CO is selectively inhibited by non-steroid anti-inflammatory drugs (NSAIDs).

Although administration of NSAIDs remains the most successful therapy to reduce symptoms of inflammation, there is a need for new initiatives, especially in the treatment of chronic inflammation. The value of NSAIDs in chronic inflammatory disease is limited since they do not reduce tissue damage. Some NSAIDs potentiate leucocyte influx into inflammatory exudates in an animal model [105] suggesting that this class of compound could indirectly exacerbate tissue damage: this is also indicated in clinical situations (e.g. [106]). As in the treatment of inflammation, the administration of NSAIDs can be deleterious for asthmatics; for example, aspirin can precipitate an asthmatic attack in some subjects which could be explained by diversion of arachidonic acid metabolism to 5-LO products (see [107] and section 3.2).

The inflammatory response is characterised by cell infiltration and the invading cells contribute to the pathological events by releasing enzymes and toxic oxygen radicals. For example, phagocytosis of immune complexes by PMNs in the rheumatoid arthritic joint can result in the release of mediators which sustain the inflammation and as a result the synovium is stimulated to proliferate as granuloma tissue or "pannus" which eventually spreads over the adjacent cartilage [108]. Thus, by-products of the phagocytic process, such as lysosomal pro-teases and reactive oxygen species, are brought into intimate contact with articular cartilage which is gradually destroyed [109]. Depending on the duration and severity of the disease, areas of cartilage may be completely lost and the underlying bone eroded by a similar process. Once this stage has been reached there is significant disability and irreversible joint damage has occurred [108]. Therefore, endogenous mediators which increase cellular infiltration may play a crucial role in the inflammatory process.

The mono-substituted 5-LO products are weak chemokinetic and che-motactic agents *in vitro* and *in vivo* for human and rabbit neutrophils [110]. However, LTB$_4$ has more powerful effects on PMN function; it is a potent chemokinetic and chemotactic agent for PMNs of several species *in vitro* and causes PMN accumulation *in vivo* (for a review see [111]). It also causes degranulation of PMNs but at higher concentra-tions than those which induce chemotaxis [112]. In the presence of a vasodilator prostaglandin (e.g. PGE$_2$) LTB$_4$ also increases plasma ex-udation [103,113,114] which is probably mediated by its effects on PMNs [103]. Other chemoattractants such as the complement frag-ment C$_{5a}$ and the synthetic peptide f-Met-Leu-Phe (FMLP) exhibit si-milar indirect activity on plasma exudation [103]. The actions of LTB$_4$ on PMNs are stereospecific and are not shared by other leukotrienes [114–117], and receptors on PMNs for LTB$_4$ have been demonstrated which are distinct from those for C$_{5a}$ and FMLP [118,119]. Clearly LTB$_4$ fulfils the first of the classic criteria used to define a mediator; i.e. (i) it possesses the appropriate biological activity at relevant con-centrations. Additional criteria as modified from those suggested by Sir Henry Dale are: (ii) the mediator must be recoverable from sites of inflammation, (iii) the mediator should be identified by various phar-macological and physicochemical tests, (iv) antagonists of the action or inhibitors of the release of the suspected mediator must reduce the inflammatory response thought to be due to that substance, and (v) in-hibition of the destruction (metabolism) of the suspected mediator should increase the magnitude and duration of the inflammatory re-sponse attributable to the substance.

The second and third criteria were satisfied in an animal model of in-flammation. LTB$_4$ was detected by specific radioimmunoassay (RIA) in inflammatory exudates produced by the subcutaneous implantation in rats of 0.5% carrageenin-soaked polyester sponges [120]. LTB_4 was not detected up to 2 h post implantation but then the concentration increased and reached a maximum 6 h after implantation; thereafter the level declined and was undetectable after 16–24 h. The peak of LTB_4 concentration correlated with the maximum rate of PMN influx into the exudate. The presence of LTB_4 was confirmed by high-pressure liquid chromatography (HPLC) of the exudate; peaks of immunoreactivity and UV absorbance (at 270 nm) eluted at the same retention time as authentic LTB_4. Additionally the material eluting at the retention time of authentic LTB_4 caused aggregation of rat PMNs *in vitro* indicating that the concentrations attained were biologically relevant. In experiments in which the animals were pre-dosed with colchicine (1 mg/kg), the concentration of LTB_4 in the exudate as well as the PMN count, was decreased. These findings suggest that the PMNs were the source of LTB_4 and probably, therefore, LTB_4 is not the initial signal for PMN infiltration, but may contribute to an amplification of the response.

Experiments using zymosan as well as carrageenin-soaked sponges have confirmed the above findings [121]. Others [122] have reported that monosodium urate crystals injected into a subcutaneous air pouch in the rat, induce an inflammatory response which is characterised by PMN accumulation, plasma leakage and increased levels of LTB_4, as well as PGE_2, 6-keto-$PGF_{1\alpha}$ and TXB_2 in the exudate.

Using animal models, LO products have also been implicated as mediators of inflammatory responses in the gastro-intestinal tract. There are no totally satisfactory animal models of human inflammatory bowel disease (IBD) but there are some which enable the investigation of the possible role of particular inflammatory cells and mediators (see [123]). One approach has been to measure the concentration of eicosanoids attained during rectal dialysis in animals in which colonic inflammation has been induced [124]; a similar type of study can be performed in man [125–127] (see section 6.1.4). There is a close relationship between the increased formation of LTB_4 and neutrophil infiltration into the colon in a variety of animal models of colitis. However, it is not certain whether the elevated levels of LTB_4 are a cause or a consequence of the influx of neutrophils. The availability of selective antagonists and/or inhibitors of synthesis will help answer this question and thereby assist in defining the precise role of leukotrienes in this and other inflammatory responses.

Raised concentrations of leukotrienes have also been detected in clinical conditions. Synovial fluids from patients with rheumatoid arthritis [128,129] and gout [130] contain elevated levels of LTB_4. Also, higher than normal concentrations of LTB_4 occur in buffer in contact with involved skin of psoriatic patients [131] and in blister fluid from patients with atopic dermatitis as well as psoriasis [132]. Intestinal mucosa obtained during surgical resection from patients suffering from IBD produces higher concentrations of 5-LO metabolites and other eicosanoids *in vitro* [133,134]. There is also *in vivo* evidence for enhanced production of LTB_4 in ulcerative colitis [126]. Thus, the above data suggest that LTB_4 could be an important mediator of leucocyte influx at sites of inflammation.

The peptido-lipid leukotrienes (LTC_4, LTD_4 and LTE_4) are biosynthesized in inflammatory cells (eg. macrophages, eosinophils) and there is some evidence that they are formed in increased amounts at inflammatory sites [135] and they do have pro-inflammatory activity. They cause dilatation of post capillary venules which leads to plasma extravasation; for example, in the skin they produce wheal and flare responses [136,137] and increase vascular permeability [138,139]. Thus, these leukotrienes could modulate the vascular responses occurring in inflammation but, since they do not have chemotactic activity, they are unlikely to affect the cellular phase.

Mono-hydroperoxy/hydroxy derivatives of arachidonic acid may also play a part in inflammatory reactions. For example, the generation of 12(R)-HETE by involved psoriatic skin may be of pathological relevance (see 2.4). Also, 15-HPETE and its possible metabolite 8(R)15(S)-diHETE potently stimulate hyperalgesia [140,141] which is a characteristic symptom of inflammation.

3.2   Role of lipoxygenase products in asthma

Although peptido-lipid leukotrienes may be involved in inflammation, most interest is directed to their role as putative mediators of the bronchoconstriction occurring in asthma and similar hypersensitivity reactions. They are major components of the bronchoconstricting activity of anaphylactic origin which was described 50 years ago [142]. Pharmacologists referred to this activity as the "slow-reacting substance of anaphylaxis" (SRS-A; [22]) because it caused slowly developing and prolonged contraction of bronchial smooth muscle. (For reviews of the biological activity of SRS-A, see [143,144]). Subsequently elucidation of the structures of the major components of SRS-A [145–148] revealed that these were also metabolites of arachidonic acid formed via 5-LO activity. These leukotrienes are released from human lung by immunological and non-immunological stimuli, and their pharmacological properties include many of the pathophysiological features of asthma (see [24,149–153]). Peptido-lipid leukotrienes are potent bronchoconstrictor substances [149] being three orders of magnitude more active than histamine on a molar basis. In addition they increase the production of mucus, impair mucociliary clearance and cause oedema because of their effects on airway vascular permeability [154–158].

When stimulated with the calcium ionophore A 23187, leucocytes from asthmatics generate more LTB_4 and LTC_4 than cells from non-asthmatics [159]. This difference was not associated with a greater total number of leucocytes nor with a change in the differential cell count in the blood of asthmatics compared to normal subjects [159]. Therefore, it appears that leucocytes from asthmatics are more responsive to A 23187 than cells from normal subjects.

Increased synthesis of peptido-lipid leukotrienes during asthmatic attacks in humans has been established by measurement of urinary LTE_4 [160]. In these studies urinary LTE_4 was determined by radioimmunoassay after extraction and purification by HPLC. Urinary LTE_4 was significantly higher after antigen challenge of atopic subjects than in controls (154 vs 24 ng LTE_4/nmol creatinine). Mean urinary LTE_4 was also higher in asthmatic patients (78 ng LTE_4/nmol creatinine) than in normal subjects but levels of LTE_4 in the urine of patients with rhinitis were within the normal range. However, the authors did comment that the data should be treated with some caution because all the patients were on combination therapy including corticosteroids, $\beta 2$ agonists, anticholinergic bronchodilators and, in some cases, methylxanthine derivatives: it is possible that such drugs may affect leukotriene biosynthesis, metabolism or urinary excretion. Later studies [161] showed that, whereas elevated levels of LTE_4 were excreted during the acute phase, no significant increase occurred during the late response. These data suggest that peptido-lipid leukotrienes may mediate early asthmatic responses but may not be involved in the late phase bronchospasm.

The presence of leukotriene-like biological activity has been reported in bronchoalveolar lavage (BAL) fluid from chronic asthmatics [162,163] although others did not detect elevated levels [164]. Leukotrienes have been detected in the sputum from patients with asthma and other respiratory disorders [165–167]. Also, leukotrienes are released into nasal washings and plasma after allergen challenge [168,169]. Leukotrienes were detected in plasma of a few patients with acute, severe asthma [170,171].

There is also evidence that LTB_4 could mediate the "late-phase" bronchopulmonary eosinophilia that occurs 6–24 h after inhalation of specific antigen. For example, the LTB_4-receptor antagonist, U-75302 (see 5.2) inhibits antigen-induced influx of eosinophils into the bronchial lumen in guinea-pigs although the number of neutrophils was not affected [172]. Increased levels of LTB_4 have been detected by HPLC and mass spectrometry in BAL from a patient with chronic pulmonary disease [173].

Products derived from the 15-LO pathway may also play a role in hypersensitivity reactions. It has been reported that *in vitro* 15-LO activity is increased in asthmatic lung [79,80] and increased levels of 15-HETE have been detected in BAL from atopic patients after local antigen challenge [164].

At the present time, asthma affects approximately 5% of the population in industrialized countries and there is evidence that both the prevalence and severity of the disease is rising despite the increased use of anti-asthma drugs. This implies that the current therapy is inadequate. As discussed above there is good evidence that the leukotrienes are mediators of asthmatic responses. Thus, pharmacological intervention of the actions of leukotrienes in the airways, which could be achieved by antagonism or inhibition of their biosynthesis, offers exciting potential for the development of new anti-asthmatic medicines. In this review, attention will be focussed on the progress of LTD_4 antagonists and inhibitors of 5-LO. However, other possibilities will be considered briefly.

3.3   Role of lipoxygenase products in other diseases

Although, the biological roles of products of 12-LO action have not been elucidated it is interesting to note that 12-HETE stimulates tumour cell adhesion to endothelial cells, subendothelial matrix and fibronectin and, therefore, it could play a part in tumour cell metastasis (see [174]). Also the 12-LO enzyme is present in nervous tissue and it has been suggested that 12-HPETE and its derivatives, as well as other lipoxygenase products, could be second messengers, possibly involved in the modulation of neurotransmitter release (see [175]).

Peptido-lipid leukotrienes are formed by brain tissue and increased synthesis occurs under various pathophysiological conditions such as ischaemic insult, concussive injury, subarachnoid haemorrhage and seizures in gerbils (see [176,177]). Therefore, it is possible that leukotrienes are involved in the pathogenesis of some brain disorders.

Elevated concentrations of leukotrienes are produced during experimental endotoxaemia and they may contribute to some of the deleterious sequelae associated with shock [178]. Indeed, several peptido-lipid leukotriene antagonists (see 5.1.2) and 5-LO inhibitors (see Section 6), significantly attenuate endotoxin-induced thrombocytopaenia and haemoconcentration [179–184].

There is preliminary data suggesting that peptido-lipid leukotrienes may mediate some symptoms of glomerular nephritis; an LTD_4-antagonist, SK & F 104353 (see 5.1.2) abrogated the reduction in glomerular ultrafiltration rate in nephritis in the rat [185].

Peptido-lipid leukotrienes have been implicated as mediators of cardiac anaphylaxis and may be involved in the resulting vasoconstriction and myocardial depression [186–188]. Some investigators have suggested that peptido-lipid leukotrienes play a role in the pathogenesis of myocardial ischaemia and reperfusion injuries since an LTD_4-antagonist, ONO-RS-411 (see 5.1.5), and several 5-LO inhibitors, including BW755C and AA–861 (see 6.2.2), have reduced infarct size in a canine coronary occlusion – reperfusion model [187–189]. However, other authors using a similar model in rats and employing a different LTD_4-antagonist, SK & F 104,353, claimed that peptido-lipid leukotrienes do not contribute to the progression of myocardial ischaemic/reperfusion injury [190]. Also, more selective inhibitors of 5-LO such as BWA4C (see 6.2.3) have no protective effect against reperfusion damage in the dog [191]. It has also been proposed that LTB_4 may contribute to symptoms associated with myocardial ischaemia: for example, LTB_4 may mediate the PMN infiltration which occurs, since the 5-LO inhibitors, BW755C and AA-861 reduced the influx of cells in models of myocardial ischaemia [187–189].

4   Leukotriene receptors
4.1   Peptido-lipid leukotriene receptors

Probably the major role of the peptido-lipid leukotrienes is in mediating symptoms associated with allergic asthma, for example, the prolonged contraction of airway smooth muscle and increased mucus secretion (see 3.2). Therefore, it is not surprising that most effort has been directed to the examination of receptors in lung tissue although other tissues have also been investigated (see [192]).

Since the leukotrienes are a familiy of agonists it may be expected that each could have its own specific class of receptor and also that each leukotriene may have the capacity to interact with subsets of these receptors. Clearly LTB_4 acts on a different receptor to that of the peptido-lipid leukotrienes (see 4.2). But there are also different receptors for LTC_4 and LTD_4 in certain tissues [193,194]: LTE_4 has a high affinity for the LTD_4 receptor but not for the LTC_4 receptor. These studies were possible due to the availability of FPL 55712, an antagonist of SRS-A [195], and also of pure samples of peptido-lipid leukotrienes. Early studies demonstrated that FPL 55712 was, in fact, a selective LTD_4 antagonist (it had negligible effect on LTC_4 receptors). The concept of multiple peptido-lipid leukotriene receptors in different tissues (particularly lung, heart and ileum) is convincing. Evidence has been obtained from both pharmacological [196–198] and radioligand-binding experiments (see below). However, it should be noted that different receptors for LTC_4 and LTD_4 have not been confirmed in human tissue; premliminary data obtained using human foetal lung tissue suggested separate receptors [195] but later data in human bronchus supports the existence of only one receptor [199]. The leukotriene antagonists discussed later (section 5) all affect the LTD_4 receptor preferentially.

Pharmacological and receptor binding studies with the leukotrienes are complicated by the fact that LTC_4 is readily converted to LTD_4 by γ-glutamyl transpeptidase present in many tissues (see 2.2). Thus, the activity, and binding to receptors, of LTC_4 in lung tissue is apparently antagonised by FPL 55712 but this is due to blocking the activity of the LTD_4 formed. Inhibition of the conversion of LTC_4 to LTD_4 by isolated guinea-pig trachea and other tissues has been accomplished satisfactorily by the addition of an L-serine-borate complex which is a transition state inhibitor of γ-glutamyl transpeptidase [200–202]. Thus, the inclusion of this inhibitor in pharmacological or ligand binding experiments enables the investigation of the LTC_4 receptor. However, it should be noted that relatively high concentrations of the inhibitor are required (ca 50 mM) and could, potentially, produce non-specific effects. Also, LTD_4 is converted to LTE_4 and this could further compromise interpretation of data: in this case the transformation can be blocked by the addition of cysteine, an inhibitor of the dipeptidase which is responsible for the metabolism of LTD_4 [203,204].

Despite the complication of having to inhibit metabolism, radioligand binding assays have been used to study the peptido-lipid leukotriene receptors in different tissues from several species. A commonly used system is the binding of high specific activity $[^3H]$-LTD_4 (or $[^3H]$-LTC_4) to a crude membrane fraction isolated from guinea-pig lung [205–210]. The separation of bound and free ligand is readily accomplished by filtration. The binding of $[^3H]$-LTD_4 to the specific binding sites reaches an equilibrium after approximately 20 min at 37 °C and 150 min at 4 °C. Measurement of the saturation equilibrium yielded K_d values of 5.5×10^{-11}M at 20 °C and 2.1×10^{-11}M at 0 °C while the number of binding sites (B_{max}) were 384 and 302 fmol/mg protein at 20 °C and 0 °C, respectively [206]. The high affinity binding is saturable, reversible and stereospecific. For several leukotriene antagonists (see Section 5), estimates of the dissociation constants obtained from binding studies and functional assays are in good agreement. The binding is dependent on the presence of divalent cations particularly Ca^{2+} and Mg^{2+}. These characteristics strongly suggest that the binding sites are physiological receptors. The radioligand studies have also revealed comparable affinities of LTD_4 and LTE_4 for the LTD_4 binding site in the guinea-pig lung which supports the suggestion that their biological effects are mediated by activity at the same receptor [206]. However, LTC_4 does not act at the LTD_4 receptor in guinea-pig lung [206,211], guinea-pig trachea [203] or rat lung [212]. Monovalent cations (i.e. Li^+, Na^+, K^+) have no effect on the binding of LTC_4 to its receptor. However, Na^+, but not K^+ or Li^+, strongly inhibits LTD_4-specific binding. GTP, but not other nucleotides, inhibits LTD_4 but not LTC_4 binding. This profile suggests that the activity of LTD_4, is associated with a depression of cyclic AMP levels (see [213]). Ligand-binding studies, followed by biochemical characterisation of the receptor transduction mechanisms, have demonstrated that the LTD_4 receptor initiates its signal via GTP-binding proteins (G-proteins) which, in most cells, are distinct from the adenylate-cyclase coupled proteins. It has been demonstrated that receptor-LTD_4 complex formation leads, via a G-protein, to the breakdown of phosphotidylinositol bisphosphate, the mobilization of Ca^{2+} and the activation of phospholipase A_2. Thus, LTD_4-binding is influenced by stable GTP analogues and by monovalent and divalent cations as well as by LTD_4 antagonists (see [214–216]).

Peptido-lipid leukotriene receptors have been demonstrated in other tissues beside lung and ileal tissue. For example, LTC_4 binding sites are present in myocardial [217] and brain tissue [202] and in a smooth muscle cell line derived from vas deferens [218].

ICI 198,615, which is one of the most potent LTD_4 antagonists (see Section 5.1.4), is available commercially in a high specific activity tritiated form. Since it has high affinity for the LTD_4-receptor and it has greater chemical and metabolic stability compared to the natural ligand, [^{3}H]-ICI 198,615 provides a useful tool for binding experiments [219].

4.2   Leukotriene B_4 receptors

The most important activity of LTB_4 is probably its affect on leucocytes: it induces chemokinesis, chemotaxis, adherence, aggregation and degranulation of PMN (see Section 3.1). The receptors for LTB_4 on PMN are present primarily on the plasma membranes; they exist in two affinity states that appear to be coupled to separate functions of PMN [119,220]. It has been suggested that occupancy of high affinity receptors mediates chemokinesis, chemotaxis and adherence while the low affinity receptors are coupled to the responses of degranulation and oxygen radical production [220]. There is evidence that the high affinity receptors are linked to a G-protein mediated transduction mechanism (see [221]).

5   Leukotriene antagonists

5.1   Antagonists of peptido-lipid leukotrienes

As noted earlier (4.1) distinct receptors for LTC_4 and LTD_4 have been identified in animals although this has not been confirmed in human tissue. LTD_4 is considered to contribute the major biological activity present in SRS-A and, therefore, antagonism of its activity is the main target: the antagonists discussed below all act preferentially on the LTD_4 receptor.

There are now many compounds which are claimed to be peptido-lipid leukotriene antagonists – in fact too many to be able to review each of them in this article. The following sections will describe the pharmacological activity of selected compounds *in vitro* and *in vivo*. Also, clinical information which is available for some compounds will be discussed (see also [152,222–224]).

As with all agents which may exert their clinical effects via a novel mechanism it is important to confirm that the effects can be attributed to that unique mode of action. Since LTD_4 antagonists are being considered primarily for use in the treatment of asthma, potential drugs have often been tested for their ability to reduce the response caused by inhaled LTD_4 in man, as well as in animals. Some of the earlier compounds which had promising activity *in vitro* failed to affect LTD_4 responses in man, probably because of poor bioavailability, and, therefore, it is not surprising that such compounds also did not have beneficial effects when tested in asthmatics. There are now several compounds which have been shown to cause rightward displacement of a dose-response curve to inhaled LTD_4 in man (see below) and, therefore, these offer an opportunity to test, confidently, the clinical efficacy of peptido-lipid leukotriene antagonists in the treatment of asthma and other diseases. One caveat is that although the selectivity of most of the new compounds has been claimed to be excellent, the tests employed are often limited; for example, the effect of compounds on cAMP phosphodiesterase is rarely mentioned and leukotriene antagonists which also inhibit phosphodiesterase could achieve anti-asthma effects by inhibition of this enzyme rather than antagonism of leukotrienes. However, there are now several compounds with excellent leukotriene antagonist properties and bioavailability with diverse chemical structures and, therefore, beneficial effects can be more confidently ascribed to antagonism of leukotrienes.

As mentioned previously, a key event in the development of leuko-triene antagonists was the demonstration that the SRS-A antagonist, FPL 55712 [195] was actually a selective LTD_4 antagonist [193,194,225]. FPL 55712 (see Fig. 3) was developed from a series of compounds related to the anti-asthma drug, disodium cromoglycate. However, lack of oral bioavailability and short biological half-life limited the therapeutic potential of this compound [226,227]. The search for bioavailable, long-lasting, potent and selective antagonists of LTD_4 activity has followed two obvious courses. Firstly, there has been major effort in capitalizing on the knowledge that FPL 55712 was an LTD_4-antagonist and, therefore, several companies have syn-thesized analogues in an attempt to identify hydroxy-acetophenones which maintain the selectivity of FPL 55712 but which are more po-tent and, above all, are effective *in vivo*. Secondly, others have synthes-ized and evaluated compounds based on the leukotriene structure. Additionally, the radioligand binding experiments described above (4.1) have been adapted for high-throughout, random screening of compounds.

An LTD_4-receptor model has been proposed [222] based on the study of the interaction of the natural ligand and analogues thereof with the binding site. The experimental data suggested that: (i) the receptor contains at least one hydrophilic site that requires a carboxylic acid functionality or equivalent; (ii) the cysteinylglycine chain binds in a polar but non-ionic state; (iii) a portion of the receptor binds to the lipophilic polyene chain; (iv) there is some recognition of the triene system, with the double bond at C-7 being most important [222]. This model may assist in the design of novel antagonists.

5.1.1   Peptido-lipid leukotriene antagonists from Eli Lilly and Company

LY-171883, a tetrazole-substituted acetophenone (see Fig. 3) is a po-tent and selective antagonist of LTD_4 in guinea-pig ileum, trachea and parenchyma [228]. When given orally to guinea-pigs, LY-171883 was able to prevent increases in tracheal pressure caused either by i.v. ad-ministration of LTD_4 or by administration of ovalbumin to sensitized animals [229]. The compound also inhibits cAMP phosphodiesterases and this may account for a direct bronchodilator activity although

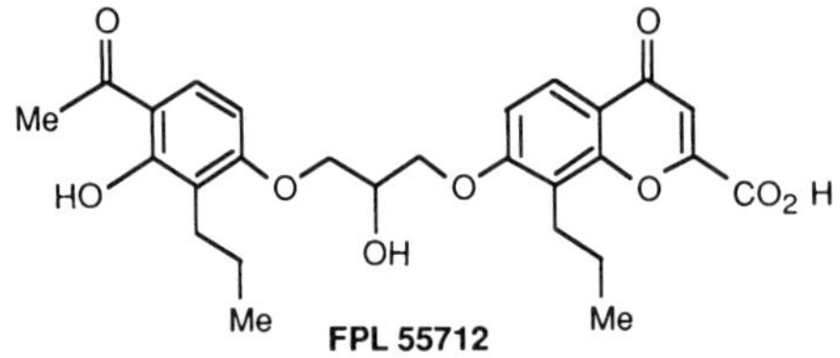

Figure 3
Structures of some leukotriene D4 antagonists.

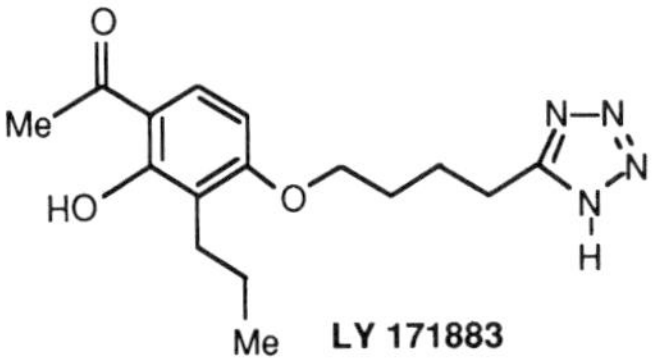

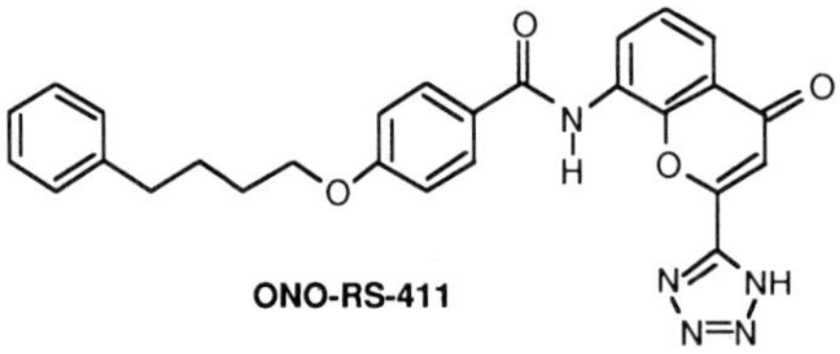

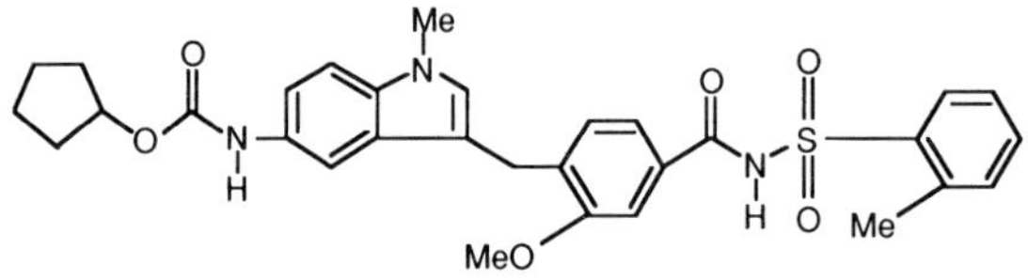

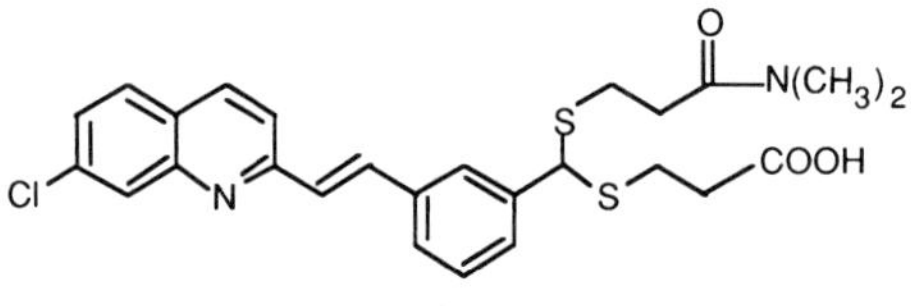

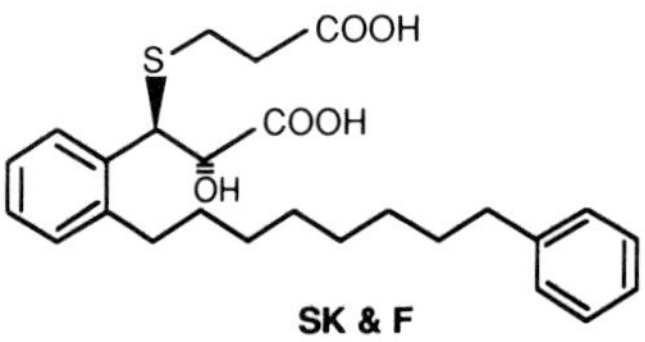

recent data indicates that inhibition of phosphodiesterases would not occur after therapeutic doses [230].

An oral dose of 400 mg LY-171883 caused a shift to the right of the inhaled LTD_4 dose-response curve in 10 out of 12 non-asthmatic subjects [231]; lower doses (50 and 200 mg) did not produce convincing effects. The activity was confirmed when LY-171883 was given to atopic subjects; 400 mg orally caused a small reduction in the response to inhaled LTD_4 [232]. In addition, the compound reduced the wheal and flare response to intradermal LTD_4 although it had no effect on this response induced by intradermal antigen [232].

The effect of LY-171883 on bronchospasm produced by challenge of asthmatic subjects with cold air has been examined using a randomized, double-blind, two phase cross-over design [233]. LY-171883 reduced the response significantly; however, the improvement was small which led the authors to suggest that either mediators other than LTD_4, had important effects in cold-air isocapnic hyperpnoea or that LTD_4 receptors were inadequately blocked. Further clinical evaluation of LY-171883 is not proceeding because of chronic toxicological effects in female mice [228].

A second generation of acetophenone-derived leukotriene receptor antagonists has been described by investigators at Eli Lilly. One of the key compounds, LY-163443, is nearly ten-fold more potent *in vitro* and has a longer biological half-life than LY-171883 [234,235].

Another series of LTD_4 antagonists was synthesized based on a proposed model of LY-171883 binding to the LTD_4/LTE_4 receptor, in which the *n*-propyl and tetrazole moieties of LY-171883 occupy those parts of the receptor to which the C 1–C 5 chain and the cysteinyl carboxyl of LTE_4 bind, respectively. Of this series, LY-203647 showed good antagonist activity with a suitable pharmacological and toxicological profile which has encouraged clinical evaluation [236].

Another tetrazole, LY-170680, has also been evaluated against LTD_4-induced effects in mild to moderate asthmatics. Pharmacological studies *in vitro* had shown that it was a potent, competitive, antagonist of LTD_4 [237]. Also, the compound was effective in various *in vivo* tests when it was given intravenously and by inhalation but was less active when given orally. The compound is metabolized by ω and β oxidation in the liver during "first-pass" after oral dosing. Therefore, an aerosol formulation was developed: a dose of 4 $\mu g/kg$ was found to reduce the effects of LTD_4 in man for 8 h. The compound was well tolerated and did not appear to affect histamine or prostaglandin release [238].

5.1.2   Peptido-lipid leukotriene antagonists from SK & F Laboratories

SK & F 88046 was shown to inhibit LTD_4 activity on the guinea-pig ileum and in several models of bronchoconstriction in guinea-pigs [239,240]. However, ligand binding experiments revealed that although it bound to an "LTC_4-binding site" [240,241] it did not displace [^{3}H]-LTD_4 from specific high affinity binding sites. It was concluded that SK & F 88046 is an "antagonist" of the indirectly mediated actions of LTD_4 which are believed to involve the synthesis and activity of CO metabolites, particularly TXA_2 (i.e., it is probably a TXA_2 antagonist) [242].

A series of desamino-2-*nor*-leukotriene analogues are potent leukotriene antagonists (e.g. SK & F 101132). Although some of the compounds were relatively selective, others also caused contractions of airway smooth muscle [243]. It is also probable that several members of this series would suffer from poor oral bioavailability and short half-lives: these properties were not reported in the initial publication.

A more potent and selective receptor antagonist of peptido-lipid leukotrienes has been developed by SK & F laboratories. The compound, SK & F 104,353 ([2(S)-hydroxy-3(R)-[(2-carboxyethyl)thio]-3-[2-(8-phenyloctyl)phenyl]-propanoic acid is a structural analogue of LTD_4 (see Fig. 3). It is a potent and selective LTD_4 receptor antagonist *in vitro* [244,245]. Also, it reduced LTD_4-induced bronchoconstriction in anaesthetised, spontaneously breathing guinea-pigs when it was administered intravenously: it was approximately 60-fold less effective when given intraduodenally [246]. SK & F 104,353 did not affect responses induced by aerosolized acetylcholine, histamine or the TXA_2-agonist, U-44069; also, it did not itself produce bronchoconstriction [246]. SK & F 104,353 has now been evaluated in man [247]. When inhaled by healthy subjects, SK & F 104,353 (100–800 μg) protected against LTD_4-induced bronchospasm when compared to placebo. There was no evidence of partial agonist activity or side effects. Therefore, it was concluded that SK & F 104,353 is a well-tolerated, potent, selective LTD_4 antagonist in normal human airways and has sufficient duration of activity after inhalation to encourage assessment of its efficacy as an anti-asthmatic in appropriately designed clinical trials.

A related compound, SK & F 106,203 (hydroxy group replaced by hydrogen) is apparently more orally bioavailable than SK & F 104,353 in animals and man [248]. Although SK & F 106,203 is less potent as a LTD_4-antagonist compared to SK & F 104,353 it may have more suitable properties for development as a medicine.

5.1.3   Peptido-lipid leukotriene antagonists from Merck, Sharpe and Dohme Research Laboratories

Investigators at the Merck-Frosst Laboratories in Canada evaluated a series of compounds which retained the hydroxy-acetophenone group present in FPL-55 712. Many were potent and selective antagonists *in vitro* and *in vivo* [249,250]. Of these, L-649,923 was identified as a suitable candidate for investigation in man. An oral dose (1 g) of L-649,923 was reported to give some protection against LTD_4-induced bronchoconstriction in normal subjects [251] and minimal protection against antigen-induced bronchoconstriction in patients with mild asthma [252]. However, the compound had undesirable side effects, (cramping abdominal pain associated with watery diarrhoea) which limited the doses which could be administered and this consequently limited the assessment of efficacy of the compound.

L-648,051, which also retains the hydroxy-acetophenone moiety, is a more potent antagonist of the LTD_4 receptor than L-649,923 in guinea-pig and human lung tissue [253–255] which was not predicted by receptor binding studies (Ki = 6.2 μM for L-648,051 versus 0.4 μM for L-649,923). It was suggested that the two antagonists may equilibrate with the leukotriene receptors in various tissues at different rates because of their distinct physical properties. L-648,051 is rapidly metabolized and eliminated *in vivo* which restricts the use of the compound to topical (i.e. inhaled) administration. Inhaled, L-648,051 (1.6, 6.0 and 12.0 mg) partially blocked LTD_4-induced bronchoconstriction in healthy male subjects [256]: there was no evidence of partial agonist activity and no effect on histamine-induced bronchospasm.

MK-571 (see Fig. 3; [257]), which was previously referred to as L-660,711 has high affinity for LTD_4 receptors on both guinea-pig and human lung parenchymal membranes (IC_{50} values 1 and 8 nM, respectively; $pA_2 = 9.4$), The compound is a potent, competitive inhibitor of LTD_4 responses in several smooth muscle preparations from both guinea-pig and man. It does not block contractions induced by a variety of other spasmogens and, therefore, it appears to be selective. The *in vivo* activity of the compound was demonstrated by its ability to reduce bronchoconstriction in sensitized animals challenged with antigen. The pre-clinical data for MK-571 encouraged clinical evaluation. Kips *et al.* [258] reported that MK-571 at doses which provided plasma concentrations of greater than 1 $\mu g/ml$ afforded complete antagonism of LTD_4-induced responses but had no effect on baseline airway function. The compound was well tolerated at doses likely to be effective in the treatment of asthma. In asthmatic men, infusions of MK-571 increased baseline airway calibre and produced shifts in the aerosolized LTD_4 dose-response curve of ≥ 80 and ≥ 40 fold at plasma concentrations of 20 and 2 $\mu g/ml$ [259]. The significant bronchodilator properties (improvements in the forced expiratory volume in one second, FEV_1) of MK-571 in asthmatics has been confirmed in another double blind, placebo controlled, randomized, cross-over study and its effects were additive with the bronchodilator β_2 agonist, salbutamol [260]. In a double-blind, randomised, crossover study, 12 subjects with stable asthma were treated with MK-571 (160 mg, i.v.) or placebo 20 min. before each of two challenges involving exercise at a level previously demonstrated to cause a fall of at least 20% in FEV_1: treatment with MK-571 attenuated exercise-induced bronchoconstriction in all subjects [260a]. Also, MK-571 appears to reduce the late phase, as well as the early phase, response to inhaled antigen [261]. All the early clinical studies with MK-571 were conducted using intravenous infusions because the investigators considered that this enabled accurate correlation of clinical efficacy with blood levels. However, it is claimed that MK-571 is also effective via the oral route. MK-571 is a racemate but both enantiomers are potent antagonists. During development some advantages of one enantiomer (referred to as MK-679) were recognised and this is the compound being developed by Merck Sharpe and Dohme (see [262]). During pharmacokinetic studies in humans it was noted that the (+) enantiomer appeared to be eliminated faster than the (−) enantiomer [263] and this could be the advantage referred to above.

5.1.4   Peptido-lipid leukotriene antagonists from ICI
Pharmaceuticals

ICI 198,615 was shown to be several orders of magnitude more potent than FPL 55712 but it lacked consistent oral bioavailability in several species [264–268]. Further studies identified a structural analogue of ICI 198,615 (see Fig. 3) which had an improved oral bioavailability profile and retained potent LTD_4 antagonism, albeit weaker than ICI 198,615; this compound is referred to as ICI 204,219.

The pre-clinical pharmacology of ICI 204,219 (see [269]) demonstrated that it was a potent, competitive antagonist of contractions of guinea-pig lung tracheal and parenchymal strips induced by LTD_4 (and LTE_4), but not by LTC_4. Radioligand binding experiments confirmed the high affinity of ICI 204,219 for the LTD_4 receptor in guinea-pig tissue and also in human lung parenchymal membranes. These experiments also revealed that the compound did not bind to a variety of other receptors (e.g. adrenergic, histamine, 5-HT, prostanoid) when tested at concentrations 1000–10000-fold higher than the apparent K_b value for peptido-lipid leukotriene receptors. When administered orally, intravenously or by aerosol to conscious guinea-pigs, ICI 204,219 provided dose-related antagonism of the airway effects of aerosolized LTD_4 on both large and small airways. Furthermore the compound inhibited or reversed antigen-induced leukotriene-dependent bronchospasm in guinea-pigs; this type of test is successfully employed by many investigators studying the effects of LT antagonists, or inhibitors of synthesis (see 6.1.3), but it should be recognized that antagonists or inhibitors of other mediators (e.g. histamine, prostaglandins, catecholamines) have to be co-administered with the test substance in order to reveal the "leukotriene-dependent" bronchoconstriction.

Additionally, ICI 204,219 inhibited other effects produced by LTD_4: for example, it reduced LTD_4-induced increases in cutaneous vascular permeability in guinea-pigs and it was approximately three orders of magnitude more potent in this test than either FPL 55712 or LY-171,883.

Clearly the pre-clinical pharmacological properties of ICI 204,219, both *in vitro* and *in vivo,* encouraged clinical evaluation of the compound. The effect of a single oral dose (40 mg) of ICI 204,219 on LTD_4-induced bronchoconstriction in normal subjects was tested using a double-blind, placebo-controlled cross-over design (see [270]). The compound had no effect on baseline pulmonary function nor did it produce any adverse effects. When given 2 h before challenge with aerosolized LTD_4 it increased by 117-fold the concentration of LTD_4 required to reduce specific airway conductance by 35%. Even when given 12 and 24 h before challenge, ICI 204,219 was able to attenuate significantly the effect of LTD_4. The inhibition of LTD_4-induced bronchoconstriction produced by ICI 204,219 was also tested in patients with mild asthma; the antagonist potency was similar to that observed in normal subjects [271]. Thus, it was demonstrated that ICI 204,219 was an effective LTD_4 receptor antagonist in normal and mildly asthmatic human subjects. Recently, the influence of a single oral dose (20 mg) of ICI 204,219 was evaluated on allergen-induced bronchoconstriction in a group of ten atopic asthmatics with documented airways hyperresponsiveness to histamine [272]. In these studies ICI-204,219 caused a marked increase in the dose of allergen required to achieve a pre-determined level of bronchoconstriction.

5.1.5 Peptido-lipid leukotriene antagonists from Ono Pharmaceutical Co.

Orally active LTD_4 antagonists have been developed by the Ono Company; the biological activity of a very extensive series of compounds was assessed *in vitro* and *in vivo*, and lead compounds were identified (ONO-RS-260, ONO-RS347 and ONO-RS-411; see Fig. 3). The most potent of these compounds were approximately three orders of magnitude more potent than FPL-55712 (e.g. pA_2 of RS-411 and FPL-55712 are 10.4 and 7.69, respectively) [273–275]. Although these compounds do not contain the hydroxy-acetophenone group present in FPL-55712 they do have an equivalent to the chromone portion present in the prototype inhibitor. In preliminary studies in man, it was reported that ONO-RS-411 (also referred to as ONO-1078) can significantly reduce symptoms such as wheezing and dyspnoea in asthmatic subjects [276]. A double-blind placebo controlled clinical study of ONO-RS-411 in asthma has commenced.

5.1.6   Peptido-lipid leukotriene antagonists from Ciba-Geigy Ltd

Investigators at Ciba-Geigy succeeded in synthesizing analogues of "1-methyl-LTD$_4$" which retained LTD$_4$ antagonist activity but which had a longer duration of action and better chemical stability in comparison to analogues containing the natural backbone [277]. Later the activity of another LTD$_4$ analogue, CGP 45715A (1R,2S)-1-hydroxy-1-(3-trifluoromethylphenyl)-10-(4-acetyl-3-hydroxy-2-propyl-phenoxy)-deca-3(E),5(Z)-diene-2yl-7-thio-4-oxo-4H-1-benzopyran-2-carboxylic acid, sodium salt) was reported: it is a potent, apparently non-competitive, LTD$_4$-antagonist *in vitro* [278]. It is also a competitive antagonist of TXA$_2$ receptors but at higher concentrations than are required to block the LTD$_4$ receptor; it is inactive against other spasmogens. It is claimed that CGP 45715A also displays potent LTD$_4$-antagonist properties (inhibition of LTD$_4$/LTE$_4$ and antigen-induced bronchoconstriction in guinea-pigs) *in vivo* when given either orally or as an aerosol. However, it is reported to also inhibit enzymic reactions at relatively low concentrations (1–10 μM), e.g. phospholipase A$_2$, prostaglandin and leukotriene synthesis, interleukin-1 synthesis. Therefore, while it may be of interest as a therapeutic agent, it is not a useful tool with which to investigate the pathophysiological role of LTD$_4$.

5.1.7   Peptido-lipid leukotriene antagonists from
          Hoffmann-La Roche Inc.

Evaluation of 3,4-dihydro-2H-1-benzopyran-2-carboxylic acids linked to the 2-hydroxy-acetophenone pharmacophore present in FPL 55712 identified Ro 23–3544 as the most potent LTD$_4$-antagonist in the series. The separate enantiomers of Ro 23–3544 exhibited similar potencies *in vitro* and *in vivo* when administered intravenously. However, the S-enantiomer was 15 times more active than the R-form at reducing LTC$_4$ and LTD$_4$-induced bronchoconstriction in the guinea-pig when the compound was administered by the aerosol route [279].
Ro 24–5913 ((E)-[3-[2[(4-cyclobutyl-2-thiazolyl)ethenyl]phenylamino]-2,2-diethyl-4-oxobutanoic acid) is a potent, competitive LTD$_4$-antagonist *in vitro* and *in vivo*. The compound was effective at inhibiting LTD$_4$ induced bronchoconstriction in guinea-pigs whether it was

by intravenous (ED_{50} 0.013 mg/kg), oral ED_{50} 0.012 mg/kg) or aerosol (ED_{50} 0.008%) routes of administration [280]. The compound was reported to have a long-lasting effect against LTD_4- and antigen-induced bronchospasm. The *in vivo* activity was claimed to be specific since intravenous doses of Ro 24–5913 up to 10 mg/kg showed no inhibitory activity towards the bronchoconstrictor effects of LTC_4, PAF or histamine. However, it would be expected that LTC_4 would be converted to LTD_4 (see 2.2) *in vivo* and, therefore, it is surprising that Ro 24–5913 did not modify the LTC_4-induced effect.

5.1.8   Peptido-lipid leukotriene antagonists from Wyeth-Ayerst Research

Wy-48,252 (1,1,1-trifluoro-N-(3-(2-quinolinyl-methoxy)phenyl) methane sulphonamide is an orally active LTD_4-antagonist [281–283]. After intraduodenal administration the compound was approximately 8 to 17 times more potent than the previously characterised compounds, Wy-45,911 and LY-171,883 at inhibiting inhaled LTD_4-induced bronchoconstriction in the guinea-pig. After intragastric administration, Wy-48,252 also inhibited antigen-induced bronchoconstriction and it was approximately 300 times more potent than LY-171,883 [284]. The anti-allergic activity of the compound was also demonstrated in sheep [285]; both early and late phase responses induced by antigen were modified by intragastric administration. However, it was reported that Wy-48,252 also inhibited both 5-LO and CO at relatively low concentrations (in macrophages IC_{50} values were 4.4 and 4.3 μM, respectively [286]). Earlier the Wyeth group had disclosed a series of selective LTD_4 antagonists exemplified by WY-46,928 [287,288].

The Wyeth group noted that a structural feature common to most of the LTD_4 antagonists and to LTD_4 itself was an acidic moiety and this encouraged them to examine the stucture-activity relationships of four series of acidic compounds [289]. The addition of carboxylic, hydroxamic, sulphonyl carboxamide and tetrazole groups to the N-[(quinolinyl-methoxy)phenyl] system present in Wy-48,252 was tested. Several compounds exhibited LTD_4-antagonist activity but none were more potent than Wy-48,252; also, these compounds inhibited 5-LO.

5.2   Antagonists of leukotriene B_4

Since LTB_4 may play a role in the pathogenesis of inflammatory disease some pharmaceutical companies have attempted to identify antagonists of its action. However, the research effort dedicated to the development of LTB_4-antagonists has been minor in comparison to that expended on the search for LTD_4 antagonists. Some examples of LTB_4 antagonists which have been reported are briefly described below.

ONO-LB-109, which was one of a series of *m*-acylaminocinnamyl alcohols synthesized, antagonised LTB_4-induced aggregation of leucocytes *in vitro,* inhibited [^{3}H]-LTB_4 binding *in vitro* and reduced LTB_4-induced neutropaenia in rats *in vivo* [290]. The group at the ONO Pharmaceutical Co. also reported that members of a series of substituted β-phenylpropionic acids (e.g. ONO-LB-457) are potent antagonists of LTB_4 [291,291 a]. SC-41 930, a potent LTB_4 receptor antagonist *in vitro* inhibited the chemotactic actions of LTB_4 when co-administered into the dermis; SC-41 930 also affected the LTB_4 response when given intravenously and orally [292]. Compound U-75,302 is another LTB_4 antagonist which exhibits activity *in vivo* [293–295]; interestingly, U-75, 302 dose-dependently inhibited antigen-induced late-phase influx of eosinophils into the bronchial lumen of guinea-pigs [296].

6   Inhibitors of leukotriene biosynthesis

The pursuit of LTD_4 antagonists has been intensive and current evidence suggests that they will be of therapeutic benefit in the treatment of asthma. However, other biologically active leukotrienes are formed during asthma attacks and inflammatory reactions which could also contribute to the pathogenesis of the disease. This suggests that a cocktail of antagonists may be required to provide effective therapy. An alternative approach is to inhibit the synthesis of the leukotrienes. There are several enzymic transformations involved in the biosynthesis of leukotrienes (see Section 2.2) and inhibition of each may offer a worthwhile therapeutic approach. However, inhibition of 5-LO is the most attractive target since this would result in reduced formation of all the leukotrienes and also of 5-HPETE and 5-HETE, which may also contribute to pathological events. In this review only inhibitors of

5-LO will be considered. An attempt has been made to describe methods for evaluating 5-LO inhibitors both *in vitro* and *in vivo* as well as reviewing some of the most interesting compounds currently available.

6.1   Evaluation of the activity of inhibitors of 5-lipoxygenase
6.1.1   Inhibition of 5-lipoxygenase *in vitro*

Several *in vitro* systems for studying inhibitors of 5-LO have been described including the use of partially purified enzymes, RBL-1 cells, neutrophils and macrophages from various species. It is possible that the enzyme from the different sources will be affected similarly by inhibitors but at Wellcome we chose to use PMN from human volunteers because this relevant source avoids the potential problem of species differences. The initial test uses an homogenate of human PMN which is incubated with exogenous arachidonic acid as described by Tateson *et al.* [297]; this is preferred to the use of whole cells since the latter would require penetration of the compound into the cell which consequently may complicate the structure-activity relationship. Also, the enzyme in whole cells requires activation, which is usually achieved experimentally by addition of the calcium ionophore, A 23 187, and this stimulus may produce data which can be misleading [298]. An isolated enzyme may be preferred but as there are technical difficulties in purification (see 2.3), this was not considered a practical option for testing many compounds. Some investigators have tested the activity of inhibitors (e. g. quercetin, phenidone, AA-861 and BW 755 C; see Section 6.2.2) on the immunoaffinity-purified 5-LO from porcine leucocytes [299]. The results indicated that the presence of inhibitors can modify the kinetics of 5-LO at the levels of the initiation of the reaction and the rate of enzyme inactivation, with variations depending on the structural class of the inhibitor and the concentration of lipid hydroperoxides. Thus, these data endorse the recommendation to use a simpler system than the purified enzyme for routine assessment of the activity of 5-LO inhibitors, and these methods are described below.

Neutrophils are separated from human blood after the sedimentation of the majority of erythrocytes by the addition of 2% methyl cellulose. The cells are sonicated in buffer containing EDTA. The compound under test is added to the homogenate and incubated at 37 °C for

5 min before the addition of arachidonic acid and calcium. Incubation is continued for a further 5 min and then the reaction is terminated by boiling. The inhibition of 5-LO is studied by monitoring the formation of LTB_4, which is measured by a specific radioimmunoassay (RIA), and compared to the value obtained in a control incubation. Alternatively, the LTB_4 formed can be monitored by an HPLC assay but this is limited by poor sensitivity compared to RIA and a lower throughput of samples. The homogenate contains the CO enzyme (mainly from contaminating platelets) and, therefore, the synthesis of a CO metabolite, TXB_2, is also determined and this provides an early indication of the selectivity of the inhibitor.

We employ human whole PMN stimulated with A 23 187 (or serum treated zymosan) in a secondary *in vitro* test to confirm that inhibitors penetrate cells and decrease the conversion of endogenous arachidonic acid to LTB_4 [297]. Also, if the objective is to inhibit leukotriene biosynthesis by preventing the translocation of the 5-LO rather than inhibit the enzyme directly, then a whole cell system must be employed (see Section 6.2.4). Other stimuli such as monosodium urate crystals could be used to stimulate LTB_4 synthesis in neutrophils [300]. An additional *in vitro* test can be used to establish that the test compound prevents leukotriene synthesis by inhibiting the 5-LO. [^{14}C]-arachidonic acid is incubated with human PMN stimulated with A 23 187, the products are extracted and separated by TLC (or HPLC). These experiments also permit assessment of the selectivity of compounds on different lipoxygenases; for example, the data illustrated in Fig. 4 shows that the anti-oxidant BW 755 C reduces the formation of 12- and 15-HETEs as well as 5-HETE and LTB_4 with a similar potency, whereas BW A 4 C selectively inhibits the generation of products of 5-LO. In fact, at low concentrations of BW A 4 C, which inhibit the synthesis of both 5-HETE and LTB_4, there is increased formation of 12- and 15-HETEs (see Fig. 4).

Finally, it is an advantage to be aware of the possibility of binding of the 5-LO inhibitors to plasma proteins which could compromise their activity. This can be easily gauged by assessing the activity of the test compound in whole blood using the procedure detailed later (Section 6.1.2). Major differences between the IC_{50} values obtained in buffer and in blood suggest an effect of protein binding; for example, L-652,343 a dual CO/LO inhibitor [301], exhibited potent 5-LO inhibi-

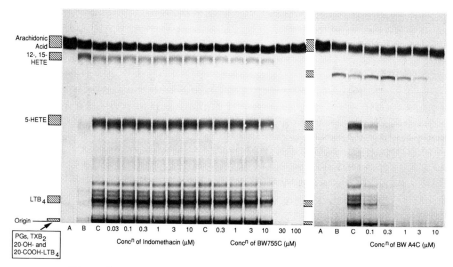

Figure 4

An autoradiogram illustrating the metabolites formed from [¹⁴C]-arachidonic acid during incubation with human neutrophils and the effects of indomethacin, BW 755 C and
BW A 4 C on the metabolism. The leucocytes (1×10^7) were incubated with 50 nCi
[¹⁴C]-arachidonic acid and the calcium ionophore A 23 187 (1 μg/ml)for 4 min at 37°C.
The products were extracted from acidified cell-free supernatant into ethyl acetate,
separated by thin-layer chromatography (solvent system: diethyl ether/hexane/acetic
acid, 60 : 40 : 1, v/v/v) and visualised by autoradiography. A, Incubation with boiled
cells; B, Incubation with unstimulated cells (no A 23 187); C, Incubation with stimulated cells in the absence of inhibitors ("control"). The indicated concentrations of inhibitors were pre-incubated with the neutrophils for 5 min at 37°C before addition of
[¹⁴C]-arachidonic acid and A 23 187. The hatched areas indicate the mobility of unla-
belled standards. Note that indomethacin does not inhibit the formation of any of the
metabolites (the radioactivity at the origin is almost exclusively 20-hydroxy and
20-carboxy LTB₄), BW 755 C inhibits the synthesis of all the products whereas BW
A 4 C inhibits selectively those metabolites formed via 5-lipoxygenase activity (i.e.
5-HETE, LTB₄ and its metabolites) – in fact the synthesis of 12- and 15-HETEs is increased by concentrations of BW A 4 C which completely inhibit 5-LO.

tory activity in cells suspended in buffer but was completely inactive
in whole blood [302].

6.1.2   Inhibition of 5-lipoxygenase *ex vivo*

The degree and duration of the inhibition of 5-LO after both oral and
intravenous administration to laboratory animals can be evaluated by
monitoring the synthesis of LTB₄ in blood stimulated *ex vivo* with the
calcium ionophore A 23 187 [297,303–305]. Blood samples are collected at frequent intervals after administration of test compound (or

vehicle), and the whole, anti-coagulated (heparin) blood is incubated with A 23 187 at 37 °C. After 30 min, the blood is centrifuged and the concentrations of both LTB_4 and TXB_2 in the diluted cell-free plasma are determined by specific RIA [297].

This simple protocol provides an excellent method of evaluating the bioavailability and duration of action of test compounds but there are some disadvantages which should be recognised. The major pitfall is the use of RIA to measure the concentration of LTB_4 without extraction and purification of the sample prior to assay. This may be valid but it should be realised that very large concentrations of 12-HETE are also generated in A 23 187-stimulated blood. Consequently if the antibody used for RIA is not very selective a significant amount of immunoreactivity may be due to the formation of 12-HETE from platelets thereby, potentially, leading to an underestimate of the inhibition of 5-LO. In our experience, the species used for the study, as well as the characteristics of the antibody, are important considerations.

The cross reaction of 12(S)-HETE in the RIA which we use is 0.2% (the cross reaction of 12(S,R) HETE is 2% [306]). Even this relatively low cross reaction can be a problem. Although rats are a convenient species in which to conduct these tests we have found that rat blood stimulated with A 23 187 produces relatively low amounts of LTB_4 (ca 25–50 ng/ml) but high concentrations of 12-HETE (ca 20 μg/ml). Thus, even when LTB_4 synthesis is inhibited completely, a residual amount of immunoreactivity can remain due to the presence of crossreacting 12-HETE. Carey *et al.* [305] have also drawn attention to the problem of employing direct RIA to monitor the synthesis of LTB_4 in A 23 187-stimulated blood from rats and mice. The ratio of LTB_4 to 12-HETE appears to be greater in other species (e.g. rabbit, dog and man). Different antibodies raised against LTB_4 have different characteristics (see [307] for review) and some may be better than others for the direct assay of LTB_4 produced by A 23 187-stimulated blood. Alternatively, the samples could be extracted and purified by HPLC or TLC prior to RIA [308–310]. However, the inclusion of the latter procedures makes the technique less attractive for routine assessment of compounds.

Additionally, we have noted relatively poor reproducibility of LTB_4 synthesis in this test system which we have attributed to varying leucocyte count and protein binding of A 23 187. However, correction of the LTB_4 data to the leucocyte count did not significantly improve the reproducibility: Borgeat et al. [308] suggested that platelet number also influences the amount of LTB_4 formed. The use of zymosan instead of A 23 187 for stimulating 5-LO activity may provide more reliable data because it affects leucocytes more selectively and, therefore, less 12(S)HETE is produced by platelets [308]. However, as long as the data are reviewed critically the simple protocol described provides a useful preliminary assessment of the activity of the test compound (see Fig. 9 later as an example). The same method can be used for monitoring the effect on ex vivo synthesis of LTB_4 in man (see 6.1.4).

A minor variant of the above procedure for assessing 5-LO inhibitory potency ex vivo is to monitor the reduction of LTB_4 synthesis by A 23 187-stimulated inflammatory exudate cells after administration of test compounds to animals [311]. Other ex vivo methods of assessing 5-LO inhibitor have included measurement of LTC_4 and/or LTB_4 produced during incubation of fragments of rat gastric corpus mucosa obtained from animals which had been given ethanol [312–314]. Ethanol induces macroscopic damage to the gastric mucosa which is accompanied by constriction of sub-mucosal venules and arterioles and stasis of blood flow. The damaged tissue produces levels of LTC_4 during incubation (20 min at 37 °C) in vitro which can be measured using RIA. Pre-treatment of animals with 5-LO inhibitors reduces the levels of LTB_4 and LTC_4 formed [312,315]. The effect of compounds on the degree of ethanol-induced damage can also be monitored, however it is not always clear whether improvements are a cause or a consequence of inhibition of 5-LO (see [316]). Some compounds at doses which inhibited completely the synthesis of leukotrienes fail to provide any protection against ethanol-induced damage and suggests that factors other than leukotrienes are involved in producing the damage ([315], see 6.2.3).

A similar approach using damaged colonic tissue has also been used successfully for monitoring the ex vivo activity of compounds [317–320]. In these experiments the damage was induced by prior treatment of guinea-pigs with trinitrobenzene sulphonic acid (TNB): other methods of inducing intestinal inflammation have been explored (see [123]).

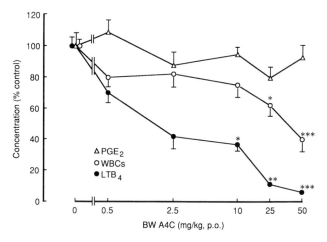

Figure 5
Effect of orally administered BW A4C on total leucocyte number (O), and the concentrations of LTB_4 (●) and PGE_2 (△) in 6 h inflammatory exudates produced by implanting carrageenin-soaked polyester sponges into rats. Each point represents the mean ± SEM of 5–15 determinations obtained on 1–3 occasions. *$p < 0.1$; **$p < 0.01$; ***$p < 0.001$. The data were reported in [393].

6.1.3 Inhibition of 5-lipoxygenase *in vivo*

The assessment of the activity of test compounds in the *ex vivo* test systems described above is valuable but a method of evaluating the compounds in a more relevant *in vivo* situation is desirable.

We have monitored the effects of compounds on the levels of mediators in a model of acute inflammation in rats. Polyester sponges which have been soaked in a solution of the irritant substance carrageenin are implanted subcutaneously into rats (see 3.1). The resulting inflammatory response is characterized by increasing concentrations of LTB_4 and prostanoids in the exudate; also, the numbers of infiltrating leucocytes increases. The level of LTB_4 is maximal at 6 h after implanting the sponge and this time was chosen to evaluate the activity of test compounds. Several compounds exhibit potent and long lasting, selective inhibition of LTB_4 synthesis in this model (as an example, see Fig. 5). Some compounds also reduced leucocyte influx but this was not a consistent finding with all inhibitors of 5-LO. For example, BW 755 C (see section 6.2.2) produced dose-related reduction of both the concentration of LTB_4 and the cell count but the two dose-response curves were not parallel; cell influx still occurred at doses of BW755C that completely inhibited the synthesis of LTB$_4$ [311]. Administration of the anti-inflammatory steroid dexamethasone produced comparable data [311], presumably because it prevented the release of arachidonic acid from phospholipids (see [321]). Leucocyte accumulation was also inhibited by high doses of the NSAIDs indomethacin and flurbiprofen but, although these drugs reduced the concentration of both PGE$_2$ and TXB$_2$ in the exudate, they did not affect LTB$_4$ levels. Similar data were also reported for benoxaprofen [322] suggesting that this drug has a mechanism of action identical to conventional NSAIDs. These data suggest that reduction of PMN accumulation by NSAIDs is mediated by a mechanism other than inhibition of LTB$_4$ synthesis. However, the mechanism by which both BW755C and dexamethasone reduce cell accumulation could be attributed in part to inhibition of the synthesis of chemotactic principles formed via 5-LO (e.g. LTB$_4$). Although LTB$_4$ may have a chemotactic role, it is not the only mediator of cell accumulation *in vivo* in this model. Others have also questioned whether PMN recruitment in this model of acute inflammation is mediated by LTB$_4$ [323]. This test does provide a useful system for evaluating the 5-LO inhibitory activity (both potency and selectivity) *in vivo* but it is probably not ideal as a model of the inflammatory response.

Similar protocols have been used by others for evaluating 5-LO inhibitors: for example, Ford-Hutchinson *et al.* [121] reported that zymosan soaked sponges produced higher concentrations of LTB$_4$ than sponges soaked in carrageenin or uric acid. Forrest *et al.* [122] evaluated the effects of BW755C on the inflammatory response and concentrations of mediators in exudate induced by injection of monosodium urate crystals into a subcutaneous air pouch in rats. In this model, BW755C significantly lowered the concentration of both LO and CO derived arachidonic acid metabolites but, although it also reduced plasma leakage, it did not affect the influx of PMN. The authors concluded that LTB$_4$ was not the mediator of PMN infiltration in this model of acute inflammation.

Other investigators have used a rat peritoneal anaphylaxis model to test compounds [324]. In this system, groups of rats are injected intraperitoneally (i.p.) with rabbit antibody to bovine serum albumin (BSA) followed 3 h later by an i.p. injection of BSA which triggers the synthesis of leukotrienes in the peritoneal cavity. The rats are killed

15 min after this challenge and the peritoneal fluids are collected and processed. The amount of immunoreactive LTC_4 in the fluid is determined by RIA. The effect of several 5-LO inhibitors have been examined in this test system (see [324]).

There is evidence that compounds that inhibit 5-LO decrease the severity of arthritic lesions in animal models. The dual inhibitors of 5-LO and CO, SK & F, 86002, SK & F 104351 and phenidone (see 6.2.2) reduced serum levels of an acute-phase protein and other symptoms in the murine, collagen-induced arthritis model [325]. These positive effects were not exhibited after treatment with selective CO inhibitors which suggests that leukotrienes or other 5-LO products may contribute to the pathological changes in this model. Therefore, this model may provide an opportunity of evaluating the efficacy of 5-LO inhibitors for the treatment of arthritis.

An anaphylactic response in actively sensitized, artificially ventilated anaesthetised guinea-pigs is often used to mimic the asthmatic reaction [326, 327]. In the absence of any drug pre-treatment, challenge with aerosolized antigen (ovalbumin) provokes intense bronchoconstriction, measured as an increase in pulmonary inflation pressure (PIP). Concomitant cardiovascular effects are minimal which illustrates the local pulmonary, rather than systemic nature, of the anaphylactic response. Pretreatment of the animals with a combination of an anti-histamine (mepyramine, 2 mg/kg i. v.) and a CO inhibitor (indomethacin, 10 mg/kg i. v.) reduces the maximum rise in PIP by approximately 45%. A significant proportion of the residual response is considered to be "leukotriene-dependent"; it has been confirmed that guinea-pigs suffering from anaphylactic shock produce LTD_4 endogenously [328]. Therefore, the activity of both LTD_4 receptor antagonists and leukotriene synthesis inhibitors can be examined.

Models of asthma in species other than guinea-pigs have been explored; for example, 5-LO inhibitors, as well as leukotriene antagonists, have been tested against an IgE-mediated bronchospasm provoked by Ascaris suum antigen in monkeys [329, 330] and in sheep [331]. The model in sheep is claimed to be particularly useful because sheep, like asthmatic patients, can be separated into those that have an acute antigen-induced-response (acute responders) and those that have antigen-induced acute and late responses (dual responders) (see [331]).

6.1.4   Inhibition of 5-lipoxygenase: Clinical assessment

It is highly desirable to be able to provide unequivocal evidence that the 5-LO is inhibited in man after administration of test compounds so that any clinical effects (or lack of) may be interpreted appropriately. Several investigators have used the *ex vivo* method of monitoring LTB_4 synthesis in A 23 187 stimulated blood as a means of confirming the effect on 5-LO (see [332–334]). This has proved a very useful procedure but it is limited to an evaluation of the drug activity in the blood compartment. It would be more appropriate if the effect on the enzyme in the effector tissue could be determined.

As discussed earlier (Section 2.2) the metabolism of the peptido-lipid leukotrienes proceeds via successive removal of amino acids and, in some species, acetylation of LTE_4. Taylor *et al.* [160] have reported that immunoreactive LTE_4 is excreted in the urine of patients suffering an asthmatic attack but the levels of immunoreactive material is negligible in normal volunteers (see section 3.2). Others [335] observed that urinary LTE_4 concentrations increased after asthmatic attacks induced by aspirin. Therefore, this suggests that the LTE_4 is derived from the lung and, consequently, this offers the opportunity of examining the activity of compounds against lung 5-LO. This type of information about the effects on the excretion of LTE_4 obtained during clinical trials with A 64 077 in asthma was critical; it was shown that efficacy was poor but also that the degree of inhibition of urinary LTE_4 was only 50% at the dose employed (see 6.2.3, [336]).

Nasal washes obtained from patients suffering from allergic rhinitis contain elevated concentrations of leukotrienes compared to control subjects (see 3.2). Therefore, the effectiveness of 5-LO inhibitors in the treatment of rhinitis can be assessed by monitoring the levels of leukotrienes in the nasal washes during clinical trials.

Bronchoalveolar lavage (BAL) fluid taken from asthmatic patients soon after an attack also contains relatively high levels of leukotrienes (see 3.2). Thus, it is possible to assess the activity of compounds by measuring the concentrations of leukotrienes in BAL. However, there are significant technical problems and, possibly, ethical concerns about obtaining samples of BAL and, therefore, this approach is less attractive than measuring urinary LTE_4 as a routine procedure.

There is considerable evidence that eicosanoids, including leukotrienes, are involved in mediating some of the symptoms of IBD (see section 3.1). However, there are significant obstacles to the measurement of eicosanoids in faecal samples (e. g. difficulties in the isolation and purification of the eicosanoids from this biological matrix prior to assay). In order to avoid these difficulties, small dialysis bags have been ingested orally and passed *per rectum* and the concentration of eicosanoids in the dialysis fluid determined [125]. Alternatively the dialysis bags can be placed in the rectum for 1–4 h (see [125–127]). The concentrations in the latter samples reflect production of eicosanoids from the lower bowel but the cellular origin of the eicosanoids is unknown. It is likely that the concentration of the eicosanoids in the dialysis fluid is a gross underestimate of the amount of the mediators produced because a high proportion of the compounds probably will be removed by venous or lymphatic drainage rather than excreted into the bowel lumen. Thus, the method does offer a suitable procedure for monitoring the effects of 5-LO inhibitors on the synthesis of leukotrienes at a relevant site *in vivo* but it may not be perfect for studying the pathology of the disease. The effectiveness of A-64 077 at inhibiting leukotriene synthesis in IBD has been assessed using the above procedure (see section 6.2.3; [337]).

Increased concentrations of LTB_4 were detected in buffer in contact with involved psoriatic skin (3.1). Therefore, measurement of LTB_4 concentration in the buffer enables assessment of the 5-LO inhibition activity of test compounds during clinical trials designed to assess the efficacy of 5-LO inhibitors in psoriasis. Data from this type of study was invaluable during clinical assessment of L-652,343 for the treatment of psoriasis. Although L-652,343 was reported to inhibit both CO and 5-LO *in vitro* [338] it failed to reduce the concentration of LTB_4 in the buffer in contact with psoriatic skin: it did, however, lower the level of PGD_2 detected [339].

Thus, there are several procedures which enable *in vivo* evaluation of the 5-LO inhibitory activity in man. However, a limitation of most of these procedures is that compounds which reduce an inflammatory response by mechanisms other than inhibition of 5-LO may also reduce the concentrations of 5-LO products. For example, this can be achieved by the anti-inflammatory compound reducing cellular influx: since the infiltrating cells are frequently the source of 5-LO, a decrease in their number will be accompanied by a decrease of leukotrienes. Therefore, although the monitoring of the *in vivo* effects on

5-LO can be very informative the data should be interpreted cautiously.

6.2   Inhibitors of 5-lipoxygenase
6.2.1   Substrate analogues and related compounds

The substrate analogue 5,8,11,14-eicosatetraynoic acid (ETYA) inhibits both CO and 12-LO approximately equally [340] but is less effective against 5-LO [10]. However, ETYA does reduce enzymic formation of LTA_4 from 5-HPETE [341] so that the concentration of LTB_4 is reduced. Other acetylenic substrate analogues, such as 5,8,11-eicosatriynoic acid [342], 4,7,10,13-eicosatetraynoic acid [343], 5,8,11,14-heneicosatetraynoic acid and 4,7,10,13-heneicosatetraynoic acid [344] also have differential effects on CO, 5-LO and other enzymes in the cascade.

Some N-hydroxyamide derivatives of arachidonic acid inhibit 5-LO [345]. This finding stimulated the synthesis and testing of other hydroxamates and related compounds as possible inhibitors of 5-LO (see 6.2.3). 4,5-dehydroarachidonic acid [346] and 5,6-benzoarachidonic acid [347] both inhibit 5-LO *in vitro*.

Analogues of LTA_4 such as 5,6-methano-LTA_4 and carba-analogues of LTA_4 block 5-LO and 12-LO [348, 349]. The carba-analogues of 5-HPETE and, particularly, LTA_4 are potent inhibitors of 5-LO [350].

Metabolites of arachidonic acid can themselves inhibit 5-LO; Vanderhoek *et al.* [351, 352] demonstrated that 15-HPETE and 15-HETE inhibit 12-HETE synthesis by platelets, and 5-HETE and LTB_4 production by rabbit PMNs. 15-HPETE and 15-HETE may be alternative substrates for these enzymes rather than inhibitors. However, Cashman *et al.* [353] claimed that the inhibition of 5-LO was not due to metabolism of 15-HPETE to 5,15-di-HPETE, nor was it attributable to chemical or enzymatic decomposition products. It is possible that inhibition of 5-LO by 15-HPETE is mediated by depletion of ATP which is an essential requirement for 5-LO activity (see [354]).

Prostaglandin E_2 and prostacyclin (or stable analogues of the latter) inhibit LTB_4 synthesis in PMNs stimulated by A 23 187 or opsonized zymosan [355, 356]. These interactions between arachidonic acid metabolites suggest the possibility of complex feedback mechanisms in the control of the biosynthesis of eicosanoids. These data may explain the finding that low doses of indomethacin reduce the concentration of PGE_2 but potentiate PMN accumulation in the sponge implant model [105]; cell influx could be mediated by increased synthesis of a LO product (e.g. LTB_4). Piriprost, (6,9-deepoxy-6, 9-phenyli-mino)-6,8-prostaglandin I_1 (U 60 257; Fig. 6) was reported to inhibit the generation of leukotrienes but not the formation of 12-HETE or CO products [357]. Piriprost has complex effects on eicosanoid synthesis and its precise mechanism of action is unclear [358]. Recently, data obtained from experiments on the oxidative response in human neutrophils suggested that piriprost behaves as a specific and apparently competitive antagonist of FMLP and this action did not seem to involve inhibition of 5-LO [359]; it was concluded that the activity of piriprost may be exerted at the level of the FMLP receptor or its associated transduction mechanism. Piriprost was evaluated as a potential anti-asthmatic drug in man but its effects were equivocal [360].

Although the above compounds provide very useful experimental tools to assist in the examination of 5-LO activity *in vitro*, they probably have limited potential as drugs because of poor metabolic stability.

6.2.2   Anti-oxidants

The anti-oxidant nordihydroguaiaretic acid (NDGA; [361]) has been used by several investigators as a selective inhibitor of 5-LO although it inhibits other lipoxygenases and also CO at higher concentrations.

Natural products such as flavonoids exhibit potent and relatively selective activity against 5-LO; quercetin, esculetin, baicalein (see Fig. 6) and cirsiliol inhibit 5- and 12-LO but not CO [362–365]. Some of these compounds are present in plant extracts which have been used for centuries in Oriental medicine for treatment of inflammatory ailments; it is tempting to speculate that the benefits of these remedies could, in part, be due to inhibition of 5-LO. Some retinoids, in particular retinol (vitamin A), are also effective inhibitors of LTB_4 synthesis [366, 367] and have been used in the treatment of psoriasis. Caffeic acid also reduces arachidonic acid metabolism via 5-LO [368].

BW 755 C (3-amino-1-[*m*-trifluoromethylphenyl]-2-pyrazoline; see Fig. 6) has been investigated extensively; it blocks LO of platelets [369] and PMNs [370, 371] at concentrations similar to those required to inhibit CO. The precise mechanism of action of BW 755 C has not been defined but the enzymic reaction is probably affected by the re-

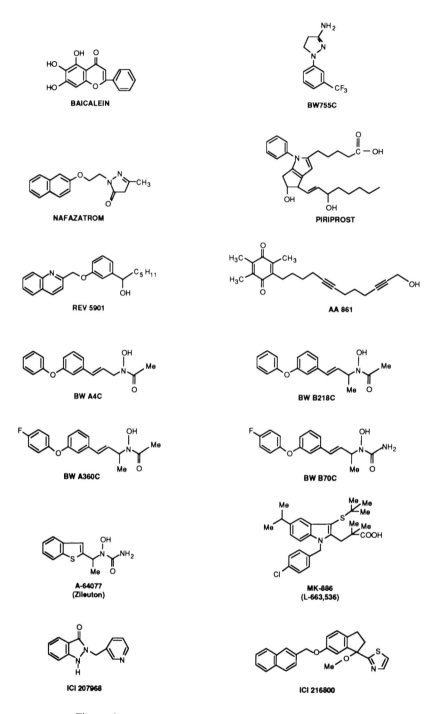

Figure 6
Structures of some inhibitiors of 5-lipoxygenase.

dox properties of the compound. Thus, BW 755 C, as well as the above phenols, quinones and flavones, probably reduce ferric to ferrous iron at the active site of the enzyme. This "dual-inhibitor" (i.e. both LO and CO are blocked) has been employed widely as an experimental tool both *in vitro* and *in vivo* to explore the role of lipoxygenase products in a variety of inflammatory and allergic reactions. However, since it is not a specific inhibitor of 5-LO, interpretation of data cannot be made with confidence. The further development of BW 755 C and related compounds was compromised by the finding that it induced methaemoglobinaemia, which may be caused by its redox properties.

Nafazatrom (BAY-G 6576: Fig. 6), originally developed as an antithrombotic agent, is a relatively selective inhibitor of 5-LO [372, 373]. Since nafazatrom is believed to be a reducing co-factor for peroxidase, it could act by increasing 15-HETE synthesis [372] which in turn may inhibit 5-LO [351]. Nafazatrom had no effect on antigen-induced bronchoconstriction in atopic asthmatics but, also there was no evidence of *ex vivo* inhibition of 5-LO [374].

A derivative of benzoquinone, AA 861 (Fig. 6), selectively inhibits 5-LO [375] and was shown to reduce allergic bronchoconstriction in guinea-pigs and to reduce carrageenin-induced paw oedema and pleurisy in rats [376]. When given at a dose of 400 mg/day for 4 days, AA 861 had no effect on airway responsiveness to acetylcholine in asthmatic subjects [377].

Many other quinones and hydroquinones have been synthesized and tested as inhibitors of 5-LO (see [222, 224]). Also, substitution of an heteroatom for one of the oxygens of a quinone/hydroquinone produces anti-oxidant compounds which inhibit 5-LO; for example L- 651,392 ([378]; see also, [222, 224]).

An extensive series of 2,3-dihydro-5-benzofuranols have been synthesized and their 5-LO inhibitory activity determined because it was suggested that this group maximises stereoelectronic effects necessary for efficient hydrogen atom abstraction by peroxyl radicals [379]. Although the compounds were not very potent inhibitors, it was claimed that the 2,3-dihydro-5-benzofuranol moiety may offer a useful template for the design of anti-oxidant-based inhibitors of 5-LO. Two of these benzofuran derivatives, L-656,224 and L-651,896, have been investigated more extensively [224, 380, 381]. When administered orally, L-656,224 inhibited antigen-induced bronchoconstriction in inbred, hyperreactive rats (ED_{50} 0.7 mg/kg) and ascaris-antigen induced bronchoconstriction in the squirrel monkey [381].

The quinoline derivative Rev 5901 (see Fig. 6) inhibits 5-LO [382, 383] and this was attributed to its structural similarity to 15-HETE, which is an endogenous inhibitor of the enzyme (see above). Rev-5901 is also an LTD_4-antagonist *in vitro* and in man [384] but it is probable that its major activity is as an inhibitor of 5-LO. It does also reduce histamine release which implies that it may not be a very selective compound. The exact mechanism of action of Rev-5901 has not been established; it may act as an anti-oxidant although there is also a suggestion that it may affect the translocation of the 5-LO enzyme (see 6.2.4).

Another quinoline (Wy-47,288; (2-[1-naphthalenyloxy)-methyl] quinoline) demonstrated topical anti-inflammatory activity in several animal models of skin inflammation which was attributed to inhibition of CO as well as 5-LO [385]. Another compound from the Wyeth-Ayerst Research Group, Wy-50,295 ((S)-α-methyl-6-(2-quinolinylmethoxy)-2-naphthaleneacetic acid) exhibited LTD_4 antagonist properties as well as inhibition of 5-LO [386].

Compound CGS 8515 (methyl 2-[3,4-dihydro-3,4-dioxo-1-naphthalenyl]-amino)-benzoate is an inhibitor of 5-LO *in vitro* and *in vivo* [387]; it inhibited LTB_4 synthesis in guinea-pig leucocytes (IC_{50} = 0.1 μM), but did not appreciably affect CO, 12-LO or 15-LO from other sources. The selective inhibitory effect was confirmed in rat whole blood. *Ex vivo* and *in vivo* studies showed that CGS 8515, at a dose of 2–50 mg/kg significantly inhibited A 23 187-induced leukotriene synthesis in blood and in the lung. Inhibitory effects of the compound on leukotriene synthesis and inflammatory responses were reported in the carrageenin-induced pleurisy and sponge models in the rat [387].

Lipoxygenation is postulated to occur via the formation of a carbon centred radical (see [224]). Therefore, compounds that inhibit the generation of this radical or trap it once formed would be expected to inhibit 5-LO. These compounds often act by formation of a lower energy radical thus diverting the intended path of the reaction [224]. This was postulated to be the mechanism of the disulphide class of 5-LO inhibitors (e.g. [388, 389]).

2-Substituted indazolinones (e.g. ICI 207 968; see Fig. 6) selectively inhibit leukotriene biosynthesis *in vitro* and *in vivo* [390]. In several systems *in vitro* ICI 207 968 exhibited similar inhibitory potency against 5-LO (IC_{50} = 1.5-6.0 μM) and it was approximately 300 times less potent against CO. Following oral administration to rats, ICI 207968 inhibited LTB_4 synthesis in A23187-stimulated blood *ex vivo;* the ED_{50} values at 1,3 and 5 h after dosing were 2.5, 10 and 25 mg/kg, respectively. Co-administration of ICI 207968 with arachidonic acid into rabbit dermis potently inhibited both extravasation and PMN infiltration induced by the fatty acid. Although these compounds may achieve inhibition of 5-LO because of their anti-oxidant properties it was demonstrated that the inhibitory potency was not directly related to the redox potential, although they could participate in redox reactions. It was suggested that an alternative mechanism of action was by iron chelation (see Section 6.2.3). Therefore, at present the precise mechanism of action of ICI 207968 is unknown.

6.2.3   Iron chelators: Hydroxamates and hydroxyureas

As noted above (6.2.1), Corey *et al.* [345] synthesized analogues of arachidonic acid containing a hydroxamic acid moiety and demonstrated that these compounds inhibited 5-LO, presumably by the hydroxamic acid portion of the molecule binding to Fe^{3+} at the catalytic site of the enzyme. A series of compounds were synthesized by Jackson *et al.* [391] in which the hydroxamic acid moiety, and other potential iron-chelating groups, were linked via a spacing group to a hydrophobic/lipophilic aryl unit. The structure-activity relationships of modifying the aryl function, the linking group and the arrangement of the iron-chelating group (e.g. straight or reversed hydroxamic acids) were studied *in vitro* [297]. Of the compounds prepared, N-(3-phenoxycinnamyl), N-(4-benzyloxybenzyl) and N-[3-(5,6,7,8-tetrahydro-2-naphthyl)prop-2-enyl] acetohydroxamic acids (BW A4C, BW A137C and BW A797C, respectively) have been studied extensively in several biological tests [297, 392, 393].

The acetohydroxamic acids were potent (IC_{50} values ca 0.05–0.2 μM) and selective inhibitors of 5-LO in human PMN *in vitro,* using both broken and whole cell tests (see Section 6.1.1), and in A23187-stimulated whole blood [297]. The acetohydroxamic acids do not reduce the binding of [³H]-LTC_4 or [³H]-LTD_4 to guinea-pig lung homogenates indicating that these compounds are not peptido-lipid leukotriene antagonists. These data encouraged further examination of several acetohydroxamic compounds and related compounds *in vivo*. Evaluation of the compounds in A23187-stimulated whole blood *ex vivo* (see

Section 6.1.2) revealed that several hydroxamic acids were orally bio-available and had satisfactory half-lives, whereas other compounds (e.g. nafazatrom) which inhibited 5-LO *in vitro* failed to affect significantly the formation of LTB_4 *ex vivo* [297]. The acetohydroxamic acids did not inhibit completely the formation of immunoreactive-LTB_4 (i-LTB_4) in rat blood because part of the i-LTB_4 was due to the synthesis of high concentrations of 12-HETE which cross reacted in the RIA: the formation of 12-HETE was not reduced at doses of acetohydroxamic acids which blocked biosynthesis of LTB_4 (see discussion in Section 6.1.2). The acetohydroxamic acids did not inhibit significantly the synthesis of TXB_2 in the stimulated blood, thereby confirming their selective action.

There is no doubt that the acetohydroxamic moiety confers the ability to bind iron; for example, the binding constant for BW A 4 C has been measured to be in the order of 10^{12}/mole. Although this property was a consideration in the initial design of this class of 5-LO inhibitor, it is probable that their mechanism of action is more complex. Electro-chemical evidence shows that BW A 4 C and the related hydroxyurea, BW B 70 C (see below), have relatively high electrode potentials (E_o ca 2 V against a normal hydrogen electrode) and are not powerful redox compounds. However, both BW A 4 C and BW B 70 C inhibited lipid peroxidation in a model system based on the oxidation of linoleic acid by a thermolabile azo compound ([394] and unpublished observations) and this property was clearly separate from the iron-chelating property of the compounds. Thus, it is possible that these compounds inhibit 5-LO by acting as site-directed peroxyl radical scavengers.

Some structural features in the series of hydroxamic acids were shown to confer increased duration of action which was presumably because of greater metabolic stability: (i) the "reversed" hydroxamic acids (acetohydroxamic acids) were longer lasting than the analogous "straight" hydroxamic acids after similar dosing to rats and rabbits (ii) the inclusion of a C = C group in a three carbon link was more meta-bolically stable than the saturated analogue (iii) the half-life was af-fected by the nature of the lipophilic group [297, 395].

The *ex vivo* method provided very useful preliminary information about the bioavailability and duration of action of compounds. How-ever, it was not ideal for detailed pharmacokinetic analysis because it had a limited linear range and it was somewhat variable, which was possibly due to fluctuating cell counts and varying plasma protein binding of A 23 187 (see 6.1.2). Therefore, a more accurate and reliable method of determining unchanged acetohydroxamic acid was developed using high pressure liquid chromatography (HPLC). The HPLC method enabled the measurement of a wide range of acetohydroxamic acids; individual assays only required minor modification of internal standard, mobile phase and detection wavelength (ultra violet absorption or fluorescence) [297].

The concentrations of unchanged acetohydroxamic acids in plasma correlated well with the inhibition of *ex vivo* synthesis of LTB$_4$, thereby providing important validation of the latter technique for a preliminary investigation of the pharmacokinetics of the compounds (e. g. see Fig. 9). The good correlation of these data also indicated that biological activity was probably not related to the formation of active metabolites. The determination of unchanged compound in plasma by HPLC suggested an explanation for the observed species differences in the degree of inhibition of leukotriene biosynthesis caused by the acetohydroxamic acids. For example, BW A 137 C inhibited leukotriene-dependent anaphylaxis in guinea-pigs more potently than was expected based on inhibition of 5-LO in rats *ex vivo;* HPLC analysis demonstrated that the peak plasma concentrations and the half-life of BW A 137 C were higher and longer, respectively, in guinea-pigs than in rats [392].

Several acetohydroxamic acids reduced the bronchoconstriction occurring in actively sensitized guinea-pigs challenged with aerosolised antigen [392]. As described earlier (Section 6.1.3), this test requires animals to be pre-treated with mepyramine and indomethacin to block the effects of histamine and CO metabolites and this results in a prolonged increase in pulmonary inflation pressure (PIP) which is "leukotriene dependent". The inhibition of the increase of PIP by the acetohydroxamic acids was both dose and time dependent [392].

The effects of BW A 4 C and BW A 797 C upon the synthesis of mediators and cell influx occurring in a model of acute inflammation described above (Section 3.1) were investigated. The concentrations of PGE$_2$ and LTB$_4$, as well as the number of leucocytes, were determined in an inflammatory exudate produced 6 h after the subcutaneous implantation in rats of a sponge impregnated with an irritant substance (carrageenin) [393]. These experiments confirmed that the acetohydroxamic acids selectively inhibited the 5-LO; the concentration of LTB$_4$ was reduced dose-dependently but PGE$_2$ was not affected (for example see Fig. 5). The infiltration of leucocytes into the exudate was also suppressed but this effect was not correlated directly with the inhibition of LTB_4 [393]. Doses of the compounds which reduced the synthesis of LTB_4 by 80–90% only lowered the leucocyte count by 50–65%. If LTB_4 is important in the initiation of cell influx, these data may indicate that the acetohydroxamic acids were not available in the relevant tissues at the beginning of the response. An alternative explanation is that LTB_4 is not the only chemotactic signal operating in this model of acute inflammation (see Section 3.1).

The acetohydroxamic acids were ineffective at reducing inflammatory responses mediated by CO metabolites. Thus, the acetohydroxamic acids did not inhibit carrageenin-induced oedema in rat paws whereas the selective CO inhibitor indomethacin, and the dual CO/LO inhibitor, BW 755 C, did reduce swelling in the period 1–4 h after injection of carrageenin [393]. The swelling of the rat paw after carrageenin also depends on the presence and activation of circulating leucocytes and, therefore, the failure of the acetohydroxamic acids to reduce the oedema in this model suggests that the leukotrienes do not contribute to increased vascular permeability either through a direct action on the vasculature or through activation of leucocytes [393].

The acetohydroxamic acids also failed to inhibit carrageenin-induced hyperalgesia and phenyl benzoquinone-induced writhing; both these effects are reduced by selective CO inhibitors [393]. However, BW A4C and BW A797C did reduce yeast induced hyperthermia, which suggested that lipoxygenase metabolites could be pyretic although subsequent experiments indicated that this was unlikely [396].

It has been suggested that leukotrienes may mediate the formation of gastric erosions; however, the acetohydroxamic acids did not reduce ulceration induced in rats by administration of ethanol, even though gastric mucosal 5-LO activity was inhibited [315]. But in contrast to the CO inhibitors, the acetohydroxamic acids did not induce the formation of ulcers [315] and this is an important advantage if these inhibitors of 5-LO do show therapeutic efficacy in asthma and/or inflammatory conditions.

The data from the initial series of acetohydroxamic acids was encouraging but, although active *in vivo* they had relatively short half-lives both in animals [297, 395] and man [333, 334]. For example, the plasma $t_{1/2}$ of BW A4C following oral administration of 400 mg to human volunteers was approximately 2 h; the inhibitory activity on 5-LO *ex vivo*

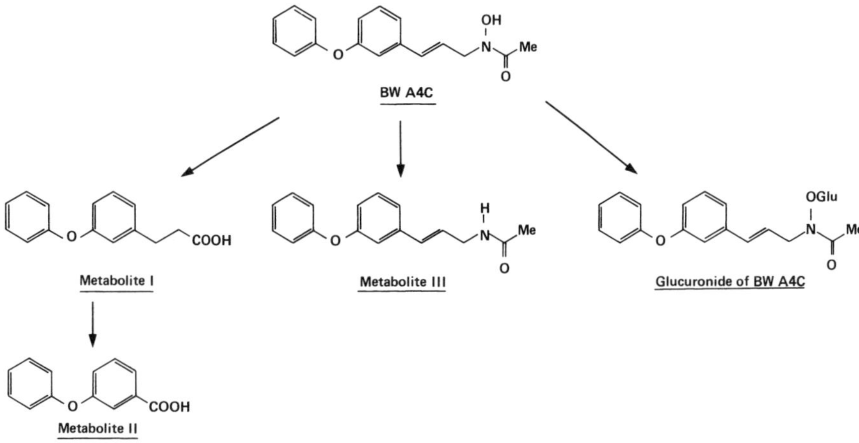

Figure 7
Major metabolic transformations of BW A4C (information from [395]).

declined with falling plasma levels of unchanged drug [333, 334]. Compounds with longer half-lives and increased bioavailability were considered to be desirable. Therefore, the major routes of elimination were elucidated and this information was used to develop a second generation of acetohydroxamic acids with enhanced metabolic stability.

Three metabolic transformations were common to all acetohydroxamic acids studied in rats and rabbits (i) oxidation of the carbon adjacent to the hydroxamic acid moiety leading to the formation of the corresponding carboxylic acid (ii) glucuronidation of the N-hydroxy and subsequent excretion in bile and urine (iii) reduction of the N-hydroxy to form the acetamide analogue [395]. These reactions of BW A4C are illustrated in Fig. 7. The enzymatic reduction of the C = C in the linking group of BW A4C probably occurs before oxidation of the α-methylene because the saturated analogue had a much shorter half-life compared to BW A4C; only the saturated carboxylic acids derived from BW A4C were detected in plasma. It should be noted that all the metabolites had little or no effect on 5-LO activity.

Other metabolic reactions occurred on specific acetohydroxamic acids. For example, in rats the benzyloxy group of BW A137C was oxidised to produce benzoic acid; the latter was not detected as such because it was conjugated with glycine to form hippuric acid which was rapidly excreted in urine. This additional metabolic transformation is the explanation for the short half-life of BW A 137 C compared to BW A 4 C.

Oxidation of the carbon adjacent to the hydroxamic moiety and glu-curonidation of the N-hydroxy group suggested that substitution of the α-methylene may confer more metabolic stability. Indeed, the α-methyl analogues reach higher plasma concentrations which are maintained for longer than the unsubstituted analogues [395] (the structure of BW B 218 C, the α-methyl analogue of BW A 4 C is shown in Fig. 6). The α-methyl analogues were slightly less potent inhibitors of 5-LO *in vitro* (2–5 times) but they were more active *ex vivo* and this activity was maintained for longer because of the higher plasma concentrations [395]. No carboxylic acid metabolites were detected after administration of α-methyl acetohydroxamic acids.

The α-methyl analogues are also more potent and longer lasting inhibitors of the "leukotriene-dependent" bronchoconstriction in the guinea-pig model described above [326, 392].

Further increases in the half-life of the acetohydroxamic acids in laboratory animals can be achieved by substitution in the 3-phenoxy group, possibly by hindering 4-hydroxylation. However, the substitution has produced compounds which exhibit relatively high plasma levels and long half-lives but which do not inhibit 5-LO *ex vivo* as effectively as would be expected based on *in vitro* results. For example, oral administration of 3'-trifluoromethyl-BW B 218 C (BW A 914 C) to rabbits (10 mg/kg) produced only 30–70% inhibition of LTB_4 synthesis *ex vivo* although it was predicted that the concentration of unchanged compound attained in plasma should have caused at least 80% inhibition based on *in vitro* data [395]. These data suggest that binding to plasma proteins of some of the substituted acetohydroxamic acids may compromise biological activity. Thus, the choice of compounds to be tested in the clinic should be influenced by the degree and affinity of binding to (human) plasma protein as well as on metabolic stability and inhibitory activity *in vitro*. Additionally, for anti-asthmatic activity, the compounds should be able to penetrate into the lungs; several of the acetohydroxamic acids have been detected in guinea-pig BAL fluid obtained in the experiments to evaluate the compounds against "leukotriene-dependent" bronchospasm. BW B 360 C, the 4-fluoro-phenoxy analogue of BW B 218 C (see Fig. 6) exhibited one of the most appropriate profiles; for example, the plasma levels attained after oral dosing to rabbits are much higher

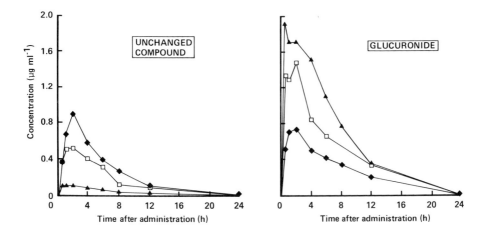

Figure 8
Concentrations of unchanged compound (left panel) and glucuronide (right panel) after oral administration (10 mg/kg) to rats of racemic BW B218C (□, (S)-BW B218C
(♦) and (R)-BW B218C (▲). Data from [395].

and maintained for longer than those of BW A4C and this is accompanied by much more effective inhibition of LTB_4 synthesis *ex vivo*
(see Fig. 9).

The α-methyl analogues were studied initially as racemic mixtures but
we were aware of the potential for stereoselective metabolism and,
therefore, the chirality of the metabolites was investigated. Unchanged compound was extracted from plasma of animals dosed
(p.o.) with BW B218C; purification was performed by reverse phase
(RP)-HPLC and then recovered material was subjected to chiral
HPLC on a Chiracel OB or OD column. Also, the glucuronide of BW
B218C was extracted from plasma and purified by RP-HPLC; incubation with β-glucuronidase liberated the aglycone which was then
subjected to chiral HPLC. In rats, rabbits and dogs more than 90% or
the unchanged compound recovered from plasma chromatographed
as the S-enantiomer [395]. Conversely, the majority of the aglycone
derived from the glucuronide chromatographed with the R-enantiomer [395]. Therefore, the glucuronidation of BW B218C and similar α-methyl acetohydroxamic acids is stereoselective.

The separate S(−) and R(+) enantiomers of BW B218C, have been
synthesized [397] and tested *in vitro* and *in vivo*. The enantiomers have
identical activity against the 5-LO *in vitro* but, as expected they exhibit

different pharmacokinetic profiles (Fig. 8). The S-enantiomer attained higher plasma concentrations which were maintained for longer than those of the R-enantiomer after similar oral administration to rabbits and this correlated with a reduced formation of the glucuronide [395]. This information suggests that the (S)-α-methyl acetohydroxamic should be preferred to the R-enantiomers for development as therapeutic agents both for scientific reasons and to satisfy the current regulatory climate. However, it should first be confirmed that stereoselective metabolism of the compounds in human tissue is similar to that in animals and that there are no pharmacological or toxicological reasons for selecting the R-enantiomer.

The above information and discussion has focussed on the experience of hydroxamic acids gained by investigators at Wellcome Research Laboratories, however, similar data have been published by the group at Abbott Laboratories [324, 398–401]. Also, the Rorer Group have reported data for N-methyl-4-benzyloxyphenyl acetohydroxamic acid (RG 6866; [186, 402]).

As noted earlier, several potential iron chelating groups have been evaluated as alternatives to hydroxamic acids. The hydroxyurea moiety provided equivalent 5-LO inhibitory potency and selectivity *in vitro* to that of the acetohydroxamic acids and, therefore, examples of this series have been test *in vivo*. The structure of the hydroxyurea analogue of a key acetohydroxamic acid, BW A 360 C, is shown in Fig. 6: the hydroxyurea is referred to as BW B 70 C. Higher plasma levels, which are maintained for longer, are attained after oral administration of BW B 70 C than after comparable dosing with BW A 360 C (see Fig. 9 [403] and this is accompanied by a longer duration of inhibition of 5-LO *ex vivo* (see Fig. 9). The difference in the pharmacokinetic profile of the hydroxyurea compared to the acetohydroxamic acid is explained by the reduced formation of glucuronide metabolites by the former. However, glucuronidation of the α-methyl hydroxyureas is stereoselective although, interestingly, the S-enantiomer, and not the R-form, is the preferred substrate in rats, rabbits and dogs *in vivo* and in human hepatocytes *in vitro* (cf hydroxamic acids, see above).

Abbott Laboratories have also developed a series of hydroxyureas and one compound, A-64077 (or Zileuton; see Fig. 6), which is also a racemate, has been investigated extensively in animals and man [336, 337, 404–409]. A-64077 is not as potent as BW B 70 C as an inhibitor of 5-LO *in vitro* and it also has a shorter duration of activity *ex vivo* after

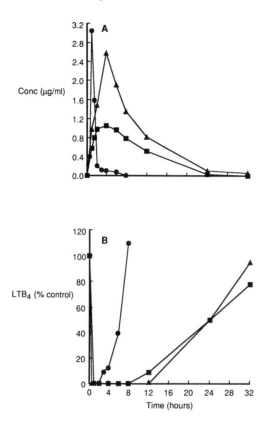

Figure 9
A Concentrations of unchanged compound in plasma after oral administration to rabbits of BW A4C, 50 mg/kg (●), BW A 360 C, 10 mg/kg (■) and BW B 70 C, 10 mg/kg (▲). *B* The formation of LTB_4 in A 23 187-stimulated whole blood *ex vivo* corresponding to the data presented in panel *A*.

oral administration to animals. However, the properties of A-64 077 in the pre-clinical studies encouraged the Abbott group to perform an early investigation of its activity in man.

The determination of plasma levels after oral administration (200–800 mg) of A-64 077 indicated that the compound was absorbed rapidly and had a half-life of 2.3 h [408]; three metabolites were also monitored, these were the N-dehydroxylated compound in plasma and diastereomeric O-glucuronides of A-64 077 in urine. *Ex vivo* inhibition of 5-LO in A 23187-stimulated blood was confirmed.

Clinical trials to ascertain the efficacy of A-64 077 in the treatment of asthma, rhinitis, inflammatory bowel disease and rheumatoid arthritis have commenced. The effects of A-64077 on both the early and late asthmatic response in mild atopic asthmatics was evaluated in a randomised, placebo-controlled, double-blind, crossover study. The response of subjects to inhaled antigen (house dust mite or mixed grass pollen) was studied on 2 days at least 2 weeks apart: the effect of the compound on the allergen-induced fall in FEV_1 was monitored for 8 h. In these studies it was noted that urinary LTE_4 was only inhibited by approximately 50% (61.4 to 30.3 ng i-LTE_4/nmol creatinine) and, therefore, it is not surprising that clinical efficacy was equivocal [336]. It was concluded that the dose of A-64077 used in these studies (800 mg) was insufficient to inhibit effectively the 5-LO in the lungs. In a randomised, double-blind, placebo-controlled, crossover study the effect of A-64077 on the bronchoconstriction induced by hyperventilation of cold, dry air in 13 patients with asthma was examined. The dose of the 5-LO inhibitor used (800 mg, p.o.) decreased the mean ionophore-induced synthesis of LTB_4 in blood *ex vivo* by 74%. It was also demonstrated that the amount of cold air (expressed as respiratory heat exchange) required to reduce FEV_1 by 10% was increased by 47% after A-64077. Similar results were obtained when minute ventilation was used as an indicator of outcome [408 a]. Administration of A-64077 (800 mg, p.o.) to patients suffering from allergic rhinitis has also been accompanied by a significant reduction in the nasal congestion provoked by challenge with allergen [406, 408 b]. In these latter studies it was demonstrated that the dose of A-64077 employed not only inhibited ionophore-induced synthesis of LTB_4 in blood *ex vivo* but also reduced significantly the peak levels of both LTB_4 and 5-HETE in nasal-rinse fluids, although levels of histamine and PGD_2 were unaffected.

Before proceeding with an assessment of the effectiveness of A-64077 in the treatment of IBD it was first established that the compound inhibited the synthesis of LTB_4 using the rectal dialysis technique described above (Section 6.1.4). Ten patients with active ulcerative colitis were given 800 mg A-64077 [337]. The median LTB_4 concentration in the rectal dialysis fluid fell significantly from 4.9 ng/ml before treatment to 1.6 and 0.7 ng/ml, 4 and 8 h after dosing, respectively, and had returned to pre-treatment levels by 28 h. The concentration of PGE_2 in the dialysate did not change significantly during the study. Subsequently the efficacy of the compound was examined in double-blind, placebo-controlled clinical trials: a dose of 800 mg b.i.d. was shown to reduce symptoms of IBD such as diarrhoea, also the endoscopic and histological scores were improved compared to patients treated with placebo [406, 409]. Further, larger scale trials are required to confirm the early promise that inhibition of 5-LO by compounds such an A-64077 will have therapeutic benefit in the treatment of IBD.

Administration of A-64077 to patients suffering from allergic rhinitis has also been accompanied by a significant reduction in symptoms (e. g. periods of sneezing) [406]. Clinical trials to assess the efficacy of A-64077 in the treatment of psoriasis and rheumatoid arthritis have commenced. Preliminary data obtained in an open study in arthritic patients are encouraging.

6.2.4   Inhibitors of 5-lipoxygenase translocation

MK-886 (previously referred to as L-663,536; see Fig. 6) has a unique mode of action. The compound reduces leukotriene synthesis in whole cells but it was demonstrated that this was not achieved by a direct effect on 5-LO. Further studies revealed that its inhibitory activity was due to inhibition of the translocation of 5-LO to the cell membrane. These findings led to the discovery of FLAP which is essential for cellular leukotriene biosynthesis (see Section 2.3) and it is now believed that MK-886 binds to FLAP thereby preventing 5-LO "docking" onto the protein [62, 63, 262]. The compound inhibits leukotriene biosynthesis in human intact PMN (IC_{50} 2.5 nM) and in human whole blood (IC_{50} 1.1 μM) but it was not effective at inhibiting rat "crude" 5-LO or a porcine purified enzyme. The reduced activity of MK-886 in blood relative to its effect on isolated cells was explained by binding to plasma proteins. At concentrations required to inhibit 5-LO, no reduction in CO or 12-LO activity was observed [410].

When administered *in vivo* MK-886 was a potent inhibitor of antigen-induced dyspnoea in inbred rats pretreated with methysergide (ED_{50} 0.036 mg/kg p.o.) and ascaris-induced bronchoconstriction in squirrel monkeys (1 mg/kg p.o.) [410]. The compound was effective at inhibiting leukotriene biosynthesis in a rat pleurisy model (ED_{50} 0.2 mg/kg p.o.), in an inflamed rat paw model (ED_{50} 0.8 mg/kg), and in the guinea-pig ear where leukotriene biosynthesis was stimulated by topical challenge with A23187 (ED_{50} 2.5 mg/kg p.o. and 0.6 μg topically) [410]. MK-886 also inhibited leukotriene excretion in bile following antigen provocation [410].

MK-886 (10 mg/kg i.v., 15 min before challenge) suppressed antigen-induced peptido-lipid leukotriene production in guinea-pigs and this was associated with a complete protection against lethal shock [411]. Dexamethasone was also evaluated in these latter studies but it was reported that even at high doses (10 mg/kg i.p. once daily for 7 days or a single dose of 10 mg/kg i.v., 3.5 h before challenge) this antiinflammatory steroid had no effect on leukotriene synthesis during anaphylaxis *in vivo,* although inhibition of both CO and 5-LO product synthesis in macrophages *ex vivo* was observed.

MK-886 has been tested in a rat model of colitis (intracolonic administration of trinitrobenzene sulphonic acid). A single dose of MK-886 (10 mg/kg) significantly inhibited for greater than 24 h colonic LTB_4 synthesis, measured after incubation of tissue samples *in vitro* and by *in vivo* equilibrium dialysis [320]. Treatment with this dose significantly reduced colonic damage, as assessed macroscopically and histologically, when the compound was given 2 h before induction of colitis and daily thereafter for 1 week. A less marked beneficial effect of MK-886 was observed when the pretreatment dose was excluded, suggesting a role for leukotrienes in the early events of the inflammatory process.

MK-886 has been given to healthy male volunteers in single oral doses from 10 to 750 mg and in multiple oral doses of 100 or 250 mg t.i.d. for 10 days: inhibition of LTB_4 synthesis *ex vivo* was confirmed. Also, the compound has shown significant attenuation of the early phase of antigen-induced bronchoconstriction in asthmatic patients [412].

6.2.5   Miscellaneous inhibitors

Benoxaprofen was claimed to be a selective inhibitor of 5-LO when evalutated by monitoring the conversion of exogenous [^{14}C]-arachidonic acid to 5-HETE and LTB_4 in PMN stimulated with A 23187 [413, 414]. Inhibition of LTB_4 synthesis from endogenous substrate in A 23187-stimulated human PMNs has been confirmed, although this compound was a more effective inhibitor of TXB_2 synthesis [298]. However, benoxaprofen was a less effective inhibitor of opsonized zymosan-induced LTB_4 synthesis by PMNs leading these authors to speculate that it may affect A 23187-induced 5-LO activity indirectly

[298]. Also, it did not inhibit synthesis of LTB_4 in a model of acute in-flammation (see Section 6.1.3), although it did reduce the concentra-tions of CO products [322] which suggested that it had a profile simi-lar to conventional NSAIDs. Support for this hypothesis is provided by reports that benoxaprofen does not inhibit LTC_4 synthesis by zy-mosan-stimulated macrophages at doses up to 10^{-4} M [415] or 5-HETE and LTB_4 synthesis in a cell-free system derived from human PMN [416]. Thus, neither the reported anti-inflammatory [417, 418] nor the toxic properties of benoxaprofen (Opren) can be attributed to inhibition of 5-LO.

ICI 216800 has a single chiral centre, as have several of the selective 5-LO inhibitors described above (e.g. BW A360C, BW B70C, A-64077; see Fig. 6). However, unlike the other compounds, it has been reported that the separate enantiomers of ICI 216800 have differen-tial effects on 5-LO; for example the IC_{50} values for inhibition of a cell free 5-LO for the racemate, (+)- and (−)-enantiomers were 0.77, 0.13 and > 20 μM, respectively [419]. The authors concluded that the com-pound exerted its 5-LO inhibitory activity by chiral interaction with the enzyme and not by either a redox or iron chelation mechanism. It was suggested that the methoxy alkyl thiazole group could interact at the active site of 5-LO. Topically applied (+) ICI 216800 produced dose-dependent inhibition of plasma extravasation induced by ara-chidonic acid. Also, the compound was effective in reducing LTB_4 synthesis in A23187-stimulated human blood in vitro but the activity after systemic exposure has not yet been reported.

Auranofin, an oral gold compound, dose-dependently inhibited A23187-induced LTB_4 and 5-HETE synthesis in rat alveolar macro-phages [420]. The authors suggested that inhibition of 5-LO could re-present an important mechanism of action of auranofin in chronic in-flammatory disorders.

6.3 Inhibition of leukotriene biosynthesis by modification of the diet

Administration of dihomo-γ-linolenic acid, which is the precursor of monoenoic prostaglandins but which cannot be converted to leuko-trienes, has been claimed to provide anti-inflammatory effects but since this is not achieved by a direct effect on the activity of leuko-trienes it will not be considered in this review.

Eicosapentaenoic acid (EPA) is a poor substrate for CO [6, 421] but is a competitive inhibitor of this enzyme. In contrast EPA is a good substrate for LO enzymes and can be converted to leukotrienes and other LO products [422–425]. One product of EPA metabolism, LTB_5, is approximately 30 times less active than the analogous metabolite of arachidonic acid (i.e. LTB_4) in affecting PMN function *in vitro* (aggregation, degranulation and chemokinesis; [424]). Furthermore, the potency of LTB_5 in potentiating bradykinin-induced plasma exudation was at least 10 times lower than that of LTB_4 [424]. Oral administration of EPA also reduced the formation of LTB_4 by rat leucocytes stimulated with A 23 187 *in vitro* [426]. These authors found that the ratio of LTB_4 to LTB_5 produced was directly correlated with the AA: EPA ratio in leucocyte phospholipids. The effect of an EPA-rich diet on leucocyte accumulation, and LTB_4 and PGE_2 levels in inflammatory exudates induced by implanting carrageenin-soaked sponges has also been evaluated [427]. Supplementation of the diet for 4 weeks with 240 mg/kg/day EPA significantly decreased the concentration of PGE_2 and TXB_2 in the exudate, indicating inhibition of CO by EPA. The concentration of LTB_4 and the total leucocyte count were also suppressed, but not significantly. In another model of acute inflammation, the rat foot carrageenin model, an EPA-rich diet caused significant reduction of oedema [427]. Also, treatment with EPA markedly reduced the severity of glomerulonephritis in NZB/NZW which is used as a model of systemic lupus erythematosus [428]. Thus, supplementation of the diet with EPA could, by reducing the synthesis of metabolites of arachidonic acid and by antagonizing the biological activity of LTB_4 be beneficial in the prevention and/or treatment of inflammatory disease.

However, the inhibition of PGE_2 synthesis by EPA may compromise the use of this dietary supplement to treat chronic inflammatory disease because PGE_2 is believed to be immunosuppressive. Indeed, Prickett *et al.* [429] reported that addition of EPA to the diet increased the incidence, although not the severity, of collagen induced arthritis in rats. However, in another study [430], supplementing a normal diet with fish oil decreased the susceptibility of mice to collagen-induced arthritis.

The biological properties of the peptido-lipid leukotrienes derived from EPA are comparable, both qualitatively and quantitatively, to those from arachidonic acid. Also, the yield of these leukotrienes from EPA and arachidonic acid are similar and, therefore, administration of EPA is unlikely to be of benefit in treatment of hypersensitivity reactions. In fact, Lee *et al.* [431] demonstrated, that in guinea-pigs, the anaphylactic reaction may be exacerbated by administration of EPA; leukotriene synthesis was increased by feeding an EPA-rich diet and this could be due to the suppression of the synthesis of modulator prostaglandins (e.g. PGE_2).

Several human studies to investigate the anti-inflammatory properties of EPA have been reported. Increased biosynthesis of LTB_5 by PMNs obtained from volunteers given an EPA rich diet was confirmed [432, 433]. Functional changes in leucocytes have been observed after 6 weeks consumption of a diet supplemented with EPA [432] although not after 3 weeks [433]. Modest anti-inflammatory activity in patients with rheumatoid arthritis has been observed after administration of EPA (434–439]. Also EPA provided some mild to moderate improvement in symptoms in patients with psoriasis [440, 441].

Thus, these results from clinical trials indicate that, at best, EPA will provide a modest improvement in symptoms and should only be considered as a possible adjunct to conventional anti-inflammatory therapy.

7   Conclusion

The biological properties of the leukotrienes coupled with the demonstration that the biosynthesis of these endogenous compounds is increased suggests that they are mediators of the symptoms of certain diseases, particularly in asthma and inflammatory conditions. The prevalence of asthma is growing despite increased intervention with current drugs, and, therefore, the availability of new medicines is awaited with considerable interest. New initiatives are also needed in the treatment of chronic inflammatory disease, such as arthritis, since current therapy may only provide symptomatic relief and does not affect the underlying pathological process. It is possible that leukotrienes mediate some of the key events in these diseases. Thus, antagonists or inhibitors of the biosynthesis of the leukotrienes may provide important improvements in therapy.

Therefore, it is not surprising that the Pharmaceutical Industry has committed considerable research effort to the discovery and development of compounds which reduce the activity of leukotrienes. Most attention has been focussed on obtaining (i) LTD_4-antagonists and (ii) inhibitors of 5-LO. The former offer potential as anti-asthmatic agents: the latter may provide additional opportunities (e. g. treatment of inflammatory disease, such as IBD, psoriasis and, possibly, arthritis) because these inhibit the biosynthesis of a wide range of leukotrienes and other putative mediators.

Many potent and relatively selective LTD_4 antagonists have now been described. Some of the earlier compounds suffered from poor bioavailability and/or short duration of activity. However, later compounds have improved pharmacokinetic profiles and have excellent LTD_4-antagonist activity in laboratory animals and in man. Clinical evaluation of the most attractive compounds (e.g. ICI 204,219, MK-571 and SK&F 104,353) is at an early stage but the preliminary data are encouraging. The fact that these compounds with diverse chemical structures, which apparently share only one common property, i.e. antagonism of LTD_4, do reduce asthmatic symptoms implies that leukotrienes are indeed important mediators of bronchoconstriction in hypersensitivity reactions. More extensive trials with leukotriene antagonists are in progress and these should provide clarification of the involvement of the leukotrienes in disease.

Inhibitors of 5-LO with qualities which have encouraged evaluation in man have also been described. The mechanism of the inhibition of the enzyme by these compounds is, in the main, poorly understood. The potential of developing compounds with anti-oxidant (e.g. BW 755 C) and iron chelating (e.g. BW B 70 C, A-64 077) properties has been explored; also compounds (e.g. MK-886) which inhibit the translocation of the enzyme have been considered. Studies in man with compounds with proven 5-LO inhibitory activity *in vivo* are limited at present. In the past some confusion has been created by inadequate assessment of compounds prior to study in animal models of human disease, or before clinical evaluation. For example, some compounds with potent *in vitro* activity against 5-LO have very short biological half-lives (e.g. ETYA, NDGA, nafazatrom, quercetin and baicalein; see Section 5.3) and, therefore data demonstrating any effects *in vivo* must be treated with scepticism. Other compounds (e.g. benoxaprofen) have been claimed to be selective inhibitors of 5-LO but subsequent studies have revealed only poor activity against the enzyme; once again, data from clinical trials must be interpreted with caution. However, clinical trials designed to assess the efficacy of A-

64077, which is a proven 5-LO inhibitor *in vivo,* for the treatment of IBD and allergic rhinitis have produced encouraging results. Also, preliminary data from limited clinical studies suggests that A-64077 may have beneficial effects in the treatment of asthma and, possibly rheumatoid arthritis.

Thus, the clinical investigations performed so far with LTD_4 antagonists and 5-LO inhibitors suggest that these classes of compounds will provide important new therapy in the treatment of asthma and some inflammatory diseases. It is to be hoped that the exciting results obtained in the early trials are confirmed in the larger, more carefully controlled studies which are presently underway.

References

The literature up to and including 1990 has been examined for the preparation of this review. Also, information available to the authors which has been accepted for publication in 1991 was considered.

1   H. van den Bosch, Biochem. Biophys. Acta *604,* 191 (1980).
2   R. F. Irvine, Biochem. J. *204,* 3 (1982).
3   R. J. Flower and G. J. Blackwell, Brit. Med. Bull *39,* 260 (1983).
4   J. R. Vane, Nature (New Biol.) *231,* 232 (1971).
5   J. R. Vane, J. Allergy Clin. Immunol. *58,* 232 (1976).
6   D. A. van Dorp, Progr. Biochem. Pharmacol. *3,* 71 (1967).
7   M. Hamberg and B. Samuelsson, J.Biol.Chem. *242,* 5329 (1967).
8   D. H. Nugteren, Biochem. Biophys. Acta *380,* 299 (1975).
9   M. Hamberg, J. Svensson, T. Wakabayashi and B. Samuelsson, Proc. Natl. Acad. Sci. USA *71,* 345 (1974).
10   P. Borgeat, M. Hamberg and B. Samuelsson, J. Biol. Chem. *251,* 7816 (1976).
11   F. A. Kuehl, H. W. Dougherty and E. A. Ham, Biochem. Pharmacol. *33,* 1 (1984).
12   F. H. Chilton, Biochem. J. *258,* 327 (1989).
13   P. Borgeat and B. Samuelsson, Proc. Natl. Acad. Sci. USA *76,* 3217 (1979).
14   P. Borgeat and B. Samuelsson, J. Biol. Chem. *254,* 2643 (1979).
15   O. Radmark, T. Shimizu, H. Jornvall and B. Samuelsson, J. Biol. Chem. *259,* 12339 (1984).
16   J. F. Evans, P. Dupuis and A. W. Ford-Hutchinson, Biochem. Biophys. Acta, *840,* 43 (1985).
17   R. C. Murphy, S. Hammarstrom and B. Samuelsson, Proc. Natl. Acad. Sci. USA *76,* 4275 (1979).
18   H. R. Morris, G. W. Taylor, P. J. Piper and J. R. Tippins, Nature (London) *285,* 104 (1980).
19   H. R. Morris, G. W. Taylor, P. J. Piper, M. N. Samhoun and J. R. Tippins, Prostaglandins *19,* 185 (1980).
20   M. E Andersson, R. D. Allison and A. Meister, Proc. Natl. Acad. Sci. USA, *79,* 1088 (1982).
21   K. Bernstrom and S. Hammarstrom, Biochem. Biophys. Res. Commun. *109,* 800, (1982).

22   W. E. Brocklehurst, Prog. Allergy 6, 539 (1962).
23   P. F. Weller, C. W. Lee, D. W. Foster, E. J. Corey, K. F. Austen and R. A. Lewis, Proc. Natl. Acad. Sci. USA 80, 7626 (1983).
24   B. Samuelsson, Science 220, 568 (1983).
25   W. R. Henderson, A. Jorg and S. J. Klebanoff, J. Immunol, 128, 2609 (1982).
26   C. W. Lee, R. A. Lewis, A. I. Tauber, M. Mehrotra, E. J. Corey and K. F. Austen, J. Biol. Chem. 258, 15004 (1983).
27   L. Orning and S. Hammarstrom, J. Biol. Chem. 255, 8023 (1980).
28   A. Foster, B. Fitzsimmons, J. R. Rokach and L. G. Letts, Biochem. Biophys. Acta 921, 486 (1987).
29   L. Orning, B. Norin, B. Gustafsson and S. Hammarstrom, J. Biol. Chem. 261, 766 (1986).
30   W. Hagman, C. Denglinger and D. Keppler, Circ. Shock 14, 223 (1984).
31   W. Hagman, C. Denglinger, S. Rapp, G. Weckbecker and D. Keppler, Prostaglandins 31, 239 (1986).
32   S. Hammarstrom, L. Orning and A. Keppler, Ann. N. Y. Acad. Sci. 524, 43 (1988).
33   A. Foster, B. Fitzsimmons, J. R. Rokach and L. G. Letts, Biochem. Biophys. Res. Commun. 148, 1237 (1987).
34   D. O. Stene and R. C. Murphy, J. Biol. Chem. 263, 2773 (1988).
35   J. Rokach, A. Foster, D. Delorme and Y. Girard, Advances in Prostglandin, Thromboxane and Leukotriene Research, vol. 19 (eds. B. Samuelsson, P. Y.-K. Wong and F. F. Sun) (Raven Press Ltd., New York 1989) p. 102.
36   R. C. Murphy and D. O. Stene, Ann. N. Y. Acad. Sci. 524, 35 (1988).
37   D. O. Stene and R. C. Murphy, Advances in Prostaglandin, Thromboxane and Leukotriene Research, vol. 19 (eds. B. Samuelsson, P. Y.-K. Wong and F. F. Sun) (Raven Press Ltd., New York, 1989) p. 108
38   K. Bernstrom and S. Hammarstrom, Arch. Biochem. Biophys. 244, 486 (1986).
39   L. Orning, L. Kaijser and S. Hammarstrom, Biochem. Biophys. Res. Commun. 130, 214 (1985).
40   G. Hansson, J. A. Lindgren, S. E. Dahlen, P. Hedqvist and B. Samuelsson, FEBS Lett. 130, 107 (1981).
41   W. S. Powell, J. Biol. Chem. 259, 3082 (1984).
42   S. Shak and I. M. Goldstein, J. Clin. Invest. 76, 1218 (1985).
43   R. T. Soberman, T. W. Harper, R. C. Murphy and K. F. Austen, Proc. Natl. Acad. Sci. USA 82, 2292 (1985).
44   W. S. Powell, S. Wainwright and F. Gravelle, Advances in Prostaglandin, Thromboxane and Leukotriene Research, vol. 19 (eds. B. Samuelsson, P. Y.-K. Wong and F. F. Sun) (Raven Press Ltd., New York, 1989) p. 112.
45   B. Samuelsson, Prog. Lipid Res. 20, 23 (1981).
46   B. Samuelsson, Science 220, 568 (1983).
47   M. Johnson, F. Carey and R. M. McMillan, Essays in Biochem. 19, 40 (1983).
48   S. Hammarstrom, Ann. Rev. Biochem. 52, 335 (1983).
49   T. Shimizu, O. Radmark and B. Samuelsson, Proc. Natl. Acad. Sci. USA 81, 689 (1984).
50   A. M. Goetze, L. Fayer, J. Bouska, D. Bornemeier and G. W. Carter, Prostaglandins 29, 689 (1985).
51   G. K. Hogaboom, M. Cook, J. F. Newton, A. Varrichio, R. G. L. Shorr, H. M. Sarrau and S. T. Crooke, Mol. Pharmacol. 30, 510 (1986).
52   C. A. Rouzer, T. Matsumoto and B. Samuelsson, Proc. Natl. Acad. Sci. USA 83, 857 (1986).
53   N. Ueda, S. Kaneko, T. Yoshimoto and S. Yamamoto, J. Biol. Chem. 261, 7982 (1986).

54   T. Shimizu, T. Izuma, Y. Seyama, K. Tadokoro, O. Radmark and B. Samu-
      elsson, Proc. Natl. Acad. Sci. USA *83*, 4175 (1986).
55   B. A. Jakschik and L. H. Lee, Nature *287*, 51 (1980).
56   B. A. Jakschik, F. F. Sun, L. H. Lee and M. M. Steinhoff, Biochem. Bio-
      phys. Res. Commun. *95*, 103 (1980).
57   C. A. Rouzer and S. Kargman, J. Biol. Chem. *263*, 10 980 (1988).
58   A. Wong, S. M. Hwang, M. N. Cook, G. K. Hogaboom and S. T. Crooke,
      Biochem. *27*, 6763 (1988).
59   T. Matsumoto, C. D. Funk, O. Radmark, J.-O. Hoog, H. Jornvall and
      B. Samuelsson, Proc. Natl. Acad. Sci. USA *85*, 26 (1988).
60   R. F. Dixon, R. E. Jones, R. E. Diehl, C. D. Bennett, S. Kargman and C. A.
      Rouzer, Proc. Acad. Sci. USA *85*, 416 (1988).
61   J. M. Balcarek, T. W. Theisen, M. N. Cook, A. Varrichio, S.-M. Hwang,
      M. W. Strohsacker and S. T. Crooke, J. Biol. Chem. *263*, 13 937 (1988).
62   D. K. Miller, J. W. Gillard, P. J. Vickers, S. Sadowski, C. Leveille, J. A.
      Mancini, P. Charleson, R. A. F. Dixon, A. W. Ford-Hutchinson, R. Fortin,
      J. Y. Gauthier, J. Rodkey, R. Rosen, C. Rouzer, I. S. Sigal, C. D. Strader
      and J. F. Evans, Nature *343*, 278 (1990).
63   R. A. F. Dixon, R. E. Diehl, E. Opas, E. Rands, P. J. Vickers, J. F. Evans,
      J. W. Gillard and D. K. Miller, Nature *343*, 282 (1990).
64   T. Schewe, S. M. Rapoport and H. Kuhn, Adv. Enzymol. *58*, 191 (1986).
65   C. R. Rouzer, N. A. Thornberry and H. G. Bull, Ann. N. Y. Acad. Sci. *524*,
      1 (1988).
66   S. Yamamoto,   N. Ueda,   H. Ehara,   T. Maruyama,   C. Yokoyama,
      S. Kaneko, T. Yoshimoto, N. Komatsu, K. Watanabe, A. Hattori, B. J.
      Fitzimmons, J. Rokach and A. R. Brash, Ann. N. Y. Acad. Sci. *524*, 12
      (1988).
67   B. Samuelsson and C. D. Funk, J. Biol. Chem. *264*, 19 469 (1989).
68   T. Yoshimoto, H. Suzuki, S. Yamamoto, T. Takai, C. Yokoyama and
      T. Tanabe, Proc. Natl. Acad. Sci. USA *87*, 2142 (1990).
69   C. D. Funk, L. Furci and G. A. Fitzgerald, Proc. Natl. Acad. Sci. USA *87*,
      5638 (1990).
70   P. M. Woollard, Biochem. Biophys. Res. Commun. *136*, 169 (1986).
71   F. M. Cunningham and P. M. Woollard, Prostaglandins *34*, 71 (1987).
72   J. F. Evans, Y. Leblanc, B. J. Fitzimmons, S. Charlessons, D. Nathaniel
      and C. Leveille, Biochem. Biophys. Acta *917*, 406 (1987).
73   J. L. Humes and E. E. Opas, Advances in Prostglandin, Thromboxane and
      Leukotriene Research, vol. 19 (eds. B. Samuelsson, P. Y.-K. Wong and
      F. F. Sun) (Raven Press Ltd., New York, 1989) p. 152.
74   J. Capdevila, L. Marnett, N. Chacos, K. A. Prough and R. W. Estabrook,
      Proc. Natl. Acad. Sci. USA *79*, 767 (1982).
75   J. Capdevila, P. Yadagiri, S. Mann and J. Falck, Biochem. Biophys. Res.
      Commun. *141*, 1007 (1986).
76   R. C. Murphy, J. R. Falck, S. Lumin, P. Yadagiri, J. Zirolli, M. Balazy,
      J. Masferrer, N. Abraham and M. Schwartzman, J. Biol. Chem. *263*, 17 197
      (1988).
77   M. Schwartzman, M. Balazy, J. Masferrer, N. Abraham, J. McGiff and
      R. C. Murphy, Proc. Natl. Acad. Sci. USA *84*, 8125 (1987).
78   P. Woollard and A. P. Padfield (personal communication).
79   M. Hamberg, P. Hedqvist and K. Radegran, Acta. Physiol. Scand. *110*, 219
      (1980).
80   M. Kumlin, M. Hamberg, E. Granstrom, T. Bjorck, B. Dahlen, H. Mat-
      suda, O. Zetterstrom and S.-E. Dahlen, Arch. Biochem. Biophys. *282*, 254
      (1990).
81   E. Sigal, D. Grunberger, C. S. Craik, G. H. Caughey and J. H. Nadel, Adv-
      ances in Prostaglandin, Thromboxane and Leukotriene Research, vol. 19

(eds. B. Samuelsson, P. Y.-K. Wong and F. F. Sun) (Raven Press. Ltd., New York 1989) p. 156.

82   J. McGee and F. A. Fitzpatrick, J. Biol. Chem. *260*, 12832 (1985).

83   N. Ohishi, T. Izumi, M. Minami, S. Kitamura, Y. Seyama, S. Ohkawa, S. Terao, H. Yotsumoto, F. Takaku and T. Shimizu, J. Biol. Chem. *262*, 10200 (1987).

84   J. Haeggstrom, T. Bergman, H. Jornvall and O. Radmark, Eur. J. Biochem. *174*, 717 (1989).

85   B. Samuelsson, C. D. Funk, S. Hoshiko, T. Matsumoto and O. Radmark, Advances in Prostaglandin, Thromboxane and Leukotriene Research, vol. 19 (eds. B. Samuelsson, P. Y.-K. Wong and F. F. Sun) (Raven Press Ltd., New York, 1989) p. 1.

86   R. J. Soberman and K. F. Austen Advances in Prostglandin, Thromboxane and Leukotriene Research, vol. 19 (eds. B. Samuelsson, P. Y.-K. Wong and F. F. Sun) (Raven Press Ltd. New York, 1989) p. 21.

87   W. F. Owen, R. J. Soberman, T. Yoshimoto, A. L. Sheffer, R. A. Lewis and K. F. Austen, J. Immunol. *138*, 132 (1987).

88   C. N. Serhan, M. Hamberg and B. Samuelsson, Biochem. Biophys. Res. Commun. *118*, 943 (1984).

89   C. N. Serhan, M. Hamberg and B. Samuelsson, Proc. Natl. Acad. Sci. USA *81*, 5335 (1984).

90   C. N. Serhan, M. Hamberg, U. Ramstedt and B. Samuelsson, Advances in Prostaglandin, Thromboxane and Leukotriene Research, vol. 16 (eds. U. Zor, Z. Naor and F. Kohen) (Raven Press Ltd., New York, 1986) p. 83

91   C. N. Serhan and B. Samuelsson, Adv. Exp. Med. Biol. *229*, 1 (1988).

92   B. Samuelsson, S.-E. Dahlen, J. A. Lindgren, C. A. Rouzer and C. N. Serhan, Science *237*, 1171 (1987).

93   S.-E. Dahlen, L. Franzen, J. Raud, C. N. Serhan, P. Westlund, E. Wikstroem, T. Bjoerck, H. Matsuda, S. E. Webber, C. A. Veale, T. Puustinen, J. Haeggstrom, K. C. Nicplau and B. Samuelsson, Adv. Exp. Med. Biol. *229*, 107 (1988).

94   S.-E. Dahlen, Advances in Prostaglandin, Thromboxane and Leukotriene Research, vol. 19 (eds. B. Samuelsson, P. Y.-K. Wong and F. F. Sun) (Raven Press Ltd., New York, 1989) p. 122

95   K. F. Badr, Advances in Prostaglandin, Thromboxane and Leukotriene Research, vol. 19 (eds. B. Samuelsson, P. Y.-K. Wong and F. F. Sun) (Raven Press Ltd., New York, 1989) p. 233.

96   S. Narumiya, J. A. Salmon, F. H. Cottee, B. C. Weatherley and R. J. Flower, J. Biol. Chem. *256*, 9583 (1981).

97   J. Capdevila, L. Marnett, N. Chacos, K. A. Prough and R. W. Estabrook, Proc. Natl. Acad. Sci. USA *79*, 767 (1982).

98   E. G. Oliw, J. A. Lawson, A. C. Brash and J. A. Oates, J. Biol. Chem. *256*, 9924 (1981).

99   F. A. Fitzpatrick and R. C. Murphy, Pharmacol. Rev. *40*, 229 (1989).

100 C. R. Pace-Asciak, Biochem. Biophys. Res. Commun. *151*, 493 (1988).

101 S. H. Ferreira, M. Nakamura and M. S. Abreu-Castro, Prostaglandins *16*, 31 (1978).

102 G. A. Higgs and S. Moncada, Advances in Pain Research and Therapy Vol. 5 (J. J. Bonica ed.) (Raven Press New York 1983) p. 617.

103 C. Wedmore and T. J. Williams, Nature *289*, 646 (1981).

104 S. H. Ferreira and J. R. Vane, Anti-inflammatory Drugs (J. R. Vane and S. H. Ferreira, eds.) (Springer-Verlag, Berlin 1979) p. 348.

105 G. A. Higgs, K. E. Eakins, K. G. Mugridge, S. Moncada and J. R. Vane, Eur. J. Pharmacol, *66*, 81 (1980).

106 C. N. Ellis, J. D. Fallon, S. Kang, E. E. Vanderveen and J. J. Vorhees, J. Am. Acad. Dermatol. *14*, 39 (1986).

107 K. Slepian, K. P. Mathews and J. A. McLean, Chest *87*, 386 (1985).
108 W. Mohr, H. Westerhellweg and D. Wessinghage Annals Rheum. Dis. *40*, 395 (1981).
109 G. J. Weissman, J. Lab. Clin. Med. *100*, 372 (1982).
110 R. M. J. Palmer, R. J. Stepney, G. A. Higgs and K. E. Eakins, Prostaglandins *20*, 411 (1980).
111 M. A. Bray, Brit. Med. Bull *39*, 249 (1983).
112 T. E. Rollins, B. Zanolari, M. S. Springer, Y. Guindon, R. Zamboni, C. K. Lau and J. Rokach, Prostaglandins *25*, 281 (1983).
113 G. A. Higgs, J. A. Salmon and J. A. Spayne, Br. J. Pharmacol. *74*, 429 (1981).
114 M. A. Bray, F. M. Cunningham, A. W. Ford-Hutchinson and M. J. H. Smith, Br. J. Pharmacol. *72*, 483 (1981).
115 C. L. Malmsten, J. Palmblad, A. M. Uden, O. Radmark, K. Engstedt and B. Samuelsson, Acta. Physiol. Scand. *110*, 449 (1980).
116 I. Hafstrom, J. Palmblad, C. L. Malmsten, O. Radmark and B. Samuelsson, FEBS Lett. *130*, 146 (1981).
117 A. W. Ford-Hutchinson, M. A. Bray, F. M. Cunningham, E. M. Davidson and M. J. H. Smith, Prostaglandins *21*, 143 (1981).
118 D. W. Goldman and E. J. Goetzl, J. Immunol. *129*, 1600 (1982).
119 R. A. Kreisle and C. W. Parker, J. Exp. Med. *157*, 628 (1983).
120 P. M. Simmons, J. A. Salmon and S. Moncada, Biochem. Pharmacol. *32*, 1353 (1983).
121 A. W. Ford-Hutchinson, G. Brunet, P. Savard and S. Charleson, Prostaglandins *28*, 13 (1984).
122 M. J. Forrest, V. Zammit and P. M. Brooks, Ann. Rheum. Dis. *47*, 241 (1988).
123 N. Boughton-Smith, Eur. J. Gastroenterol. Hepatol. *1*, 140 (1989).
124 R. D. Zipser, C. C. Nast, M. Lee, H. Kao and R. Duke, Gastroenterol. *90*, 1705 (1986).
125 K. Lauritsen, J. Hansen, P. Bytzer, K. Bukhave and J. Rask-Madsen, Gut *25*, 1271 (1984).
126 K. Lauritsen, I. S. Laursen, K. Bukhave and J. Rask-Madsen, Gastroenterol. *91*, 837 (1986).
127 D. S. Rampton, G. E. Sladen and L. J. F. Youlten, Gut *21*, 591 (1979).
128 L. B. Klickstein, J. Shapleigh and E. J. Goetzl, Arth. Rheum. *23*, 704 (1980).
129 E. M. Davidson, S. A. Rae and M. J. H. Smith, J. Pharm. Pharmacol. *34*, 410 (1982).
130 S. A. Rae, E. M. Davidson and M. J. H. Smith, Lancet *ii*, 1122 (1982).
131 S. D. Brain, R. D. R. Camp, P. M. Dowd, A. K. Black, P. M. Woollard, A. I. Mallett and M. W. Greaves, Lancet *ii*, 762 (1982).
132 T. Ruzicka, T. Simmet, B. A. Peskar and J. Ring, J. Invest. Dermatol. *86*, 105 (1986).
133 N. K. Boughton-Smith, C. J. Hawkey and B. J. R. Whittle, Gut *24*, 1176 (1983).
134 P. Sharon and W. F. Stenson, Gastroenterol. *86*, 452 (1984).
135 H. Bisgaard, A. W. Ford-Hutchinson, S. Charleson and E. Taudorf, Prostaglandins *27*, 369 (1984).
136 R. D. R. Camp, A. A. Coutte, M. B. Greaves, A. B. Kay and M. J. Walport, Br. J. Pharmacol, *75*, 168P (1982).
137 J. Bisgaard, J. Kristenson and J. Sondergaard, Prostaglandins *23*, 797 (1982).
138 S. E. Dahlen, J. Bjork, P. Hedqvist, K.-E. Arfors, S. Hammarstrom, J. A. Lindgren and B. Samuelsson, Proc. Natl. Acad. Sci. USA *78*, 3887 (1981).
139 A. W. Ford-Hutchinson and A. Rackman, Brit. J. Dermatol. *109*, 26 (1983).

140   R. L. Follenfant, M. Nakamura-Craig and L. G. Garland, Br. J. Pharmacol. *99*, 289P (1990).

141   J. D. Levine, D. Lam, Y. O. Taiwo, P. Donatoni and E. J. Goetzl, Proc. Natl. Acad. Sci. USA *83*, 5331 (1986).

142   W. Feldberg and C. H. Kellaway, J. Physiol. (London) *94*, 187 (1938).

143   K. F. Austen, J. Immunol. *121*, 793 (1978).

144   R. P. Orange and K. F. Austen, Adv. Immunol. *10*, 105 (1969).

145   E. J. Corey, D. A. Clark, G. Goto, A. Marfat, C. Mioskowski and B. Samuelsson, J. Am. Chem. Soc. *102*, 1436 (1980).

146   H. R. Morris, G. W. Taylor, P. J. Piper and J. R. Tippins, Nature (London) *285*, 104 (1980).

147   H. R. Morris, G. W. Taylor, P. J. Piper, M. N. Samhoun and J. R. Tippins, Prostaglandins *19*, 185 (1980).

148   R. C. Murphy, S. Hammarstrom and B. Samuelsson, Proc. Natl. Acad. Sci. USA *76*, 4275 (1979).

149   S. E. Dahlen, P. Hedqvist, S. Hammarstrom and B. Samuelsson, Nature *288*, 484 (1980).

150   R. A. Lewis, J. M. Drazen, J. C. Figueiredo, E. J. Corey and K. F. Austen, Int. J. Immunopharmacol. *4*, 85 (1982).

151   P. J. Piper, Physiol. Rev. *64*, 744 (1984).

152   N. Barnes, J. Evans, J. Zakrzewski, P. Piper and J. Costello, Ann. N. Y. Acad. Sci. *524*, 369 (1988).

153   P. M. O'Byrne, Ann. N. Y. Acad. Sci. *524*, 282 (1988).

154   M. C. Holroyd, R. E. C. Altounyan, M. Cole, M. Dixon and E. V. Elliot, Lancet *ii*, 17 (1981).

155   T. Ahmed, D. W. Greenblatt, S. Birch, B. Marchette and A. Wanner, Am. Rev. Respir. Dis. *124*, 110 (1981).

156   W. J. Weiss, J. M. Drazen, E. R. McFadden, P. Weller, E. J. Corey, R. A. Lewis and K. F. Austen, J. Am. Med. Assoc. *249*, 2814 (1982).

157   C. Marom, J. H. Shelhamer, M. K. Bach, D. R. Morton and M. Kaliner, Am. Rev. Respir. Dis. *126*, 449 (1982).

158   D. F. Woodward, B. Weichmann, C. A. Gill and M. A. Wasserman, Prostaglandins *25*, 131 (1982).

159   A. P. Sampson, J. M. Evans, L. G. Garland, P. J. Piper and J. F. Costello, Pulmon. Pharmacol. *3*, 111 (1990).

160   G. W. Taylor, I. Taylor, P. Black, N. H. Maltby, N. Turner, R. W. Fuller and C. T. Dollery, Lancet *i*, 584 (1989).

161   P. J. Manning, J. Rokach, J. L. Malo, D. Ethier, A. Cartier, Y. Girard, S. Charleson and P. M. O'Byrne, Am. Rev. Resp. Dis. *139*, A92 (1990).

162   A. M. Karnik, K. P. Bhargava, S. M. Diab, O. Thulesius and F. F. Fenech, Med. Sci. Res. *16*, 19 (1988).

163   S. Lam, H. Chan, J. C. Leriche, M. Chang-Yeung and H. Salari, J. Allergy. Clin. Immunol. *81*, 711 (1988).

164   J. J. Murray, A. B. Tonnel, A. R. Brash, J. L. Roberts, P. Gosset, C. R. Workman, A. Capron and J. A. Oates, N. Engl. J. Med. *315*, 800 (1986).

165   J. T. Zakrzewski, N. C. Barnes, P. Piper and J. F. Costello, Br. J. Clin. Pharmacol. *19*, 549P (1985).

166   J. T. Zakrzewski, N. C. Barnes, P. Piper and J. F. Costello, Prostaglandins *33*, 663 (1987).

167   J. T. Zakrzewski, A. T. Sampson, J. Evans, N. C. Barnes, P. Piper and J. F. Costello, Br. J. Pharmacol. *93*, 108 (1987).

168   R. J. Shaw, P. Fitzharris, O. Cromwell, A. J. Wardlaw and A. B. Kay, Allergy *40*, 1 (1985).

169   P. S. Creticos, S. P. Peters, N. F. Adkinson, R. M. Naclerio, E. C. Hayes, P. C. Norman and L. M. Lichtenstein, New Engl. J. Med. *310*, 1626 (1984).

170 H. R. Morris, G. W. Taylor, P. M. Clinton, P. J. Piper, J. R. Tippins, K. Barnett, J. Costello, L. Dunlop, A. Henderson and R. Heaton, Advances in Prostaglandin and Thromboxane Research vol. 11 (eds. B. Samuelsson, R. Paoletti and P. Ramwell (Raven Press Ltd., New York 1983) p. 221.

171 T. Okubo, H. Takahashi, M. Sumitomo, K. Shindo and S. Suzuki, Int. Arch. Allergy Appl. Immunol. *84*, 149 (1987).

172 I. M. Richards, R. L. Griffin, J. A. Oostveen, J. Morris, D. G. Wishka and C. J. Dunn, Am. Rev. Respir. Dis. *140*, 1712 (1989).

173 J. Y. Wescott, K. R. Stenmark and R. C. Murphy, Prostaglandins *31*, 227 (1986).

174 K. V. Honn, I. M. Grossi, B. W. Steinert, H. Chopra, J. Onoda, K. K. Nelson and J. D. Taylor, Advances in Prostaglandin, Thromboxane and Leukotriene Research, vol. 19 (eds. B. Samuelsson, P. Y.-K. Wong and F. F. Sun) (Raven Press Ltd., New York 1989) p. 439.

175 D. Piomelli and P. Greengard, Trends Pharmacol. Sci. *11*, 367 (1990).

176 T. S. Simmet, W. Luck, W. K. Delank and B. A. Peskar, Advances in Prostaglandin, Thromboxane and Leukotriene Research, vol. 19 (eds. B. Samuelsson, P. Y.-K. Wong and F. F. Sun) (Raven Press Ltd., New York 1989) p. 402.

177 M. Ban, T. Tonai, T. Kohno, K. Matsumoto, T. Horie, S. Yamamoto, M. A. Moskowitz and L. Levine, Stroke *20*, 248 (1989).

178 W. Hagman, C. Denzlinger and D. Keppler, FEBS Lett. *180*, 309 (1985).

179 J. A. Cook, W. C. Wise and P. V. Halushka, J. Pharmacol. Exp. Ther. *235*, 470 (1985).

180 C. E. Hoock and A. M. Lefer, Circ. Shock *17*, 263 (1985).

181 E. F. Smith, L. B. Kinter, M. Jugus, M. A. Wassermann, R. D. Eckardt and J. F. Newton, Circ. Shock *25*, 21 (1988).

182 E. F. Smith, L. B. Kinter, M. Jugus, R. D. Eckardt and J. F. Newton, Eicosanoids *2*, 101 (1989).

183 H. Bitterman, B. A. Smith and A. M. Lefer, Circ. Shock *24*, 159 (1988).

184 G. Matera, J. A. Cook, R. A. Hennigar, G. E. Temple, W. C. Wise, T. D. Oglesby and P. V. Halushka, J. Pharmacol. Exp. Ther. *247*, 363 (1988).

185 K. F. Badr, G. F. Schreiner, M. Wasserman and I. Ichikawa, J. Clin. Invest. *81*, 1702 (1988).

186 S. R. Jolly, J. Travis and R. G. van Inwegen, Pharmacol. *38*, 352 (1989).

187 K. M. Mullane and S. Moncada, Prostaglandins, *24*, 255 (1982).

188 K. M. Mullane, N. Read, J. A. Salmon and S. Moncada, J. Pharmacol. Exp. Ther. *228*, 510 (1984).

189 Y. Toki, N. Hieda, T. Torii, H. Hashimoto, T. Ito, K. Ogawa and T. Satake, Prostaglandins *35*, 555 (1988).

190 J. W. Egan, D. E. Griswold, L. M. Hillegass, J. F. Newton, R. D. Eckardt, M. J. Slivjak and E. F. Smith, Prostaglandins *37*, 597 (1989).

191 M. P. Maxwell, C. Marston, M. R. Hadley, J. A. Salmon and L. G. Garland, J. Cardiovasc. Pharmacol. (1991). J. Cardiovasc. Pharmacol. *17*, 539.

192 J. H. Fleisch, L. E. Rinkema and W. S. Marshall, Biochem. Pharmacol. *33*, 3919 (1984).

193 J. M. Drazen, K. F. Austen, R. A. Lewis, D. A. Clark, G. Goto, A. Marfat and E. J. Corey, Proc. Natl. Acad. Sci. USA *77*, 4354 (1980).

194 R. D. Krell, L. Osborn, K. Vickery, M. Falcone, M. O'Donnell, J. Gleason, C. Kinsig and D. Bryan, Prostaglandins *22*, 387 (1981).

195 J. Augstein, J. B. Farmer, T. B. Less, P. Sheard and M. L. Tattersall, Nature (New Biol.) *245*, 215 (1973).

196 R. A. Lewis, C. W. Lee, L. Levine, R. A. Morgan, J. W. Weiss, J. M. Drazen, H. Oh, D. Hoover, E. J. Corey and K. F. Austen, Advances in Prostaglandin, Thromboxane and Leukotriene Research, vol. 11 (eds.

B. Samuelsson, R. Paoletti and P. Ramwell) (Raven Press Ltd., New York 1983) p. 15.

197   M. A. Lewis, S. Mong, R. L. Vessella, G. K. Hogaboom, H.-L. Wu and S. T. Crooke, Prostaglandins 27, 961 (1984).

198   M. A. Lewis, S. Mong, R. L. Vessella and S. T. Crooke, Biochem. Pharmacol. 34, 4311 (1985).

199   R. M. Muccitelli, S. S. Tucker, D. W. Hay, T. J. Torphy and M. A. Wasserman, J. Pharmacol. Exp. Ther. 243, 467 (1987).

200   S. S. Tate and A. Meister, Proc. Natl. Acad. Sci. USA 75, 4806 (1978).

201   D. W. Snyder, M. Barone, M. P. Morissette, P. R. Bernstein and R. D. Krell, Pharmacologist 25, 205 (1983).

202   J. B. Cheng and R. G. Townley, Biochem. Biophys. Res. Commun. 119, 612 (1984).

203   D. W. Snyder and R. D. Krell, J. Pharmacol. Exp. Ther. 231, 616 (1984).

204   D. E. Sok, J. K. Pai, V. Atrache and C. J. Sih, Proc. Natl. Acad. Sci. USA 77, 6481 (1980).

205   R. F. Bruns, W. J. Thomsen and T. A. Pugsley, Life Sci. 33, 645 (1983).

206   S.-S. Pong and R. N. Dehaven, Proc. Natl. Acad. Sci. USA 80, 7415 (1983).

207   J. B. Cheng and R. G. Townley, Biochem. Biophys. Res. Commun. 118, 20 (1984).

208   J. B. Cheng and R. G. Townley, Biochem. Biophys. Res. Commun. 122, 949 (1984).

209   S. Mong, H.-L. Wu, M. A. Clark, J. M. Stadel, J. G. Gleason and S. T. Crooke, Prostaglandins 28, 805 (1984).

210   S. Mong, H.-L. Wu, G. K. Hogaboom, M. A. Clark, J. M. Stadel and S. T. Crooke, Eur. J. Pharmacol. 106, 241 (1985).

211   G. K. Hogaboom, S. Mong, H.-L. Wu and S. T. Crooke, Biochem. Biophys. Res. Commun. 116, 1136 (1983).

212   S.-S. Pong, R. N. Dehaven, F. A. Kuehl and R. W. Egan, J. Biol. Chem. 258, 9616 (1983).

213   F. A. Kuehl, R. N. Dehaven and S.-S. Pong, J. Allergy Clin. Immunol. 74, 378 (1984).

214   S. T. Crooke, S. Mong, M. Clark, G. K. Hogaboom, M. Lewis and J. L. Gleason, Biochemical Actions of Hormones (ed. G. Litwick) (Academic Press, New York, 1987) p. 81.

215   S. T. Crooke, S. Mong, H. M. Sarau, J. D. Winkler and V. K. Vegesna, Ann. N. Y. Acad. Sci. 524, 153 (1988).

216   S. T. Crooke, M. Mattern, H. M. Sarau, J. D. Winkler, J. Balcarek, A. Wong and C. F. Bennett, Trends Pharmacol. Sci. 10, 103 (1989).

217   G. K. Hogaboom, S. Mong, J. M. Stadel and S. T. Crooke, Molec. Pharmacol. 27, 236 (1985).

218   S. Krilis, R. A. Lewis, E. J. Corey and K. F. Austen, J. Clin. Invest. 72, 1516 (1983).

219   D. Aharony, R. C. Falcone, Y. K. Yee, B. Hesp, R. E. Giles and R. D. Krell, Ann. N. Y. Acad. Sci. 524, 162 (1988).

220   D. W. Goldman and E. J. Goetzl, J. Exp. Med. 159, 1027 (1984).

221   C. H. Koo, J. W. Sherman, L. Baud and E. Goetzl, Advances in Prostaglandin, Thromboxane and Leukotriene Research, vol. 19 (eds. B. Samuelsson, P. Y.-K. Wong and F. F. Sun) (Raven Press Ltd., New York 1989) p. 191.

222   J. Rokach and R. N. Young, Adv. Exp. Med. Biol. 259, 75 (1989).

223   N. C. Barnes, J. Evans, J. T. Zakrzewski, P. J. Piper and J. F. Costello, Agents Actions 28, 305 (1989).

224   B. J. Fitzsimmons and J. Rokach, Leukotrienes and Lipoxygenases: Chemical, Biological and Clinical Aspects (ed. J. Rokach) (Elsevier, New York, 1989) p. 427.

225 R. D. Krell, B. S. Tsai, A. Berdoulay, M. Barone and R. E. Giles, Prosta-
     glandins 25, 171 (1983).
226 P. Sheard, T. B. Lee and M. L. Tattersall, Monogr. Allergy 12, 245 (1977).
227 B. L. Mead, L. H. Patterson and D. A. Smith, J. Pharm. Pharmacol. 33, 682
     (1981).
228 J. H. Flesich, M. C. Cloud and W. S. Marshall, Ann. N. A. Acad. Sci. 524,
     356 (1988).
229 J. H. Fleisch, L. E. Rinkema, K. D. Haisch, D. Swanson-Bean, T. Good-
     son, P. P. K. Ho and W. S. Marshall, J. Pharm. Exp. Ther. 233, 148 (1985).
230 L. E. Rinkema, C. R. Roman, W. L. Russell, S. M. Spaethe, K. G. Bemis,
     D. P. Henry, W. S. Marshall and J. H. Fleisch, J. Pharm. Pharmacol. 42,
     620 (1990).
231 G. D. Phillips, P. Rafferty, C. Robinson and S. T. Holgate J. Pharm. Exp.
     Ther. 246, 732 (1988).
232 R. W. Fuller, P. N. Black and C. T. Dollery, J. Allergy Clin. Immunol. 83,
     939 (1989).
233 E. Israel, E. F. Juniper, J. T. Callaghan, P. N. Mathur, M. M. Morris, A. R.
     Dowell, G. G. Enas, F. E. Hargreave and J. M. Drazen, Am. Rev. Respir.
     Dis. 140, 1348 (1989).
234 J. H. Fleisch, L. E. Rinkema, K. D. Haisch, D. McCullough, F. P. Carr and
     R. D. Dillard, Naunyn-Schmiedeberg's Arch. Pharmacol. 333, 70 (1986).
235 R. D. Dillard, F. P. Carr, D. McCullough, K. D. Haisch, L. E. Rinkema
     and J. H. Fleisch, J. Med. Chem. 30, 911 (1987).
236 W. S. Marshall, S. K. Sigmund, C. A. Whitesitt, S. L. Lifer, C. R. Roman,
     L. E. Rinkema, R. A. Hahn and J. H. Fleisch, Agents Actions 27, 309
     (1989).
237 J. R. Boot, A. Bond, R. Gooderham, A. O'Brien, M. Parsons and K. H.
     Thomas, Br. J. Pharmacol, 98, 259 (1989).
238 R. Wood-Baker, G. A. Turner, B. Lucas and S. T. Holgate, Am. Rev. Re-
     spir. Dis. 141, A115 (1989).
239 F. E. F. Ali, J. G. Gleason, O. T. Hill, R. D. Krell, C. H. Kruse, P. G. La-
     nanchy and B. W. Volpe, J. Med. Chem. 25, 1235 (1982).
240 J. G. Gleason, R. D. Krell, B. M. Weichmann, F. E. Ali and B. Berkowitz,
     Advances in Prostaglandin, Thromboxane and Leukotriene Research,
     vol. 9 (eds. B. Samuelsson and R. Paoletti) (Raven Press, New York, 1982)
     p. 243.
241 G. K. Hogaboom, S. Mong, J. M. Stadel and S. T. Crooke, Molec. Pharma-
     col. 27, 236 (1984).
242 B. M. Weichman, M. A. Wasserman and J. G. Gleason, J. Pharm. Exp.
     Ther. 228, 128 (1984).
243 C. D. Perchonock, I. Uzinskas, T. W. Ku, M. E. McCarthy, W. E. Bondi-
     nell, B. W. Volpe, J. G. Gleason, B. M. Weichman, R. M. Muccitelli, J. F.
     Devan, S. S. Tucker, L. M. Vickery and M. A. Wasserman, Prostaglandins
     29, 75 (1985).
244 D. W.P. Hay, R. M. Muccitelli, S. S. Tucker, L. M. Vickery-Clark, K. A.
     Wilson, P. E. Malo, J. G. Gleason, M. A. Wasserman and T. J. Torphy, J.
     Pharmacol. Exp. Ther. 243, 474 (1987).
245 M. A. Wasserman, T. J. Torphy, D. W. P. Hay, R. M. Muccitelli, S. S.
     Tucker, K. Wilson, R. R. Osborn, L. Vickery-Clark, R. F. Hall, K. R. Er-
     hard and J. G. Gleason, Advances in Prostaglandin, Thromboxane and
     Leukotriene Research, vol. 17 (eds. B. Samuelsson, R. Paoletti and
     P. Ramwell) (Raven Press, New York, 1987) p. 532.
246 T. J. Torphy, J. F. Newton, M. A. Wasserman, L. Vickery-Clark, R. R. Os-
     born, L. S. Bailey, L. A. Yodis, D. C. Underwood and D. W. Hay, J.
     Pharmacol. Exp. Ther. 249, 430 (1989).

247 J. M. Evans, P. J. Piper and J. F. Costello, Advances in Prostaglandin, Thromboxane and Leukotriene Research, vol. 21 A (eds. B. Samuelsson, P. Ramwell, R. Paoletti, G. Folco and E. Granstrom) (Raven Press Ltd., New York 1990) p. 469.

248 J. Gleason, R. Hall, D. Hay, J. Newton, T. Torphy, H. Sara, M. Hayhurst, C. Broom and H. Helfrich, Proceedings of New Drugs for Asthma IU-PHAR Symposium (1991) In press.

249 T. R. Jones, R. Young, E. Champion, L. Charette, D. Denis, A. W. Ford-Hutchinson, R. Frenette, J. Y. Gauthier, Y. Guindon, M. Kakushima, P. Masson, C. McFarlane, H. Piechuta, J. Rokach, R. Zamboni, R. N. De-haven, A. Maycock and S. S. Pong, Can. J. Physiol. Pharmacol. 64, 1068 (1986).

250 R. N. Young, T. R. Jones, J. G. Atkinson, P. Belanger, E. Champion, D. Denis, R. N. Dehaven, A. W. Ford-Hutchinson, R. Fortin, R. Frenette, J. Y. Gauthier, J. Gillard, Y. Guindon, M. Kakushima, P. Masson, A. Maycock, C. S. McFarlane, H. Piechuta, S. S. Pong, J. Rokach, H. Williams, C. Yoakim and R. Zamboni, Advances in Prostaglandin, Thromboxane and Leukotriene Research, vol. 17 (eds. B. Samuelsson, R. Paoletti and P. Ramwell) (Raven Press, New York, 1987) p. 544.

251 N. Barnes, P. J. Piper and J. Costello, J. Allergy Clin. Immunol. 79, 816 (1987).

252 J. R. Britton, S. P. Hanley and A. E. Tattersfield, J. Allergy Clin. Immunol. 79, 811 (1987).

253 T. R. Jones, Y. Guindon, R. Young, E. Champion, L. Charette, D. Denis, D. Ethier, R. Hamel, A. W. Ford-Hutchinson, R. Fortin, G. Letts, P. Masson, Y. Yoakim, R. N. Dehaven, A. Maycock and S. S. Pong, Can. J. Physiol. Pharmacol. 64, 1535 (1986).

254 T. R. Jones and D. Denis, Can. J. Physiol. Pharmacol. 66, 762 (1988).

255 R. N. Young, Agents and Actions Suppl. 23, 113 (1988).

256 J. M. Evans, N. C. Barnes, J. T. Zakrzewski, D. G. Sciberras, E. G. Stahl, P. J. Piper and J. F. Costello, Br. J. Clin. Pharmacol. 28, 125 (1989).

257 T. R. Jones, R. Zamboni, M. Belley, E. Champion, L. Charette, A. W. Ford-Hutchinson, R. Frenette, J.-Y. Gauthier, S. Leger, P. Masson, C. S. McFarlane, H. Piechuter, J. Rokach, H. Williams, R. N. Young, R. N. Dehaven and S. S. Pong, Can. J. Physiol. 67, 17 (1989).

258 J. C. Kips, G. Joos, D. Margolskee, I. Delepeleire, J. D. Rogers, R. Pauwels and M. van der Straeten, Am Rev. Respir. Dis. 139, A 63 (1989).

259 J. Kips, G. Joos, D. Margolskee, I. Delepeleire, R. Pauwels and M. van der Straeten, Eur. Resp. J. 8, 789S. (1989).

260 J. Gaddy, R. K. Bush, D. Margolskee, V. C. Williams and W. Busse, J. Allergy Clin. Immunol. 85, 197A (1990).

260a P. J. Manning, R. M. Watson, D. J. Margolskee, V. C. Williams, J. I. Schwartz and P. M. O'Byrne, N. Engl. J. Med. 323, 1736 (1990).

261 L. Hendeles, D. Davison, K. Blake, E. Harman, R. Cooper and D. Margolskee, J. Allergy. Clin. Immunol. 85, 197A (1990).

262 A. W. Ford-Hutchinson, Advances in Prostaglandin, Thromboxane and Leukotriene Research, vol. 21 A (eds. B. Samuelsson, P. Ramwell, R. Paoletti, G. Folco and E. Granstrom) (Raven Press Ltd., New York 1990) p. 9.

263 A. van Hecken, P. J. de Schepper, D. J. Margolskee, J. Y. K. Hsieh, R. S. Robinette, A. Buntinx and J. D. Rogers, Eur. J. Clin. Pharmacol. 36, Suppl. (1989).

264 D. W. Snyder, R. E. Giles, R. A. Keith, Y. K. Yee and R. D. Krell, J. Pharmacol. Exp. Ther. 243, 548 (1987).

265 R. D. Krell, R. E. Giles, Y. K. Yee and D. W. Snyder, J. Pharmacol. Exp. Ther. 243, 557 (1987).

266 R. D. Krell, E. J. Kusner, D. Aharony, E. J. Kusner and R. E. Giles, Eur. J. Pharmacol. *159*, 73 (1989).

267 D. Aharony, R. C. Falcone and R. D. Krell, J. Pharmacol. Exp. Ther. *243*, 921 (1987).

268 D. Aharony, R. C. Falcone, Y. K. Yee, B. Hesp, R. E. Giles and R. D. Krell, Ann. N. Y. Acad. Sci. *524*, 162 (1988).

269 R. D. Krell, D. Aharony, C. K. Buckner, R. A. Keith, E. J. Kusner, D. W. Snyder, P. R. Bernstein, V. G. Matassa, Y. K. Yee, F. J. Brown, B. Hesp and R. E. Giles, Am. Rev. Respir. Dis. *141*, 978 (1990).

270 L. J. Smith, S. Geller, L. Ebright, M. Glass and P. T. Thyrum, Am. Rev. Respir. Dis. *141*, 988 (1990).

271 L. J. Smith, S. Geller, L. Ebright, M. Glass and P. T. Thyrum, Am. Rev. Respir. Dis. *141*, A33 (1990).

272 S.-E. Dahlen, B. Dahlen, E. Eliasson, H. Johansson, T. Bjorck, M. Kumlin, K. Boo, J. Whitney, S. Binks, B. King, R. Stark and O. Zetterstrom and P. Borgeat, Advances in Prostaglandin, Thromboxane and Leukotriene Research, vol. 21 A (eds. B. Samuelsson, P. Ramwell, R. Paoletti, G. Folco and E. Granstrom) (Raven Press Ltd., New York 1990) p. 461.

273 M. Toda, H. Nakai, S. Kosuge, M. Konno, Y. Arai, T. Miyamoto, T. Obata, N. Katsube and A. Kawasaki, Advances in Prostaglandin, Thromboxane and Leukotriene Research, vol. 15 (eds. O. Hayaishi and S. Yamamoto) (Raven Press, New York, 1985) p. 307.

274 T. Obata, N. Katsube, T. Miyamoto, M. Toda, T. Okegawa, H. Nakai, S. Kosuge, M. Konno, Y. Arai and A. Kawasaki, Advances in Prostaglandin, Thromboxane and Leukotriene Research, vol. 15 (eds. O. Hayaishi and S. Yamamoto) (Raven Press, New York, 1985) p. 229.

275 H. Nakai, M. Konno, S. Kosuge, S. Sakuyama, M. Toda, Y. Arai, T. Obata, N. Katsube, T. Miyamoto, T. Okegawa and A. Kawasaki, J. Med. Chem. *31*, 84 (1988).

276 T. Nakagawa, Y. Mizushima, A. Ishii, F. Nambu, M. Motoishi, Y. Yul, T. Shida and T. Miyamoto, Advances in Prostaglandin, Thromboxane and Leukotriene Research, vol. 21 A (eds. B. Samuelsson, P. Ramwell, R. Paoletti, G. Folco and E. Granstrom) (Raven Press Ltd., New York 1990) p. 465.

277 A. von Sprecher, W. Breitenstein, A. Beck, W. Anderson, M. A. Bray and F. Marki, Advances in Prostaglandin, Thromboxane and Leukotriene Research, vol. 19 (eds. B. Samuelsson, P. Y.-K. Wong and F. F. Sun) (Raven Press Ltd., New York 1989) p. 647.

278 M. A. Bray, W. H. Anderson, N. Subramanian, U. Niederhauser, M. Kuhn, M. Erard and A. von Sprecher, Advances in Prostaglandin, Thromboxane and Leukotriene Research, vol. 21 A (eds. B. Samuelsson, P. Ramwell, R. Paoletti, G. Folco and E. Granstrom) (Raven Press Ltd., New York 1990) p. 503.

279 N. Cohen, G. Weber, B. L. Banner, R. J. Lopresti, B. Schaer, A. Focella, G. B. Zenchoff, A.-M. Chiu, L. Todaro, M. O'Donnell, A. F. Welton, D. Brown, R. Garippa, H. Crowley and D. W. Morgan, J. Med. Chem. *32*, 1842 (1989).

280 M. O'Donnell, H. J. Crowley, B. Yaremko and A. F. Welton, Abstract to 7th International Conference on Prostaglandins and Related Compounds, Florence (1990) Abstract book, p. 40.

281 J. M. Hand, M. A. Auen, J. Chang and I. M. Englebach, Int. Arch. Allergy Appl. Immunol. *89*, 78 (1989).

282 J. M. Hand, S. F. Schwalm, M. A. Auen, A. F. Kreft, J. H. Musser and J. Chang, Prostaglandins, Leukot. Essent. Fatty Acids *37*, 97 (1989).

283 J. Chang, P. Borgeat, R. P. Schleimer, J. H. Musser, A. F. Kreft, L. A. Marshall and J. M. Hand, Eur. J. Pharmacol. *151*, 506 (1988).

284   J. H. Musser, A. F. Kreft, R. H. W. Bender, D. M. Kubrak, J. Chang, A. J. Lewis and J. M. Hand, J. Med. Chem. *32*, 1176 (1989).

285   W. M. Abraham. J. S. Stevenson and R. Garrido, Prostaglandins *35*, 733 (1988).

286   J. Chang, P. Borgeat, R. P. Schleimer, J. H. Musser, A. F. Kreft, L. A. Marshall and J. M. Hand, Eur. J. Pharmacol. *148*, 131 (1988).

287   J. H. Musser, D. M. Kubrak, R. H. W. Bender, A. F. Kreft, S. T. Nielson, A. M. Lefer, J. Chang, A. J. Lewis and J. M. Hand, J. Med. Chem. *30*, 2087 (1987).

288   J. H. Musser, Agents Actions *22*, 59 (1987).

289   J. H. Musser, A. F. Kreft, R. H. W. Bender, D. M. Kubrak, D. Grimes, R. P. Carlson, J. M. Hand and J. Chang, J. Med. Chem. *33*, 240 (1990).

290   M. Konno, T. Nakae, N. Hamanaka, T. Miyamoto and A. Kawasaki, Abstract to 7th International Conference on Prostaglandins and Related Compounds, Florence (1990) Abstract book, p. 177

291   M. Konno, S. Sakuyama, T. Nakae, N. Hamanaka, T. Miyamoto and A. Kawasaki, Advances in Prostaglandin, Thromboxane and Leukotriene Research, vol. 21 A (eds. B. Samuelsson, P. Ramwell, R. Paoletti, G. Folco and E. Granstrom) (Raven Press Ltd., New York 1990) p. 411.

291 a   K. Kishikawa, N. Matsunaga, T. Maruyama, R. Seo, M. Toda, T. Miyamoto and A. Kawasaki, Advances in Prostaglandin, Thromboxane and Leukotriene Research, vol. 21 A (eds. B. Samuelsson, P. Ramwell, R. Paoletti, G. Folco and E. Granstrom) (Raven Press Ltd., New York 1990) p. 407.

292   D. J. Fretland, S. Levin, B.S. Tsai, S.W. Djuric, D. L. Widomski, J. M. Zemaitis, R. L. Shone and R. F. Bauer, Agents Actions *27*, 395 (1989).

293   B. M. Taylor, C. I. Czuk, M. N. Brunden, D. G. Wishka, J. Morris and F. F. Sun, Advances in Prostaglandin, Thromboxane and Leukotriene Research, vol. 19 (eds. B. Samuelsson, P. Y.-K. Wong and F. F. Sun) (Raven Press Ltd., New York 1989) p. 195.

294   A. H. Lin, J. L. Morris, D. G. Wishka and R. R. Gorman, Ann. N. Y. Acad. Sci. *524*, 196 (1988).

295   J. L. Morris and D. G. Wishka, Tetrahed. Lett. *29*, 143 (1988).

296   I. M. Richards, R. L. Griffin, J. A. Oostveen, J. Morris, D. G. Wishka and C. J. Dunn, Am. Rev. Resp. Dis. *140*, 1712 (1989).

297   J. E. Tateson, R. W. Randall, C. H. Reynolds, W. P. Jackson, P. Bhattacherjee, J. A. Salmon and L. G. Garland, Br. J. Pharmacol. *94*, 528 (1988).

298   J. A. Salmon, L. C. Tilling and S. Moncada, Prostaglandins, *29*, 377 (1983).

299   D. Riendeau, J. P. Falgueyret, D. J. Nathaniel, J. Rokach, N. Ueda and S. Yamamoto, Biochem. Pharmacol. *38*, 2313 (1989).

300   C. N. Serhan, U. Lundberg, G. Weissman and B. Samuelsson, Prostaglandins *27*, 563 (1984).

301   P. J. Bailey, A. L. Dallob, D. L. Allison, R. L. Anderson, T. Bach, P. L. Durette, K. M. Hand, S. L. Hopple, S. Luell, R. Meurer, R. Rosa, A. M. Tischler, B. E. Witzel and M. M. Goldenberg, Arzneim.-Forsch. *38*, 372 (1988).

302   P. Gresele, J. Arnout, H. Deckmyn and J. Vermylen, Biochem. Pharmacol. *36*, 3529 (1987).

303   R. M. McMillan, A. J. Millest, K. E. Proudman and K. B. Taylor, Br. J. Pharmacol, *87*, 53P (1986).

304   P. Gresele, J. Arnout, M. C. Coehne, H. Deckmyn and J. Vermylen, Biochem. Biophys. Res. Commun. *137*, 334 (1986).

305   F. Carey, R. A. Forder, K. H. Gibson and D. Haworth, Prostaglandins, Leukotrienes & Essent. Fatty Acids *36*, 57 (1989).

306   J. A. Salmon, P. M. Simmons and R. M. J. Palmer, Prostaglandins *24*, 255 (1982).

307   R. N. Young and Y. Girard, Leukotrienes and Lipoxygenases. Chemical, Biological and Clinical Aspects (ed. J. Rokach) (Elsevier Science Publishing Co. Inc., New York, 1989) p. 209.

308   A. Odeimat, P. E. Poubelle and P. Borgeat, Advances in Prostaglandin, Thromboxane and Leukotriene Research, vol. 21 A (eds. B. Samuelsson, P. Ramwell, R. Paoletti, G. Folco and E. Granstrom) (Raven Press Ltd., New York 1990) p. 311.

309   P. Patrignani and R. Canete-Soler, Prostaglandins *33*, 539 (1987).

310   F. J. Sweeney, J. D. Eskra and T. J. Carty, Prostaglandins Leukotrines Med. *28*, 73 (1987).

311   J. A. Salmon, P. M. Simmons and S. Moncada, J. Pharm. Pharmacol. *35*, 808 (1983).

312   B. M. Peskar, K. Lange, U. Hoppe and B. A. Peskar, Prostaglandins *31*, 283 (1986).

313   B. M. Peskar, Advances in Prostaglandin, Thromboxane and Leukotriene Research, vol. 19 (eds. B. Samuelsson, P. Y.-K. Wong and F. F. Sun) (Raven Press Ltd., New York 1989) p. 552.

314   N. K. Boughton-Smith and B. J. R. Whittle, Gastroenterol. *90*, 1325 (1987).

315   N. K. Boughton-Smith and B. J. R. Whittle, Br. J. Pharmacol. *95*, 155 (1988).

316   N. K. Boughton-Smith and B. J. R. Whittle, Pharmacol. Res. Commun. *20*, 919 (1988).

317   N. K. Boughton-Smith, J. L. Wallace, G. P. Morris and B. J. R. Whittle, Br. J. Pharmacol. *94*, 65 (1988).

318   J. L. Wallace, G. P. Morris and W. K. MacNaughton, Inflammatory Bowel Disease; Current Status and Future Approach (ed. R. P. MacDermott) (Elsevier, New York, 1988) p. 279.

319   J. L. Wallace, W. K. MacNaughton, G. P. Morris and P. L. Beck, Gastroenterol. *96*, 29 (1989).

320   J. L. Wallace and C. M. Keenan, Am. J. Physiol. *258*, G527 (1990).

321   G. J. Blackwell and L. Parente, Lymphokines *11*, 187 (1985).

322   J. A. Salmon, L. C. Tilling and S. Moncada, Biochem. Pharmacol. *23*, 2928 (1984).

323   S. J. Foster, M. E. McCormick, A. Howarth and D. Aked, Biochem. Pharmacol. *35*, 1709 (1986).

324   J. B. Summers, B. P. Gunn, H. Mazdiyasni, A. M. Goetze, P. R. Young, J. B. Bouska, R. D. Dyer, D. W. Brooks and G. W. Carter, J. Med. Chem. *30*, 2121 (1987).

325   D. G. Griswold, L. M. Hillegass, P. C. Meunier, M. J. Dimartino and N. Hanna, Arth. Rheum. *31*, 1406 (1988).

326   A. N. Payne and G. De Nucci, J. Pharmacol. Meth. *17*, 83 (1987).

327   D. W. Snyder, N. J. Lierati and M. M. McCarthy, J. Pharmacol. Meth. *19*, 219 (1988).

328   A. Keppler, L. Orning, K. Bernstrom and S. Hammarstrom, Proc. Natl. Acad. Sci. USA *84*, 5903 (1987).

329   R. Patterson, J. J. Pruzansku and K. E. Harris, J. Allergy Clin. Immunol. *61*, 444 (1981).

330   H. G. Johnson, M. L. McNee, M. K. Bach and H. W. Smith, Int. Arch. Allergy Appl. Immunol. *70*, 169 (1983).

331   W. H. Abraham, Ann. N. Y. Acad. Sci. *524*, 260 (1988).

332   G. W. Carter, P. R. Young, D. Albert, J. Bouska, R. D. Dyer, P. E. Malo, R. L. Bell, J. B. Summers, D. W. Brooks, P. Rubin and J. Kesterson, Ab-

tract to 7th International Conference on Prostaglandins and Related Compounds, Florence (1986). Abstract book, p. 192.

333   A. N. Payne, W. P. Jackson, J. A. Salmon, A. Nicholls, M. Yeadon and L. G. Garland, Proceedings of New Drugs for Asthma IUPHAR Symposium (1991) In press.

334   A. Nicholls and J. Posner, Br. J. Pharmacol. (1991) In press.

335   P. E. Christie, P. Tagari, A. W. Ford-Hutchinson, S. Charlesson, P. Chee, J. P. Arm and T. H. Lee, Abstract to 7th International Conference on Prostaglandins and Related Compounds, Florence (1990) Abstract book, p. 317.

336   K. P. Hui, I. K. Taylor, N. C. Barnes and P. J. Barnes, Am. Rev. Resp. Dis. 141, A32 (1990).

337   L. Staerk-Laursen, J. Naesdal, K. Bukhave, L. Lauritsen and J. Rask-Madsen, Lancet 335, 683 (1990).

338   P. Bailey, A. Dallob, H. Dougherty, R. Bonney, J. Humes, J. Tischler, P. Davies, M. Goldenberg and B. Moore, Abstract to 6th International Conference on Prostaglandins and Related Coumpounds, Florence (1986) Abstract book, p. 406.

339   R. M. Barr, A. K. Black, P. M. Dowd, O. Koro, K. Mistry, J. L. Isaacs and M. W. Greaves, Br. J. Clin. Pharmacol. 25, 23 (1988).

340   M. Hamberg and B. Samuelsson, Proc. Natl. Acad. Sci. USA 71, 3400 (1974).

341   G. M. Bokoch and P. M. Reed, J. Biol. Chem. 256, 4156 (1981).

342   S. Hammarstrom, Biochem. Biophys. Acta 487, 517 (1977).

343   F. F. Sun, J. C. McGuire, D. R. Morton, J. E. Pike, H. Sprecher and W. H. Kuman, Prostaglandins 21, 333 (1981).

344   J. E. Wilhelm, S. K. Sankarappa, M. van Rollins and H. Sprecher, Prostaglandins 21, 323 (1981).

345   E. J. Corey, J. R. Cashman, S. S. Kantner and S. W. Wright, J. Am. Chem. Soc. 106, 1503 (1984).

346   E. J. Corey, S. Kantner and P. T. Landsbury, Tetrahed. Lett. 24, 265 (1983).

347   J. R. Pfister and D. V. K. Murthy, J. Med. Chem. 26, 1099 (1983).

348   Y. Koshihara, S. Murota, N. Petasis and K. C. Nicolaou, FEBS Lett. 143, 13 (1982).

349   Y. Arai, K. Shimoji, M. Konno, Y. Konishi, S. Okuyama, S. Iguchi, M. Hayashi, T. Miyamoto and M. Toda, J. Med. Chem. 26, 72 (1983).

350   Y. Arai, M. Konno, K. Shimoji, Y. Konishi, H. Niwa, M. Toda and M. Hayashi, Chem. Pharm. Bull. 30, 379 (1982).

351   J. Y. Vanderhoek, R. W. Bryant and J. M. Bailey, J. Biol. Chem. 255, 5996 (1980).

352   J. Y. Vanderhoek, R. W. Bryant and J. M. Bailey, J. Biol. Chem. 255, 10064 (1980).

353   J. R. Cashman, C. Lambert and E. Sigal, Biochem. Biophys. Res. Commun. 155, 38 (1988).

354   M. Peters-Golden and C. Shally, J. Immunol. 140, 1958 (1988).

355   H.-E. Claesson, U. Lundberg and C. Malmsten, Biochem. Biophys. Res. Commun. 99, 1230 (1981).

356   E. A. Ham, M. E. Soderman, M. W. Zanetti, H. W. Dougherty, H. W. McCauley and F. A. Kuehl, Proc. Natl. Acad. Sci. USA 80, 4349 (1983).

357   M. K. Bach, J. R. Brashler, H. W. Smith, F. A. Fitzpatrick, F. F. Sun and J. C. McGuire, Prostaglandins 23, 759 (1982).

358   R. J. Smith, F. F. Sun, B. J. Bowman, S. S. Iden, H. W. Smith and J. C. McGuire, Biochem. Biophys. Res. Commun. 109, 943 (1982).

359   J. Flament, L. Schandene and J. M. Boeynaems, Prostaglandins Leukot. Essent. Fatty Acids 34, 175 (1988).

360   J. S. Mann, C. Robinson, A. Q. Sheridan, P. Clement, M. K. Bach and S. T. Holgate, Thorax *41*, 746 (1986).

361   M. Hamberg, Biochem. Biophys. Acta *431*, 651 (1976).

362   K. Sekiya and H. Okuda, Biochem. Biophys. Res. Commun. *105*, 1090 (1982).

363   J. Baumann, F. V. Bruchausen and G. Wurm, Prostaglandins *23*, 797 (1980).

364   W. C. Hope, A. F. Welton, C. Fiedler-Nagy, C. Batula-Bernardo and J. W. Coffey, Biochem. Pharmacol. *32*, 367 (1983).

365   T. Neichi, Y. Koshihara and S. Murota, Biochim. Biophys. Acta *753, 130* (1983).

366   M. A. Bray, Eur. J. Pharmacol. *98*, 61 (1984).

367   R. W. Randall, J. E. Tateson, J. Dawson and L. G. Garland, FEBS Lett. *214*, 167 (1987).

368   Y. Koshihara, T. Neichi, S. Murota, H. Lao, Y. Fujmoto and T. Tatsuno, Biochem. Biophys. Acta *792*, 92 (1984).

369   G. A. Higgs, R. J. Flower and J. R. Vane, Biochem. Pharmacol *28*, 1959 (1979).

370   R. W. Randall, K. E. Eakins, G. A. Higgs, J. A. Salmon and J. E. Tateson, Agents Actions *10*, 553 (1980).

371   O. Radmark, C. Malmsten and B. Samuelsson, FEBS Lett. *110*, 213 (1980).

372   M. Mardin and W.-D. Busse, In "Leukotrienes and Other Lipoxygenase Products" (P. J. Piper, ed.) (Research Studies Press, Chichester, 1983) p. 263.

373   S. Fischer, M. Struppler, B. Bohlig, C. Bernutz, W. Wober and P. C. Weber, Circulation *68*, 821 (1983).

374   R. W. Fuller, N. Maltby, R. Richmond, C. T. Dollery, G. W. Taylor, W. Ritter and E. Philipp, Br. J. Clin Pharmacol. *23*, 677 (1987).

375   T. Yoshimoto, M. Furukawa, S. Yamamoto, T. Horie and S. Watanabe-Kohno, Biochem. Biophys. Res. Commun. *116*, 612 (1983).

376   Y. Ashida, T. Saijo, H. Juriki, H. Makino, S. Terao and Y. Maki, Prostaglandins *26*, 955 (1983).

377   M. Fujimura, F. Sasaki, Y. Nakatsumi, Y. Takahashi, S. Hifumi, K. Taga, J.-I. Mifune, T. Tanaka and T. Matsuda, Thorax *41*, 955 (1986).

378   Y. Guindon, Y. Girard, A. Maycock, A. W. Ford-Hutchinson, J. G. Atkinson, P. C. Belanger, A. Dallob, D. Desousa, H. Dougherty, R. Egan, M. M. Goldenberg, E. Ham, R. Fortin, P. Hamsel, C. K. Lau, Y. Leblanc, C. S. McFarlane, H. Piechuta, M. Therien, C. Yoakim and J. Rokach, Advances in Prostaglandin, Thromboxane and Leukotriene Research, vol. 21 A (eds. B. Samuelsson, P. Ramwell, R. Paoletti, G. Folco and E. Granstom) (Raven Press Ltd., New York 1990) p. 554.

379   M. L. Hammond, I. E. Kopka, R. A. Zambias, C. G. Caldwell, J. Boger, F. Baker, T. Bach, S. Luell and D. E. MacIntyre, J. Med. Chem. *32*, 1006 (1989).

380   M. L. Hammond, R. A. Zambias, M. N. Chang, N. P. Jensen, J. McDonald, K. Thompson, D. A. Boulton, I. E. Kopka, K. M. Hand, E. E. Opas, S. Luell, T. Bach, P. Davies, D. E. MacIntyre, R. J. Bonney and J. L. Humes, J. Med. Chem. *33*, 908 (1990).

381   C. K. Lau, P. C. Belanger, J. Scheigetz, C. Dufresne, H. W. Williams, A. L. Maycock, Y. Guindon, T. Bach, A. L. Allob, D. Denis, A. Ford-Hutchinson, P. H. Gale, S. L. Hopple, L. G. Letts, S. Luell, C. S. McFarlane, E. MacIntyre, R. Meurer, D. K. Miller, E. Piechuta, D. Riendeau, J. Rokach and C. Rouzer, J. Med. Chem. *32*, 1190 (1989).

382   S. M. Coutts, A. Khandwala, R. van Inwegan, U. Chakraborty, J. Musser, J. Bruens, N. Jariwafa, V. Dally-Medd, R. Ingram, T. Pruss, H. Jones,

E. Neiss and I. Weinryb, Prostaglandins, Leukotrienes and Lipoxins (ed. L. J. M. Bailey) (Plenum Press, New York, 1985) p. 627.

383 C. M. Tennant, J. P. Seale and D. M. Temple, J. Pharm. Pharmacol. *39*, 309 (1987).

384 J. Evans, N. C. Barnes, P. J. Piper and J. F. Costello, Brit. J. Clin. Pharmacol. *25*, 111 P (1988).

385 R. P. Carlson, L. O'Neill-Davis, W. Calhoun, L. Datko, J. H. Musser, A. F. Kreft and J. Y. Chang, Agents and Actions *26*, 319 (1989).

386 J. Berkenkopf, R. Carlson, J. Chang, D. Grimes, R. Heaslip, A. Kreft, A. Lewis, L. Marshall, J. Musser, R. Sturm and B. Weichman, Am. Rev. Resp. Dis. *141*, A 15 (1990).

387 E. C. Ku, A. Raychaudhuri, G. Ghai, E. F. Kimble, W. H. Lee, C. Colombo, R. Dotson, T. D. Oglesby and J. W. F. Wasley, Biochim. Biophys. Acta *959*, 332 (1988).

388 R. W. Egan, A. N. Tischler, E. M. Baptista, E. A. Ham, D. D. Soderman and P. H. Hale, Advances in Prostaglandin, Thromboxane and Leukotriene Research, vol. 11 (eds. B. Samuelsson, R. Paoletti, P. Ramwell). (Raven Press Ltd., New York 1983), p. 151.

389 R. W. Egan and P. H. Gale, J. Biol. Chem. *260*, 11 554 (1985).

390 S. J. Foster, P. Bruneau, E. R. H. Walker and R. M. McMillan, Br. J. Pharmacol. *99*, 113 (1990).

391 W. P. Jackson, P. J. Islip, G. Kneen, A. Pugh and P. J. Wates, J. Med. Chem. *31*, 499 (1988).

392 A. N. Payne, L. G. Garland, I. W. Lees and J. A. Salmon, Br. J. Pharmacol. *94*, 540 (1988).

393 G. A. Higgs, R. L. Follenfant and L. G. Garland, Br. J. Pharmacol. *94*, 547 (1988).

394 V. M. Darley-Usmar, A. Hersey and L. G. Garland, Biochem. Pharmacol. *38*, 1465 (1989).

395 J. A. Salmon, W. P. Jackson and L. G. Garland, Therapeutic Approaches to Inflammatory Disease (eds. A. J. Lewis, N. S. Doherty and N. R. Ackerman) (Elsevier Science, Amsterdam, 1989) p. 137.

396 J. Davidson, A. S. Milton, D. Rotondo, J. A. Salmon and G. Watt, Brit. J. Pharmacol, *100*, 447 P (1990).

397 W. P. Jackson, P. J. Islip, A. Pugh and P. J. Wates, To be published.

398 J. B. Summers, H. Mazdiyasni, J. H. Holms, J. D. Ratajczyk, R. D. Dyer and G. W. Carter, J. Med. Chem. *30*, 574 (1987).

399 J. B. Summers, B. P. Gunn, J. G. Martin, H. Mazdiyasni, A. O. Stewart, P. R. Young, A. M. Goetze, J. B. Bouska, R. D. Dyer, D. W. Brooks and G. W. Carter, J. Med. Chem. *31*, 3 (1988).

400 J.B. Summers, B. P. Gunn, J. G. Martin, M. B. Martin, H. Mazdiyasni, A. O. Stewart, P. R. Young, J. B. Bouska, A. M. Goetze, R. D. Dyer, D. W. Brooks and G. W. Carter, J. Med. Chem. *31*, 1960 (1988).

401 J. B. Summers, K. H. Kim, H. Mazdiyasni, J. H. Holms, J. D. Ratajczyk, A. O. Stewart, R. D. Dyer and G. W. Carter, J. Med. Chem. *33*, 992 (1990).

402 G. W. Carnathan, D. M. Sweeney, J. J. Travis, R. J. Gordon, C. A. Sutherland, N. Jariwala, M. Clearfield, S. O'Rourke, F. C. Huang and R. G. van Inwegan, Agents Actions *28*, 204 (1989).

403 J. A. Salmon, W. P. Jackson and L. G. Garland, Advances in Prostaglandin, Thromboxane and Leukotriene Research, vol. 21 A (eds. B. Samuelsson, P. Ramwell, R. Paoletti, G. Folco and E. Granstrom) (Raven Press Ltd., New York 1990), p. 109.

404 P. R. Young, E. M. Roberts, J. Barlow, S. Culbertson, W. Rach, J. Bouska, J. B. Summers, D. W. Brooks and G. W. Carter, Fourth International Conference of the Inflammation Research Association (1988). Abstract 61.

405 R. L. Bell, D. H. Albert, J. B. Bouska, R. D. Dyer, W. S. Rach, E. R. Otis, J. B. Summers, D. W. Brooks and G. W. Carter, Fourth International Conference of the Inflammation Research Association (1988). Abstract 135.

406 G. W. Carter, P. R. Young, D. Albert, J. Bouska, R. D. Dyer, P. E. Malo, R. L. Bell, J. B. Summers, D. W. Brooks, P. Rubin and J. Kesterson, Abstract to 7th International Conference on Prostaglandins and Related Compounds, Florence (1990). Abstract book p. 192.

406b G. W. Carter, P. R. Young, D. H. Albert, J. Bouska, R. Dyer, R. L. Bell, J. B. Summers and D. W. Brooks, J. Pharm. Exp. Ther. (1991) In press.

407 E. Israel, R. M. Dermarkarian, M. A. Rosenberg, P. Rubin and J. M. Drazen, Am. Rev. Resp. Dis. *141*, A175 (1990).

408 A. Rene, G. Braeckman, R. Granneman, P. R. Rubin and J. W. Kesterson, J. Clin. Pharmacol. *29*, 837 (1989).

408a E. Israel, R. M. Dermarkarian, M. A. Rosenberg, R. Sperling, G. Taylor, P. Rubin and J. M. Drazen, N. Engl. J. Med. *323*, 1740 (1990).

408b H. R. Knapp, N. Engl. J. Med. *323*, 1745 (1990).

409 K. Lauritsen, L. S. Laursen, J. Rask-Madson, O. Jacobsen, J. Naesdal, W. Stenson, D. Cort, H. Goebell, B. Peskar, S. Hanauer, P. Rubin, L. Swanson and J. Kesterson, Gastroenterol. *98*, A185 (1990).

410 J. A. Gillard, A. W. Ford-Hutchinson, C. Chan, S. Charleson, D. Denis, A. Foster, R. Fortin, S. Leger, C. S. McFarlane, H. Morton, H. Piechuta, D. Riendeau, C. A. Rouzer, J. Rokach, R. Young, D. E. MacIntyre, L. Peterson, T. Bach, G. Eiermann, S. Hopple, J. Humes, L. Hupe, S. Luell, J. Metzger, R. Meurer, D. K. Miller, E. Opas and S. Pacholok, Can. J. Physiol. Pharmacol. *67*, 456 (1989).

411 A. Guhlmann, A. Keppler, S. Kastner, H. Kreiter, U. B. Bruckner, K. Messmer and D. Keppler, J. Exp. Med. *170*, 1905 (1989).

412 E. H. Bel, W. Tanaka, R. Spector, B. Friedman, H. von De Veen, J. H. Dijkman and P. J. Sterk, Am. Rev. Respir. Dis. *141*, A31 (1990).

413 J. R. Walker and W. Dawson, J. Pharm. Pharmacol. *31*, 778 (1979).

414 J. Harvey, H. Ho, P. P. K. Parish, J. R. Boot and W. Dawson, J. Pharm. Pharmacol, *35*, 44 (1983).

415 J. L. Humes, S. Sadowski, M. Galavage, M. Goldenberg, E. Subers, F. Kuehl and R. Bonney, Biochem. Pharmacol. *32*, 2319 (1983).

416 D. J. Masters and R. M. McMillan, Br. J. Pharmacol, *81*, 70 P (1984).

417 E. C. Huskinson and J. Scott, Rheumatol. Rehab. *18*, 110 (1979).

418 K. Kragballe and T. Herlin, Arch. Dermatol. *119*, 548 (1983).

419 R. M. McMillan, J.-M. Girodeau and S. J. Foster, Br. J. Pharmacol. *101*, 501 (1990).

420 M. Peters-Golden and C. Shelly, Biochem. Pharmacol. *38*, 1589 (1989).

421 P. Needleman, A. Raz, M. Minkes, J. A. Ferrendelli and H. Sprecher, Proc. Natl. Acad. Sci. USA *76*, 944 (1979).

422 B. A. Jakschik, A. R. Sams, H. Sprecher and P. Needleman, Prostaglandins *20*, 401 (1980).

423 R. C. Murphy, W. C. Pickett, B. R. Culp and W. E. M. Lands, Prostaglandins *22*, 13 (1981).

424 T. Terano, J. A. Salmon and S. Moncada, Prostaglandins, *27*, 217 (1984).

425 C. Yokoyama, K. Mizuno, H. Mitachi, T. Yoshimoto, S. Yamamoto and C. R. Pace-Asciak, Biochem. Biophys. Acta. *750*, 237 (1983).

426 T. Terano, J. A. Salmon and S. Moncada, Biochem. Pharmacol. *33*, 3071 (1984).

427 T. Terano, J. A. Salmon, G. A. Higgs and S. Moncada, Biochem. Pharmacol. *35*, 779 (1986).

428 J. D. Prickett, D. R. Robinson and A. D. Steinberg, Arth. Rheum. *26*, 133 (1983).

429 J. D. Prickett, D. E. Trentham and D. R. Robinson, J. Immunol. *132*, 725 (1984).
430 C. A. Leslie, W. A. Gonnerman, M. D. Ullman, K. C. Hayes, C. Franzblau and E. S. Cathcart, J. Exp. Med. *162*, 1336 (1985).
431 T. H. Lee, F. Austen, A. G. Leitch, E. Israel, D. R. Robinson, R. A. Lewis, E. J. Corey and J. M. Drazen, Am. Rev. Respir. Dis. *132*, 1204 (1985).
432 T. H. Lee, R. L. Hoover, J. D. Williams, R. I. Sperling, J. Ravalese, B. W. Spur, D. R. Robinson, E. J. Corey, R. A. Lewis and K. F. Austen, New Engl. J. Med. *312*, 1217 (1985).
433 S. M. Prescott, G. A. Zimmerman and A. R. Morrison, Prostaglandins *30*, 209 (1985).
434 J. M. Kremer, J. Iganoette, A. V. Michalek, L. Lininger, C. Huyck, J. Igauotte, M. A. Timchalk, R. I. Rynes, J. Zieminski and L. E. Bartholomew, Lancet *i*, 184 (1985).
435 J. M. Kremer, W. Jubiz, A. Michale, R. I. Rynes, L. E. Bartholomew, J. Bigaouette, M. Timchalk, D. Beeler and L. Lininger, Ann. Int. Med. *106*, 497 (1987).
436 R. L. Sperling, M. Weinblatt, J. L. Robin, J. Ravalese, R. L. Hoover, F. House, J. S. Coblyn, P. A. Fraser, B. W. Spur, D. W. Robinson, R. L. Lewis and K. F. Austen, Arth. Rheum. *30*, 988 (1987).
437 L. G. Cleland, J. K. French, W. H. Betts and G. A. Murphy, J. Rheum. *15*, 1471 (1988).
438 J. J. F. Belch, D. Ansell, R. Madhok, A. O'Dowd and R. D. Sturrock, Ann. Rheum. Dis. *47*, 96 (1988).
439 J. J. F. Belch, A. O'Dowd, D. Ansell and R. D. Sturrock, Scand. J. Rheum. *18*, 213 (1989).
440 V. A. Ziboh, K. A. Cohen, C. N. Ellis, C. Miller, T. A. Hamilton, K. Kragballe, C. R. Hydrick and J. J. Vorhees, Arch. Dermatol. *122*, 1277 (1986).
441 S. B. Bittiner, W. F. G. Tucker, I. Cartwright and S. S. Bleehen, Lancet, 1, *378* (1988).

Bacterial resistance to antibiotics: The role of biofilms

By Brian D. Hoyle and J. William Costerton

Biofilm Group, Department of Biological Sciences, University of Calgary, Calgary, Alberta, Canada T2N 1N4

1   Summary

Bacteria adhere to natural and synthetic, medically important surfaces within an extracellular polymer generically termed the glycocalyx. This quasi-structure is a biofilm. The enhanced antibiotic resistance of biofilm bacteria, relative to floating (planktonic) bacteria, encourages the establishment of chronic bacterial infections. Resistance mechanisms include the hinderance of antibiotic diffusion by the glycocalyx, the physiology of the bacteria and the environment conditions of the niche in which the biofilm resides.

2   Introduction

Examination of hundreds of surfaces in natural, industrial and pathogenic ecosystems has unequivocably established that alive and inert surfaces are colonized by bacteria [1–4]. Scanning and transmission electron microscopy examination of the surfaces of many prosthestic devices has revealed that the adherent (sessile) bacteria are frequently buried within an amorphous polysaccharide matrix [2–4]. This quasi-structure has been termed a biofilm [2].

Within the confines of the hospital biofilms are undeniably important. For example, skin flora such as *Staphylococcus aureus* and *S. epidermidis* can be spread upon contact with the surfaces of implanted devices [5], which contributes to the 100,000 to 200,000 new cases of device-related infections occurring annually in the United States. The economic and clinical consequences of biofilm formation are significant. Pneumonias, which are the second leading cause of death from nosocomial infection in the United States, exact more than one billion dollars in direct medical costs each year. Clinicians certainly appreciate the difficulty attendant in the treatment of infected biomaterials and tissue surfaces *in situ*. Acute inflammation and bacteremia can be controlled by the administration of high levels of antibiotics, leaving a chronic indolent infection. Cessation of antibiotic therapy prompts a "flare-up" of the acute events [2, 6].

The molecular bases of the antibacterial resistance of biofilms have not yet been defined. Over the past five years, however, the picture has become clearer. In the present review we have endeavoured to condense the considerable body of relevant research on the antibiotic resistance of biofilms into a lucid format. We have focussed on amino-

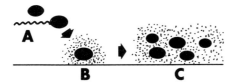

Figure 1
Generalized representation of the mechanism and temporal sequence of bacterial adhesion and biofilm formation. Reversible attachment by motile and nonmotile bacteria (A) precedes irreversible adhesion (B). Division and glycocalyx production produces a biofilm (C).

glycoside and β-lactam antibiotics, since they have been examined most intensively. Investigations with other classes of antibiotics, such as quinolones, are as yet few. Their exclusion from this review should not diminish their potential value in the treatment of biofilm-related chronic infections.

3   Formation of biofilms

A biofilm is the culmination of a series of processes (Fig. 1), which begins when floating (planktonic) bacteria encounter a surface. This can occur actively involving motility or chemotaxis by the bacteria, or because of the passive diffusion of the bacteria, or because of convective flow [7]. Hydrophobic [8] and Van der Waals [9] forces position the bacteria near the surface, which facilitates adherence. For the plastic or metal surfaces of prosthetic devices adherence can be instantaneous [7, 10–12]. With the elaboration of a glycocalyx by the bacteria adhesion becomes irreversible [2, 10, 13]. Continued growth and division of the sessile bacteria and the recruitment of other bacteria from the bulk fluid produces a biofilm of glycocalyx-enclosed microcolonies or regions of confluency [2, 4, 13].
Glycocalyx generically describes extracellular homo- or heteropolysaccharide which is intimately or loosely associated with the delimiting membrane of a bacterium [14]. While diverse in composition [15] most glycocalyces, such as the uronic acid-containing alginate of *Pseudomonas aeruginosa*, are anionic [15]. Accordingly, cationic molecules such as ruthenium red will bind to a glycocalyx polymer (Fig. 2).

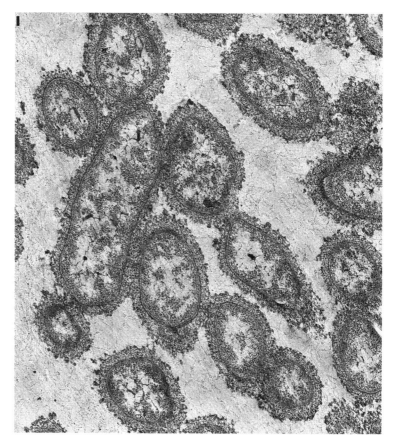

Figure 2
Transmission electron micrograph of a section of a ruthenium red-stained preparation of cells of *Bacteroides thetaiotaomicron* strain 464–74 which were treated with homologous antiserum. The extensive (about 200 nm) glycocalyx surrounding the bacteria has been stabilized in the form of an integrally-associated network which constitutes the effective outer surface of the bacteria. Scale bar = 0.1 μm.

4   Medical relevance of biofilms

Biofilms have been detected on a myriad of viable and inert surfaces within the human body [2]. Table 1 provides a partial list. The establishment of a biofilm habitually preludes the establishment of a chronic infection [2, 6]. An inert surface such as catheter latex is prone to bacterial colonization and biofilm formation [4, 5, 19] markedly in-

Table 1
Occurrence of biofilms in pathogenic ecosystems.

Site of biofilm formation	References
Urinary catheter polyvinylchloride	[16, 17]
Endotracheal polyvinylchloride	[18]
Tenckhoff catheters	[19–21]
Intravascular catheters	[22, 23]
Orthopedic protheses	[24]
Cardiac prosthetic valves and pacemakers	[25]
Intrauterine contraceptive devices	[26]
Sutures and staples	[27, 28, 29]
Tissue adhesive	[30]
Urine droppers and drainage bags	[31]
Vascular grafts	[32]
Ileal conduits	[33]
Endoscopic biliary stents	[34]
Kidney stones	[35, 36]
Vaginal epithelial tissue	[37]
Endocarditis	[38]
Peritonitis	[39]
Osteomyelitis	[40]
Prostatitis	[41]
Bovine pneumonic pasteurellosis	[42]
Lung tissue	[43]
Gut epithelial tissue	[44]
Murine corneal tissue	[45]

creasing the chance of acquiring a bacterial infection for each day of catheterization [2]. On a viable surface, such as the lung tissue of individuals afflicted with cystic fibrosis (CF), the formation of *P. aeruginosa* biofilms [2, 44] is the "harbinger of death" [46].

When cocooned within the fabric of the glycocalyx, the sessile bacteria are better able to withstand the hosts' erradication mechanisms. Complement and immunoglobulin resistance has been correlated with the presence of capsular glycocalyx in both gram-negative and gram-positive bacteria [47–49]. Sessile *P. aeruginosa* recovered from CF sputum and the urinary tract express outer membrane proteins which function to scavenge and sequester iron [50, 51], equipping the cells for survival in the low iron environment of the host. Resistance of glycocalyx-producing bacteria to host cellular defense mechanisms such as polymorphonuclear neutrophil- and alveolar macrophage-mediated phagocytosis, and antibody formation has been demonstrated [52, 53]. *P. aeruginosa* CF isolates produce an elastase which cleaves IgGs [54]. Cleaved and intact antibodies formed to the alginate of *P. aeruginosa* may ultimately be more damaging to the host than to the bacteria due to the formation and deposition of immune complexes on the host tissue [55, 56].

5   Antibiotic resistance of biofilms
5.1   Contribution of the glycocalyx

Those features of a biofilm which govern its resistance to host-mediated factors likely contribute to the antibiotic resistance of the biofilm. The biofilm mode of growth protects the sessile bacteria *in vitro* from concentrations of antibiotics which swiftly kill their planktonic counterparts [10, 13, 57–59]. In 1985, Curtis Nickel and his colleagues performed an elegant experiment which directly implicated the *P. aeruginosa* alginate in the tobramycin resistance of biofilms [13 and Table 2]. Urinary catheter latex was colonized by biofilms of a *P. aer-*

Table 2
The effect of tobramycin on the survival of sessile *Pseudomonas aeruginosa* bacteria growing within biofilms on catheter latex material.

Tobramycin Concn (mg·ml^{-1})	Viable cells at time:		
	0 h	8 h	12 h
0[a]	4.7×10^8	2.3×10^9	2.7×10^9
[b]	1.1×10^9	9.8×10^8	1.4×10^9
100[a]	5.8×10^8	5.3×10^7	4.2×10^7
[b]	9.0×10^8	0	0
1000[a]	2.0×10^8	1.1×10^7	6.1×10^6

This table has been modified from Tables 1 and 2 of [13]. Total cell numbers, as determined by epifluorescence microscopy, remained constant.
[a] Viable sessile cells·cm^{-2} of latex material.
[b] Viable planktonic cells·ml^{-1}.

uginosa urinary tract isolate. Viable densities to 10^9 bacteria·cm^{-2} were achieved. Following the colonization period the flow of sterile medium containing up to 1000 μg·ml^{-1} of tobramycin was commenced. Even after 12 h more than 10^6 viable bacteria·cm^{-2} were recovered. The survivors, when dispersed from the biofilm directly into tobramycin-containing medium, were inhibited by the same concentration of tobramycin as both planktonic and sessile populations recovered immediately before the addition of the antibiotic. The lack of an inherent tobramycin resistance by the sessile bacteria prompted the suggestion that the glycocalyx contributed directly to the antibiotic resistance of the sessile cells by virtue of its polyanionic charge. A positively-charged molecule such as tobramycin would bind to the glycocalyx, retarding its inward diffusion [60]. Subsequent observations have been consistent with this interpretation [61–63]. In order to be effective against sessile populations an aminoglycoside antibiotic such as tobramycin would have to be present at high, saturating concentrations $(mg \cdot ml^{-1})$ for extended periods of time (hours). Tobramycin concentrations in either the serum or bronchial fluid rarely achieves $1.0\ \mu g \cdot ml^{-1}$ [64, 65]. The reduced penetration of aminoglycosides into bronchial secretions [66] would also reduce the effective concentrations of the particular antibiotic. Furthermore, unless the antibiotic was administered continuously, a marked and rapid decrease in these levels would occur. Thus, bactericidal concentrations of aminoglycoside antibiotics may be difficult to achieve throughout the biofilm. While some sessile bacteria will be killed, complete eradication of the population may not be feasible.

5.2   Contribution on the sessile bacteria

The aforementioned role of the glycocalyx as a diffusion barrier is less than satisfactory in explaining the *in vitro* resistance of sessile bacteria to antibiotics which are negative or neutral in net charge. β-lactam antibiotics, for example, would not be expected to be avidly bound by a negatively-charged glycocalyx [63]. The piperacillin and ticarcillin resistance observed with *P. aeruginosa* and *Escherichia coli* biofilms was thus attributed to the bacteria themselves, particularly to their reduced growth rate [67–70], or the production and/or localization of degradative enzymes within the confines of the biofilm [67]. An investigation employing a chemostat unequivocably established that a slower growth rate of planktonic *E. coli* was of primary influence in the resistance of the bacteria to β-lactam antibiotics [71]. Techniques have been developed which have been claimed to allow the control of sessile growth rate [72]. The suggested correlation of a slow sessile growth rate with resistance to tobramycin, quinolone, and quaternary compounds is intriguing and certainly warrants further research.

It is entirely possible that the slower growth rate of the sessile bacteria is a consequence of the presence of the glycocalyx [73]. Bacteria resident on a surface are in an environment which is different from that of planktonic bacteria in the bulk fluid because of surface diffusion limitation [74]. The nutrient concentration of the bulk fluid and the environment within the biofilm will differ with the sessile bacteria experiencing a restriction of nutrients such as iron [50, 51] and of oxygen [75]. Accordingly, adherent and planktonic bacteria display phenotypic differences [50, 51, 76–80]. As well, the restricted entry of antibiotics (section 5.1) may produce an environment where the sessile bacteria perceive subgrowth-inhibitory concentrations (SICs) of the antibiotics. It is known that sessile bacteria exposed to SICs of aminoglycosides, β-lactams and quinolones are phenotypically different from untreated bacteria [81, 82]. Some of these differences, such as reduced glycocalyx production [82], and the cessation of exotoxin production [83, 84] have been produced when the biofilms were allowed to form under SIC conditions. Clinically, this might not occur. Presentation of symptoms following the establishment of biofilms would alert the clinician to the need for antibiotic therapy. Thus, we might rather expect the bacteria within pre-formed biofilms to experience SICs of antibiotics. In this regard, two studies warrant mention. Dunne has demonstrated that biofilms formed by clinical isolates of slime-producing, coagulase-negative staphylococci became thicker when exposed to SICs of vancomycin and cefamandole [85]. In the second investigation the flow of SICs of β-lactam antibiotics past intact *P. aeruginosa* biofilms increased the production of β-lactamase by the sessile bacteria [86]. In these two investigations the biofilms may have become more resiliant because of the administration of the antibiotics. Thus, unless the antibiotic of concern can be efficiently delivered to the entire sessile population at a bactericidal concentration, the biofilm may "respond" by retarding the access of the antibiotic and/or initiating physiological adaptations to the antibiotic.

5.3   Contribution of host components

Implanted foreign surfaces can potentiate infection [87]. It is generally accepted that the formation of biofilms on the surface of implanted material is important in the pathogenesis of implant-related infections [4, 6, 88]. Along with the difficulty attendant in eradicating the sessile bacteria, the biofilm layer may actually slide off the surface during removal of an implant and so remain within the host tissue [89].

In a rabbit peritoneal model, Buret *et al.* [89] have documented that silastic colonized with 10^5 viable *P. aeruginosa* per cm^2 provided a nidus for the formation of massive biofilms after 42 days. These viable numbers remained approximately the same from days 1–42 and the bacteria constituted only about 10% of the volume of the biofilm (A. B. Buret, personal communication). The bulk of the biofilm was host-generated, consisting primarily of phagocytes, fibrin and vascularized connective tissue.

The prolonged recovery of viable *P. aeruginosa* from the biofilms despite the massive host inflammatory response suggests that the inactivated leucocytes and fibrin mesh within the biofilm may have shielded the bacteria from live phagocytes. It is conceivable that the diffusion of antibiotics through this "crust" might also be hindered.

5.4   Contribution of the environment

Planktonic bacteria pheno- and genotypically respond to environmental fluctuations [90]. An analogous phenotypic behaviour of sessile bacteria has also been demonstrated [50, 51, 90]. Until recently the response of bacterial glycocalyx to chemical fluctuations was not considered, since the glycocalyx was regarded as being homogeneous in construction and static in its structure. It is now recognized that glycocalyces are not structurally static, but rather are responsive to the chemical composition of the surrounding milieu [73, 91, 92]. For example, cations influence the structure of *P. aeruginosa* alginate [73, 91, 92 and Fig. 3].

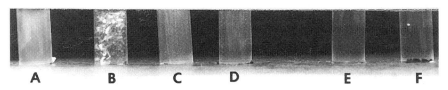

Figure 3
Effect of the addition of Ca^{2+} to mucoid and non-mucoid *Pseudomonas aeruginosa* suspensions. Phenotypically mucoid and non-mucoid bacteria recovered from Pseudomonas Isolation Agar were suspended 10 mM hydroxyethylpiperazine ethanesulfonic acid (HEPES) pH 7.0 to a final viable density of 10^8 bacteria·ml^{-1}. (A) Mucoid strain, no Ca^{2+}; (B) Mucoid strain, 2.5 mM Ca^{2+}; (C) Non-mucoid strain, no Ca^{2+}; (D) Non-mucoid strain, 2.5 mM Ca^{2+}; (E) HEPES, no Ca^{2+}; (F) HEPES, 2.5 mM Ca^{2+}.

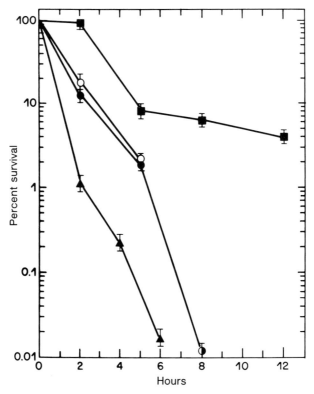

Figure 4

Viability of planktonic and sessile populations of *P. aeruginosa* upon exposure to tobramycin. Triplicate planktonic and sessile populations consisting of, respectively,
$10^8 \cdot ml^{-1}$ and $10^6 \cdot cm^{-2}$ of viable bacteria were recovered before and during tobramycin treatment. Viable and total counts were performed on each sample. Planktonic bacteria grown in a chemically-defined medium (M-56) containing 0.02 mM Ca^{2+} (▲) or
biofilms formed in M-56 containing 0.02 mM Ca^{2+} (●) or 2.5 mM Ca^{2+} (○) were exposed to 250 $\mu g \cdot ml^{-1}$ tobramycin. In the final experiment (■) biofilms formed in M-56
containing 0.02 mM Ca^{2+} were then exposed to sterile M-56 containing 2.5 mM Ca^{2+}
for 2 h prior to the addition of tobramycin. The total bacterial counts obtained
throughout all the experiments remained constant.

Studies in our laboratory have begun to address the significance of
such a structural alteration of the alginate to the antibiotic resiliency
of *P. aeruginosa*. Biofilms of a CF isolate were transiently exposed to
a concentration of calcium (Ca^{2+}; 2.5 mM) which is physiologically-
relevant in CF extracellular fluids [93] as well as in the urine of
non-CF individuals [13]. Ca^{2+} dramatically enhanced the survival of
the sessile bacteria upon a 12-h exposure to 250 $\mu g \cdot ml^{-1}$ of tobramycin (Fig. 4). When the surviving bacteria were dispersed from their al-

ginate matrix into tobramycin-containing medium, the bacteria did not survive exposure to 0.62 μg·ml^{-1} of the antibiotic [62]. In another experiment purified alginate from the same strain, untreated or treated with Ca^{2+}, received 1.0 μCi of ^{3}H-tobramycin. These samples were dialyzed and the efflux of the labeled antibiotic from the inner, alginate-containing fluid to the outer chamber fluid was evaluated

Table 3
Ratio of the counts per minute given by 1.0 μCi ^{3}H tobramycin in the outer and inner fluids following the dialysis (4°C, 24 h) of untreated or Ca^{2+} treated *Pseudomonas aeruginosa* alginate.

Inner chamber sample + 1.0 μCi ^{3}H tobramycin	Count ratio[a]
Deionized distilled water	1.0 ± 0.5
Untreated alginate	24.3 ± 0.5
Ca^{2+}-treated alginate	
0.1 mM	23.0 ± 2.0
0.5 mM	22.5 ± 1.0
1.0 mM	2.0 ± 1.0
2.5 mM	1.0 ± 0.5
5.0 mM	1.0 ± 0.1
10.0 mM	1.0 ± 0.5
25.0 mM	1.0 ± 0.1

[a] Mean $\pm$ standard error from six samples. Following dialysis, 15 μl was withdrawn from each outer and inner fluid pair. The counts per minute due to the ^{3}H tobramycin were determined. For each sample the outer count was divided by the inner count to obtain a ratio. A ratio approximating 1.0 indicated that equilibration of the radiolabel had occurred.

(Table 3). Equilibration of tobramycin occurred at Ca^{2+} concentrations of 1.0 mM and above, as evidenced by the approximately equal number of outer fluid and inner fluid radioactive counts (Table 3). Precipitation of the alginate also occurred in samples treated with 1.0 mM or more of Ca^{2+}, similar to the samples shown in figure 3. Thus, the structural alteration of the alginate by Ca^{2+} was correlated with an inhibition of tobramycin binding to the polymer.

The observations obtained with the CF isolate suggest that Ca^{2+}-induced crystallization of the glycocalyx results in the decreased permeability of the alginate to molecules even as small as tobramycin (molec. wt 800). CF pulmonary fluids, urine, and bile are elevated in cations, particularly Ca^{2+}. Biofilms which form in these locales may adopt a hitherto unrecognized three-dimensional structure which may influence their antibiotic resistance.

6   Outlook

It is clear that biofilms are protective for the bacteria residing within. Both the bacteria and the glycocalyx matrix in which the cells are enmeshed contribute to antibiotic resistance. Despite this awareness, our knowledge concerning the mechanism(s) of this resistance has remained elusive. One reason has been the testing of antibacterial compounds on planktonic bacteria cultured in nutritionally-competent media. It is prudent to suggest that in order to rationally assess the effect of antibiotics on chronic bacterial infections relevant, defined conditions must be employed. Cellular growth rate, nutritional limitation, the ionic composition of the fluid surrounding the tissue or implant, and the biofilm mode of growth must be incorporated into experimental designs. Ultimately, we will require a greater understanding of the structure and functional activities of the biofilms which form in the presence of host components.

In vivo models, combined with the data obtained from rationally-designed *in vitro* experiments, will immeasurably broaden our understanding of the nature of the barrier presented by biofilms to antibiotics. Hopefully, the ultimate manifestation of such research will be the selection of antibiotics and/or the design of other therapeutic strategies which will actually cure biofilm-related infections, not just mollify them.

Acknowledgements

Dr. Costerton is the holder of a National Science and Engineering Research Council (NSERC) Biofilm Industrial Research Chair. Dr. Hoyle is a Research Associate with the Biofilm Group. The research work described in this paper was supported by operation grants from the Natural Sciences and Engineering Research Council of Canada and from the Medical Research Council of Canada to J. W. Costerton.

References

1   G. G. Geesey, R. Mutch, J. W. Costerton and R. B. Green: Limnol. Oceanogr. *23*, 1214 (1978).
2   J. W. Costerton, K.-J. Cheng, G. G. Geesey, T. I. Ladd, J. C. Nickel, M. Dasgupta and T. J. Marrie: Ann. Rev. Microbiol. *41*, 435 (1987).

3   J. W. Costerton, R. T. Irvin and K.-J. Cheng: Ann. Rev. Microbiol. *35*, 299 (1982).
4   M. Jacques, T. J. Marrie and J. W. Costerton: Microb. Ecol. *13*, 173 (1987).
5   G. M. Dickinson and A. L. Bisno: Antimicrob. Agents Chemother. *33*, 597 (1989).
6   T. Khoury and J. W. Costerton: Elsevier, The Netherlands (1988) p. 2.
7   M. C. M. van Loosdrecht, J. Lyklema, W. Norde and A. J. B. Zehnder: Microbiol. Rev. *54*, 75 (1990).
8   G. W. Jones and R. E. Isaacson: Crit. Rev. Microbiol. *10*, 229 (1982).
9   R. M. Pashley, P. M. McGuiggan, B. W. Ninham and D. F. Evans: Science *229*, 1088 (1985).
10   H. Anwar, M. Dasgupta, K. Lam and J. W. Costerton: J. Antimicrob. Chemother. *24*, 647 (1989).
11   P. M. Stanley: Can. J. Microbiol. *29*, 1493 (1983).
12   E. Vanhaecke, J.-P. Remon, M. Moors, F. Raes, D. DeRudder and A. van Peteghem: Appl. Environ. Microbiol. *56*, 788 (1990).
13   J. C. Nickel, I. Ruseska, J. B. Wright and J. W. Costerton: Antimicrob. Agents Chemother. *27*, 619 (1985).
14   C. Whitfield: Can. J. Microbiol. *39*, 243 (1988).
15   I. W. Sutherland: Ann. Rev. Microbiol. *39*, 243 (1985).
16   J. C. Nickel, S. K. Grant and J. W. Costerton: Urology *26*, 369 (1985).
17   J. C. Nickel, P. Feero, J. W. Costerton and E. Wilson: Can. J. Surg. *32*, 131 (1989).
18   F. D. Sottile, T. J. Marrie, D. S. Prough, C. D. Hobgood, D. J. Gower, L. X. Webb, J. W. Costerton and A. G. Gristina: Crit. Care Med. *14*, 265 (1986).
19   T. J. Marrie, M. A. Noble and J. W. Costerton: J. Clin. Microbiol. *18*, 1388 (1983).
20   R. R. Read, P. Eberwein, M. K. Dasgupta, S. K. Grant, K. Lam, J. C. Nickel and J. W. Costerton: Kidney Internat. *35*, 614 (1989).
21   M. K. Dasgupta, M. Larabie, K. Lam, K. B. Bettcher, D. L. Tyrrell and J. W. Costerton: Am. J. Nephrol. *28*, 883 (1990).
22   T. R. Franson, N. K. Sheth, H. D. Rose and P. G. Sohnle: J. Infect. Dis. *149*, 116 (1984).
23   T. J. Marrie and J. W. Costerton: J. Clin. Microbiol. *19*, 687 (1984).
24   A. G. Gristina and J. W. Costerton: Infect. in Surg. *(Sept.)* 655 (1984).
25   T. J. Marrie and J. W. Costerton: J. Clin. Microbiol. *19*, 911 (1984).
26   M. Jacques, M. E. Olson and J. W. Costerton: Am. J. Obst. Gyn. *154*, 648 (1986).
27   B. Blomstedt, B. Osterberg and A. Bergstrand: Acta Chir. Scand. *143*, 71 (1977).
28   A. G. Gristina, J. L. Price, C. D. Hobgood, L. X. Webb and J. W. Costerton: Surg. *98*, 12 (1985).
29   S. Katz, M. Izhar and D. Mirelman: Ann. Surg. *194*, 35 (1981).
30   M. E. Olson, I. Ruseska and J. W. Costerton: J. Biomed. Mat. Res. *22*, 485 (1988).
31   T. J. Marrie and J. W. Costerton: Appl. Environ. Microbiol. *45*, 1018 (1983).
32   O. Goeau-Brissoniere, J. C. Pechere, R. Guidoin, H. P. Noel and J. Couture: Can. J. Surg. *26*, 540 (1983).
33   R. C. Y. Chan, G. Reid, A. W. Bruce and J. W. Costerton: Appl. Environ. Microbiol. *48*, 1159 (1984).
34   A. G. Speer, P. B. Cotton, J. Rode, A. M. Seddon, C. R. Neal, J. Holton and J. W. Costerton: Annls Inter. Med. *108*, 546 (1988).
35   R. J. C. McLean, J. C. Nickel, T. J. Beveridge and J. W. Costerton: J. Med. Microbiol. *29*, 1 (1989).

36   L. Clapham, R. J. C. McLean, J. C. Nickel, J. Downey and J. W. Coster-
      ton: J. Chrystal Growth *104*, 475 (1990).
37   K. Sadhu, P. A. G. Domingue, A. W. Chow, J. Nelligan, K. Bartlett and
      J. W. Costerton: Microb. Ecol. Health Dis. *2*, 99 (1989).
38   J. Mills, L. Pulliam, L. Dall, J. Marzouk, W. Wilson and J. W. Costerton:
      Infect. Immun. *43*, 359 (1984).
39   T. J. Marrie and J. W. Costerton: J. Clin. Microbiol. *22*, 924 (1985).
40   A. G. Gristina, M. Oga, L. X. Webb and C. D. Hobgood: Science *228*, 990
      (1985).
41   J. C. Nickel, M. E. Olson, A. Barabas, H. Benediktsson, M. K. Dasgupta
      and J. W. Costerton: Brit. J. Urol. *65*, (In Press) (1990).
42   D. W. Morck, J. W. Costerton, D. O. Bolingbroke, H. Ceri, N. D. Boyd
      and M. E. Olson: Can. J. Vet. Res. *54*, 139 (1990).
43   J. S. Lam, R. Chan, K. Lam and J. W. Costerton: Infect. Immun. *28*, 546
      (1980).
44   J. W. Costerton, K.-J. Cheng and K. R. Rozee: Attachment of Microorgan-
      isms to the Gastrointestinal Mucosal Surface. CRC Press. (1983) p. 189.
45   A. Singh, L. D. Hazlett and R. S. Berk: Infect. Immun. *58*, 1301 (1990).
46   G. Pier: J. Infect. Dis. *151*, 575 (1985).
47   J. B. Woolcock: Virulence Mechanisms of Bacterial Pathogens. Am. Soc.
      Microbiol., Washington (1988) p. 73.
48   J. M. Tomas, V. J. Benedi, B. Ciurana and J. Jofre: Infect. Immun. *54*, 85
      (1986).
49   C. Vermeulen, A. Cross, W. R. Byrne and W. Zollinger: Infect. Immun. *56*,
      2723 (1988).
50   H. Anwar, M. R. W. Brown, A. Day and P. Weller: FEMS Microbiol. Lett.
      24, 235 (1984).
51   M. R. W. Brown, H. Anwar and P. A. Lambert: FEMS Microbiol. Lett. *21*,
      113 (1984).
52   C. J. Czuprynski: Virulence Mechanisms of Bacterial Pathogens. Am. Soc.
      Microbiol., Washington (1988) p. 141.
53   A. Fomsgaard, N. Hoiby, G. H. Shand, R. S. Conrad and C. Galanos: In-
      fect. Immun. *56*, 2270 (1988).
54   R. B. Fick, Jr., R. S. Baltimore, S. U. Squier and H. Y. Reynolds: J. Infect.
      Dis. *151*, 589 (1985).
55   D. E. Woods and L. E. Bryan: J. Infect. Dis. *151*, 581 (1985).
56   N. Hoiby, G. Doring and P. O. Schiotz: Ann. Rev. Microbiol. *40*, 29 (1986).
57   R. C. Evans and C. J. Holmes: Antimicrob. Agents Chemother. *31*, 889
      (1987).
58   A. G. Gristina, C. D. Hobgod, L. X. Webb and Q. N. Myrvik: Biomat. *8*,
      423 (1987).
59   C. J. Holmes and R. C. Evans: J. Antimicrob. Chemother. *24*, 84 (1989).
60   J. W. Costerton: Rev. Infect. Dis. *6*, 608 (1984).
61   H. Anwar, T. van Biesen, M. Dasgupta, K. lam and J. W. Costerton: J. An-
      timicrob. Chemother. *24*, 1824 (1989).
62   B. D. Hoyle and J. W. Costerton: FEMS Microbiol. Lett. *60*, 339 (1989).
63   C. A. Gordon, N. Hodges and C. Marriott: J. Antimicrob. Chemother. *22*,
      667 (1989).
64   J. E. Pennington and H. Y. Reynolds: Antimicrob. Agents Chemother. *4*,
      299 (1973).
65   B. R. Smith and J. F. LeFrock: Chest *83*, 904 (1983).
66   G. A. Wong, T. H. Peirce, E. Goldstein and P. D. Hoeprich: Am. J. Med.
      59, 219 (1975).
67   W. W. Nichols, M. J. Evans, M. P. E. Slack and H. L. Walmsley: J. Gen
      Microbiol. *135*, 1291 (1989).
68   M. R. W. Brown, D. G. Allison and P. Gilbert: J. Antimicrob. Chemother.
      22, 777 (1988).

69 P. Gilbert, P. J. Collier and M. R. W. Brown: Antimicrob. Agents Chemother. *34*, 1865 (1990).
70 D. G. Allison, D. J. Evans, M. R. W. Brown and P. Gilbert: J. Bacteriol. *172*, 1667 (1990).
71 E. Tuomanen, R. Cozens, W. Tosch, O. Zak and A. Tomasz: J. Gen. Microbiol. *132*, 1297 (1986).
72 P. Gilbert, D. G. Allison, D. J. Evans, P. S. Handley and M. R. W. Brown: Appl. Environ. Microbiol. *55*, 1308 (1989).
73 B. D. Hoyle, J. Jass and J. W. Costerton: J. Antimicrob. Chemother. *26*, 1 (1990).
74 W. G. Characklis, M. H. Turakhia and N. Zelver: Biofilms. John Wiley & Sons, Inc., New York 1990, p. 316.
75 L. P. Nielson, P. B. Christensen, N. P. Revsbech and J. Sorensen: Microb. Ecol. *19*, 63 (1990).
76 D. E. Woods, M. S. Schaeffer, H. R. Rabin, G. D. Campbell and P. A. Sokal: J. Clin. Microbiol. *24*, 260 (1980).
77 A. L. Cheung and V. A. Fischetti: Infect. Immun. *56*, 1061 (1988).
78 P. Williams, S. P. Denyer and R. G. Finch: FEMS Microbiol. Lett. *50*, 29 (1988).
79 B. L. Masecar, R. A. Celesk and N. J. Robillard: Antimicrob. Agents Chemother. *34*, 281 (1990).
80 L. Dagostino, A. E. Goodman and K. C. Marshall: Biofouling (In Press) (1991).
81 T. Geers and N. R. Baker: J. Antimicrob. Chemother. *19*, 561 (1987).
82 G. Morris and M. R. W. Brown: Ps. Newslett. *13*, 18 (1988).
83 K. Grimwood, M. To, H. R. Rabin and D. E. Woods: Antimicrob. Agents Chemother. *33*, 41 (1989).
84 R. L. Warren, N. R. Baker, J. Johnson and M. J. Stapleton: Antimicrob. Agents Chemother. *27*, 468 (1985).
85 W. M. Dunne, Jr.: Antimicrob. Agents Chemother. *34*, 390 (1990).
86 B. Giwercman, E. T. Jensen, S. S. Pedersen, N. Hoiby and A. Kharazmi: Abstract A-153, Am. Soc. Microbiol. Ann. Meet. (1990), p. 26.
87 S. D. Elek and P. E. Cowen: Br. J. Exp. Pathol. *38*, 573 (1957).
88 S. H. Dougherty: Rev. Infect. Dis. *10*, 1102 (1988).
89 A. Buret, K. H. Ward, M. E. Olson and J. W. Costerton: J. Biomed. Mat. Res. (In Press) (1991).
90 J. W. Costerton: Can. J. Microbiol. *34*, (1988).
91 J. R. W. Govan and S. Glass: Rev. in Med Microbiol. *1*, 19 (1990).
92 N. J. Russell and P. Gacesa: Molec. Aspects Med. *10*, 1 (1988).
93 J. P. Kilbourn: Curr. Microbiol. *11*, 19 (1984).

Pharmacological properties of the natural polyamines and their depletion by biosynthesis inhibitors as a therapeutic approach

By Nikolaus Seiler

Marion Merrell Dow Research Institute, 16 rue d'Ankara,
67009 Strasbourg Cédex, France

1   Introduction

The structures of the natural aliphatic di-, tri- and tetramines, which are commonly designated "polyamines", are shown in Figure 1. From a chemical point of view this designation is incorrect, because the natural polyamines are in fact small molecules.

In the following the term "polyamine" will be used to designate putrescine (1,4-butanediamine), spermidine (N-[3-aminopropyl]-1,4-butanediamine) and spermine (N,N'-bis-[3-aminopropyl]-1,4-butanediamine). Cadaverine (1,5-pentanediamine) and 1,3-propanediamine also occur in nature as such and in the form of homologs of spermidine and spermine, or in conjugated form. They are, however, not considered further, because of their relative unimportance in the vertebrate organism.

It is not without irony that the polyamines have been neglected until recently by most biochemists, molecular biologists, and pharmacologists, in spite of a remarkable history, and in view of a number of long-known facts which suggest functions of basic importance for these biogenic amines.

(1) Polyamines occur in all cells. Prokaryotes normally contain putrescine and spermidine; eukaryotic cells in addition spermine. Archaebacteria, algae and also some higher plants may contain homologs and analogs of putrescine, spermidine and spermine. The ubiquity of the polyamines suggests their appearance at an early stage of evolution, and their persistence during the entire evolutionary development.

(2) Depletion of cellular spermidine prevents proliferation of eukaryotic cells and decreases the growth rate of prokaryotes.

(3) The polyamines are formed by rather demanding synthetic reactions. Their cellular concentrations are intricately regulated, and adapted to physiological needs, respectively.

Accounts on polyamine metabolism and biological functions can be found in recent reviews and books [1–10].

In normal (non-growing) rat tissues putrescine concentrations range from less than 10 nmol $\cdot$ g^{-1} (brain) to 44 nmol $\cdot$ g^{-1} (spleen). Spermidine and spermine concentrations range from 70 nmol $\cdot$ g^{-1} (skeletal muscle) to 1600 nmol $\cdot$ g^{-1} (spleen). Secretory organs (pancreas, prostate, hypophysis, lactating mammary gland etc.) have spermidine concentrations of 5000–9000 nmol $\cdot$ g^{-1}. There are species differences, but the order of magnitude of the polyamine concentrations is the same in all vertebrates. Rapidly proliferating cells and tissues (embryos, tumors, etc.) usually have higher putrescine and spermidine concentrations than the corresponding non-growing tissues.

At physiological pH the amino groups of the polyamines are protonated. From a structural point of view they are flexible molecules with positive charges distributed along the aliphatic carbon chain. (Inorganic polycations, such as Mg^{2+} and Ca^{2+} represent point-like charges). Their positive charges enable the polyamines to form ion-pairs with negatively charged molecules. Binding energy increases with the number of charges (putrescine < spermidine < spermine). Electrostatic interaction with DNA, RNA, proteins and negatively charged membrane constituents are the basis for most functions of the polyamines.

Electrostatically bound and free polyamines are in a dynamic equilibrium. The intracellular concentration of the free polyamines cannot be determined at present, but there is no doubt that they constitute only a small fraction of total spermidine and spermine. Most probably, the free, not the total polyamines, are essential in the regulation of biosynthesis, degradation, uptake and release.

In addition to electrostatic interactions, polyamines form covalent bonds with amino acids and proteins. Spider toxins, for example, contain amides of the natural polyamines or their derivatives [11–13]. These toxins turned out to be useful tools in the exploration of the elements of excitatory amino acid neurotransmission. Transglutaminase-catalyzed post-translational modifications of proteins may have a role in the regulation of growth and differentiation, but also in pathological processes, such as the formation of psoriatic plaques [14]. In the present review the focus is entirely on non-covalently-bound polyamines. Covalently bound polyamines represent only a small proportion of the total polyamines in vertebrate tissues.

Disregarding some earlier work, pharmacological interest in the polyamines was initiated after it had been recognized that spermine has marked renal toxicity [15]. It was this observation which also induced the biochemical exploration of the polyamines by H. and C. W. Tabor. During the last 15 years, pharmacological aspects have remained outside the main stream of polyamine research. This is presumably the reason why no recent overview exists of this topic. The early work was reviewed by H. and C. W. Tabor [16]. Shaw [17] and Sakurada et al. [18] gave accounts mainly of their own work. The rather original thesis of J. Buss [19] remained widely unnoticed. This is presumably the reason why part of his work was repeated later by others.

In earlier work toxicological and general pharmacological properties of the polyamines were explored. More recently, interest has focused on two functional aspects:

a) The role of polyamines in growth processes. Research in this direction led to the development of a number of inhibitors of polyamine biosynthetic enzymes, some of which have potentials in cancer chemotherapy and in the treatment of protozoan diseases [7].

b) The potential role of polyamines in Ca^{2+} transport [20] and its role in the allosteric regulation of the N-methyl-D-aspartate (NMDA) receptor [21].

2   A brief account of polyamine metabolism in the vertebrate organism

For the understanding of the involvement of polyamines in physiological processes, knowledge of their formation, degradation and regulation is essential. In the following, a brief account of the most conspicuous metabolic aspects of the polyamines is given. More complete reviews can be found in references [1–5] and [9].

Most cells of the vertebrate organism produce the polyamines they normally require; with one exception: anuclear red blood cells have no capacity to form polyamines. They accumulate polyamines by uptake and binding, and participate in the transport of the polyamines from one organ or tissue to another, and in polyamine excretion.

Ornithine (Fig. 1) is the exclusive precursor of putrescine in the vertebrate organism, from which it is formed by decarboxylation (Fig. 2).

In order to produce the aminopropyl residues that are required for the formation of spermidine and spermine, methionine first reacts with ATP to form S-adenosylmethionine (AdoMet). This is decarboxylated to decarboxy-S-adenosylmethionine (dAdoMet). This latter compound donates the aminopopyl residues which are transferred to putrescine, to form spermidine, or to spermidine, to form spermine. Spermidine synthase and spermine synthase are the two enzymes which catalyze the transfer of the aminopropyl residues. The second product of dAdoMet, 5'methylthioadenosine, is formed in equimolar amounts during the production of spermidine and spermine. It can be reused for the formation of ATP.

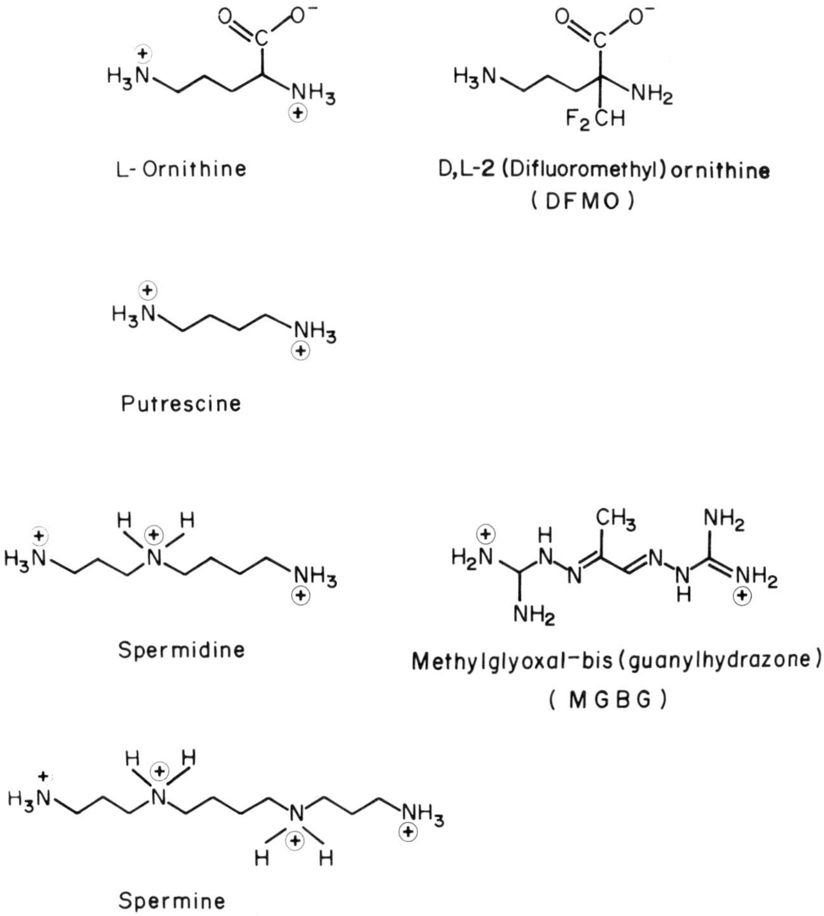

L- Ornithine

D,L-2 (Difluoromethyl) ornithine
(DFMO)

Putrescine

Spermidine

Methylglyoxal-bis (guanylhydrazone)
(MGBG)

Spermine

Figure 1
Structural formulae of ornithine, of the natural polyamines, of 2-(difluoromethyl)orni-
thine (DFMO) (an inactivator of ornithine decarboxylase) and of methyl-
glyoxal-bis(guanylhydrazone) (MGBG) (an inhibitor of S-adenosylmethionine decarboxylase).

As depicted in Fig. 2 a reaction sequence produces spermidine from
spermine, and putrescine from spermidine. In this case the monoacetyl derivatives of spermidine and spermine are first generated,
whereby acetyl-CoA is the acetyl group donor. In Fig. 3 the naturally
occurring acetyl derivatives of the polyamines are shown. They are
substrates of polyamine oxidase (PAO). This enzyme splits the
N^1-acetylpolyamines into an aldehyde (3-acetamidopropanal) which
represents the part of spermidine and spermine that originates from

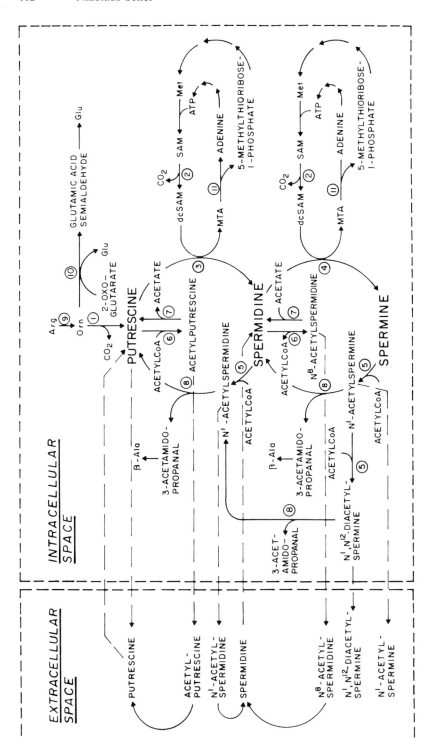

methionine. This aldehyde is oxidized to β-alanine. The spermidine and putrescine which are formed by this degradative process, can be reutilized for de novo polyamine synthesis. Thus polyamine metabolism is a cyclic process which allows the transformation of putrescine into spermidine and spermine, and vice versa, according to physiological requirements. This so-called interconversion cycle is essential for the regulation of cellular polyamine turnover.

Three enzymes, ornithine decarboxylase (ODC), S-adenosylmethionine decarboxylase (AdoMetDC), and acetyl CoA: spermidine/spermine N^1-acetyltransferase (cSAT), i.e. the cytosolic acetyltransferase which is involved in the formation of N^1-acetylspermidine and N^1-acetylspermine, are the key enzymes that regulate polyamine metabolism.

Rate-limiting enzymes are recognized by their low activity. The above-mentioned three enzymes have the lowest activities among the enzymes involved in polyamine metabolism. In order to be useful as regulatory proteins, there must be mechanisms by which the activity of the rate-limiting enzymes can be rapidly changed. This is usually achieved by induction. Physiological (hormones, growth factors) or non-physiological (tumor promotors, toxic agents) stimuli may lead to the expression of the appropriate gene which then produces mRNA. This in turn may enhance the formation of the enzyme protein. For example, treatment of female rats with testosterone stimulates ODC formation in the kidney 25-fold, with a proportional increase of ODC mRNA. Under these conditions, the ODC protein formation amounts up to 1 % of total protein synthesis [22].

<   Figure 2
Reactions involved in polyamine metabolism and polyamine exchange between intracellular and extracellular compartments. (Oxidative deaminations of the polyamines have not been included in this scheme.)
Enzymes:
(1) Ornithine decarboxylase (ODC)
(2) S-adenosylmethionine decarboxylase (AdoMetDC)
(3) Spermidine synthase
(4) Spermine synthase
(5) AcetylCoA: polyamine N^1-acetyltransferase (cytosolic; cSAT)
(6) AcetylCoA: spermidine N^8-acetyltransferase (nuclear; nSAT)
(7) N^8-Acetylspermidine deacetylase
(8) Polyamine oxidase (FAD-dependent)
(9) Arginase
(10) Ornithine aminotransferase
(11) 5'-Methylthioadenosine (MTA) phosphorylase.

A second requirement of regulatory proteins is a short half-life (rapid turnover). The three regulatory enzymes of polyamine metabolism have biological half-lives between 20–40 min, and thus belong to the group of proteins with the highest turnover rates.

Rapid induction of rate-limiting biosynthetic decarboxylases and a high rate of inactivation (by yet unknown mechanisms) permits spurts of polyamines to be produced.

A decrease of cellular polyamines leads to the induction of the biosynthetic decarboxylases which in turn are again repressed as polyamines re-accumulate. In order to rapidly deplete polyamines in cells with elevated concentrations, the induction of cSAT is required.

Polyamines regulate their own formation and degradation not only (at transcriptional level) by affecting the formation of mRNA. They also affect the rate at which the enzyme proteins are formed at the level of the translation of the genetic information. In addition, the polyamines have post-translational regulatory effects. For example, in vertebrates putrescine enhances the formation of AdoMetDC from a larger pro-enzyme [23], and it is at the same time an allosteric regulator of AdoMetDC [24].

Sustaining high putrescine concentrations may induce the formation of a protein called antizyme which binds to ODC and inactivates it [25].

In contrast to the regulatory decarboxylases and the acetyltransferase, spermidine and spermine synthase are usually present in cells and tissues at excessive activity. They are stable proteins with biological half-lives of several days. Their activity determines the maximum possible rate of polyamine formation. PAO is also a stable enzyme.

In addition to regulation by synthesis and degradation, uptake and release are important features of both cellular and global polyamine regulation. In many cells putrescine, spermidine and spermine share the same energy-dependent Na^+-activated transport system. The intracellular concentration of the free polyamines controls uptake, in analogy to the control of synthetic rates [26].

Uptake of polyamines from the bloodstream can substitute intracellular biosynthesis (Fig. 2). Circulating polyamines may originate from various organs, either released from tissue physiologically, or as a consequence of cell death. Polyamines can also enter circulation from the gastrointestinal tract. Gastrointestinal polyamines seem to be of special importance when the body has limited access to endogenous

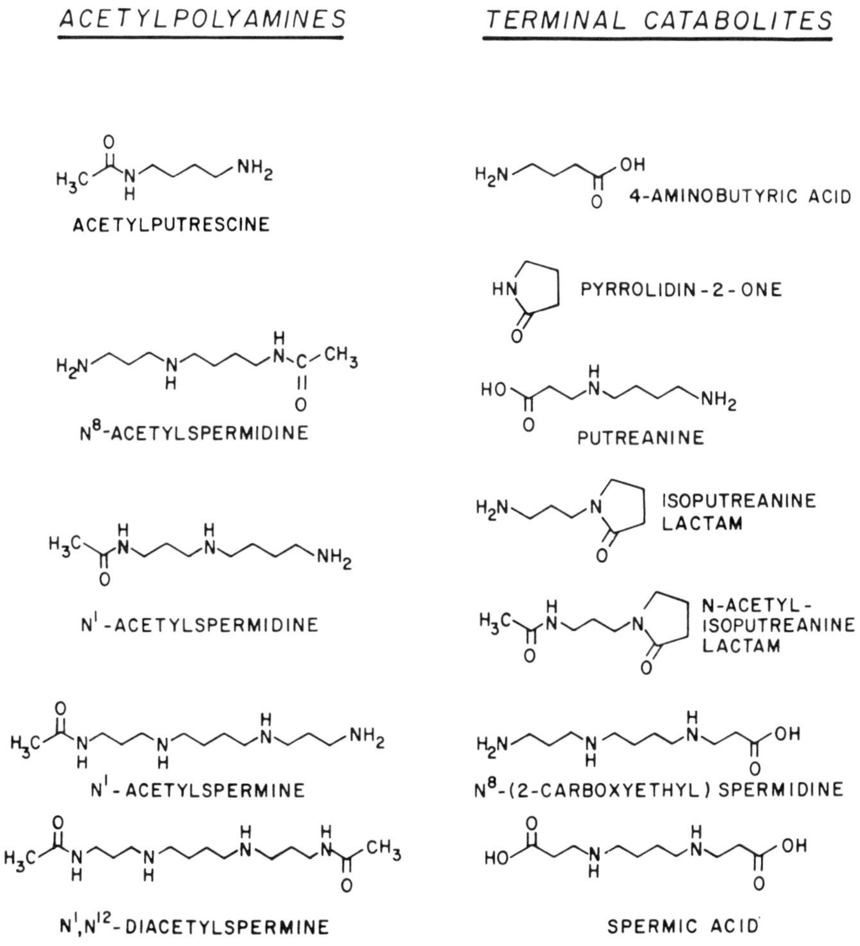

ACETYLPOLYAMINES

TERMINAL CATABOLITES

Figure 3
Structural formulae of intermediates of polyamine metabolism and terminal catabolic products of the natural polyamines.

polyamines, for example, due to inhibition of polyamine biosynthesis [27].

Acetylation removes a positive charge and decreases the electrostatic interaction of the polyamines with negatively charged binding sites. Thus, polyamine acetylation (see Fig. 2) is a means to displace polyamines from electrostatic binding sites. Release of the polyamines in the form of acetylated products is, therefore, not unexpected. Humans excrete the polyamines nearly exclusively as monoacetyl derivatives. In other species, putrescine and spermine are also excreted as such.

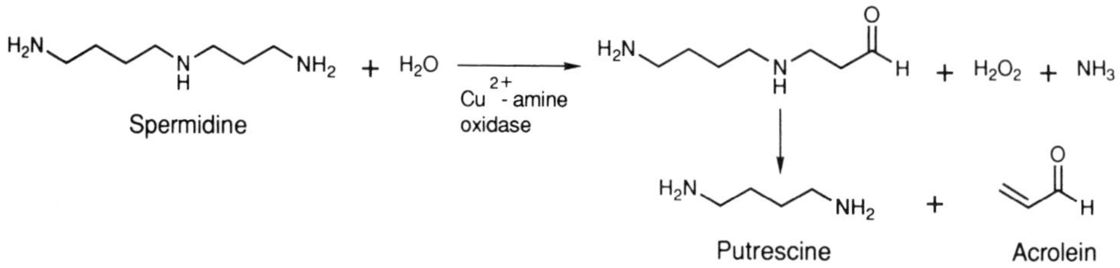

Figure 4
Oxidative deamination of spermidine by diamine oxidase or by serum amine oxidase.
(The formation of acrolein by β-elimination is a spontaneous reaction.)

Spermine is essentially an intracellular compound and is excreted only in traces.

From the constant urinary excretion of polyamines one may conclude that, normally, the vertebrate organism has more than enough polyamines. In addition to polyamines and their acetylderivatives, amino acids which are formed by oxidative deamination of the polyamines, and the intermediates of the interconversion cycle (Fig. 3) are normal excretory products [28]. Presumably all vertebrate Cu^{2+}-containing amine oxidases (diamine oxidase, serum amine oxidase and related enzymes) which are responsible for the oxidative deamination of the polyamines use 6-hydroxydopa, incorporated into the peptide chain at the active site of the enzyme, as cofactor. Evidence for the presence of this new prosthetic group in serum amine oxidase has recently been published [29]. Cu^{2+}-containing amine oxidases are unevenly distributed in the vertebrate organism. Diamine oxidase, for example, for which putrescine and probably also spermidine and spermine, are natural substrates, has a very high activity in small intestine and placenta [30]. Since the reaction products of the oxidative deaminations cannot be reconverted into polyamines, they were termed terminal catabolites [31].

From the uneven distribution of the Cu^{2+}-containing amine oxidases, it is evident that terminal catabolic reactions, in contrast to the interconversion cycle do not participate in the regulation of cellular polyamine levels in general. However, these reactions may have regulatory functions in specialized tissues, such as the intestinal mucosa [32], or during specific physiological events, such as pregnancy [33].

Oxidative deaminations of the polyamines are major catabolic events, if exogenous polyamines are administered to a vertebrate organism.

The reaction products of the oxidative deaminations are aldehydes, hydroperoxide and ammonia. These aldehydes are usually further metabolized. In the absence of a suitable aldehyde dehydrogenase, the chemically rather reactive aldehydes may react in various ways. For example from the aldehydes deriving from spermidine and spermine, the rather toxic acrolein may be formed by spontaneous β-elimination (Fig. 4) [34]. Within cells, suitable aldehyde dehydrogenases (or oxidases) usually exist, which rapidly transform the aldehydes into the corresponding amino acids, and thus avoid the accumulation of the toxic aldehydes.

Putrescine rapidly forms 4-aminobutyric acid (GABA), and its lactam, respectively [35]. GABA may be further metabolized by transamination. Injected spermine is transformed into a mono- and a dicarboxylic acid [36, 37], and spermidine into putreanine [36–38] and isoputreanine lactam [39] (Fig. 3). Pharmacologic properties of these amino acids (except that of GABA) are not known at present. It is therefore not possible to exclude the possibility that some of the effects which are ascribed to exogenous polyamines are due to their transformation into a metabolite.

The oxidative deamination of the polyamines can be prevented by pretreatment with aminoguanidine [34, 38]. Thus we have a means in our hand to avoid ambiguity in the interpretation of experiments with exogenous polyamines, ambiguity which derives from the transformation of the polyamines into aldehydes and amino acids.

3   General pharmacological properties of the polyamines in the intact animal

3.1   Acute toxicity

Administration of lethal doses of spermidine and spermine causes hypothermia, reduces spontaneous movement and tachycardia within one hour [18, 19]; after sufficiently high doses the animals usually die from respiratory arrest [40]. Buss [19] explains the acute respiratory arrest by a curare-like ganglion blocking action of the polyamines, with complete muscle relaxation. At lower, but still lethal doses lethargy and ataxia gaits may last as long as 7 days [18, 19].

LD50 values are summarized in Table 1. After intoxication with spermidine the heart revealed a deeply cyanotic myocardium, suggesting hypoxia and hypercarbia. The lungs showed no signs of edema,

Table 1
Acute toxicity of the polyamines

Species	Polyamine	Route of administration	LD_{50} mmol·kg^{-1}	Reference
Rat	Putrescine	i.v.	4.7	43
		s.c.	7.6	43
Mouse	Spermidine	i.p.	2.4 (2.0–3.0)	18
		i.v.	0.5*	41
	Spermine	i.p.	0.9 (0.6–1.4)	18

* Mean value of maximal and minimal diurnal values.
i.v. intravenous; s.c. subcutaneous, i.p. intraperitoneal.

and no pathology was evident in the rest of the organism [41]. Tabor and Rosenthal [42] suggested that a nephrotoxic effect, for which they determined an LD50 (i.p.) of 0.13 mmol · kg^{-1}, was a reason for the retarded lethal effect of spermine.

After lethal doses of putrescine internal hemorrhages and necrosis at the injection site were reported [43].

It appears that acute spermidine toxicity shows considerable diurnal variations: It is most toxic during the light phase (LD50 [i.v.] 0.36 ± 0.01 mmol · kg^{-1}) and least toxic (LD50 [i.v.] 0.56 ± 0.07 mmol · kg^{-1}) during the transition from light to dark, when motor activity and brain spermidine and histamine concentrations were found to be the highest [41].

Clearly, toxicity increases considerably from putrescine to spermidine to spermine. Behavior after intoxication is identical if appropriate amounts of spermidine or spermine are injected either systemically or i.c.v. [39, 44, 45]. This may indicate that polyamines are capable of crossing the blood brain barrier, but poorly. Direct measurements are in support of this idea [46]. One should, however, bear in mind that based on the presently available information it is not possible to rule out completely that polyamine metabolites are in fact responsible for the observed effects.

3.2   Central effects of the polyamines after sublethal doses

There is much agreement between the different investigators concerning the central actions of spermidine and spermine. The same effects were found, independent of the route of administration, when the doses were appropriately chosen [17–19, 44, 45]. Table 2 summarizes

Table 2
Some central pharmacologic effects of spermidine and spermine

Pharmacologic effect	ED_{50} (mmol $\cdot$ kg^{-1} i.p.)	
	Spermidine	Spermine
Depression of spontaneous motor activity	0.7 (0.4–1.3)	0.2 (0.08–0.3)
Motor incoordination	1.7 (1.3–2.1)	0.6 (0.3–1.2)
Potentiation of pentobarbital sleeping time	0.2 (0.1–0.4)	0.03 (0.02–0.04)
Blockade of conditioned avoidance	–	0.2 (0.1–0.3)
Depression of rectal temperature by 2 °C	0.9	0.2

Data from Sakurada et al. [18].

observations made after i.p. injections of spermidine and spermine [18]. In order to achieve comparable effects by intracerebroventricular (i.c.v.) injections on body temperature as are shown in Table 2, about 70 nmol of spermine and 200 nmol of spermidine have to be administered [44, 45]. Hypothermia and sedation last about 2–3 h after these doses [44]; 24 h after dosing increased spontaneous motor activity was observed; it lasted for many days [45]. Anderson et al. [44] also describe the development of extreme hyperexcitability of mice, and convulsions, which are sometimes lethal.

Spermine (1.1 μmol) injected i.c.v. in chicks produced similar effects as in mice. Hypothermia, decreased motor activity, behavioral sedation, and synchronization of the electrocortical activity were reported [47]. Since 30 min after spermine administration an increase in whole brain GABA concentration and glutamate decarboxylase (GAD) activity was observed, the authors suggest interactions of spermine with the brain GABA metabolic system.

In rats, putrescine produced marked hypothermia if given in a dose range from 1.2 to 2.5 mmol $\cdot$ kg^{-1} (i.p.), and it antagonized dose dependently pyrogen-induced fever [48]. A rather extensive study on behavioral and electrocortical changes in rats after local infusions into various brain regions of putrescine was published by De Sarro et al. [49]. When applied into the caudate nucleus, thalamus, substantia nigra and amygdala and other nuclei at a dose of 0.25 μmol, putrescine caused stereotyped behavior (licking, chewing, grooming, sniffing), followed after 5–20 min by epileptiform activity, first ipsilaterally, and then propagating to the contralateral limbic structures and cortex. Initially, the animals were almost sedated, but later showed wet dog shakes and masticatory movements. At higher doses

(0.5–1 μmol) putrescine produced initially tachypnoea, piloerection, hunched back and wet dog shakes, followed by rearing, tremor and myoclonic movements of limbs and head. Generalized tonic-clonic convulsions and wild running crisis were observed, especially after putrescine administration into the 3rd ventricle, hippocampus or amygdala. If putrescine was given at 0.5 μmol into the S. nigra pars compacta mild contralateral turning and circling were observed; injections into the pars reticulata caused ipsilateral turning and circling. Antiepileptic drugs (phenytoin, ethosuximide, diazepam etc.), but also GABA-related drugs (muscimol, sodium valproate, benzodiazepines) and N-methyl-D-aspartate (NMDA) receptor antagonists counteracted the epileptic phenomena elicited by intracerebral putrescine infusions. It appears that putrescine increases excitatory activity more or less in all parts of the brain. These can be antagonized by enhancing inhibitory mechanisms (or decreasing the excitatory activity by blockade of glutamate receptors).

The effects of spermidine and spermine were much the opposite of those produced by putrescine: Sedation and synchronization of electrocortical activity were the most conspicuous phenomena.

In chicks putrescine also produced behavioral effects which are opposite to those observed after i.c.v. administration of spermine: increased locomotor activity with episodes of circling and escape responses, continuous vocalization, head-neck jerks, tachypnea, ataxia. Electrocortical activity was characterized by high-voltage continuous spike activity. As a consequence of decreased GAD activity, putrescine caused a significant depletion of GABA in the diencephalon [50] which may be a basis for the explanation of the observed behavioral effects in chicks and rats.

Putrescine (in rats) (dose range 1.2–2.5 mmol · kg^{-1} [i.p.]) [51] spermidine (0.3–0.7 mmol · kg^{-1} [i.p.]) and spermine (in mice) (dose range 0.03–0.07 mmol · kg^{-1} [i.p.]) [18] seem to have significant analgesic effects. An i.p. dose of 1.2 mmol · kg^{-1} putrescine produced a 50 % increase of the basal threshold between 90 and 150 min after dosing, using the hot plate (55 °C) test. A statistically significant increase in the pain threshold was also observed after i.c.v. administration of 1 μmol putrescine to rats [51].

From the fact that pretreatment with naloxone (3 mg · kg^{-1} [i.p.]) did not antagonize the analgesic effect of putrescine one may conclude that putrescine is neither interacting directly with opiate receptors, nor via mobilization of endogenous opiates.

After doses of putrescine which were shown to be analgesic, rats developed wet-dog shaking behavior [52] which typically occurs as a result of morphine withdrawal [53]. Histologic examination of the brains of putrescine-treated rats showed edema and extravasation of proteins. Pretreatment with morphine (20 mg · kg^{-1} [s.c.]) prevented both wet-dog shaking behavior and the increase of brain vascular permeability. Naloxone (5 mg · kg^{-1} [s.c.] 5 min before putrescine) did not reduce wet-dog shakes, but prevented the antagonizing effect of morphine on blood vessel permeability.

Another striking effect of spermidine (0.2 μmol [i.c.v.]) is an immediate severe fall in food and water consumption, which is accompanied by a decrease in body weight [44]. Five days after treatment the mice still showed no sign of recovery so that by the 5th day the animals were paralyzed and emaciated and had a body temperature of 16 °C. These results were in essence confirmed by Sakurada et al. [45]. Interestingly, an i.c.v. dose of 0.1 μmol spermine had less dramatic effects; by day 5 the body weight had normalized [45].

What causes the long-lasting central effects? Nearly all authors involved in the evaluation of central effects of the polyamines report whole brain polyamine concentrations, and find increased spermidine and spermine concentrations after putrescine [44, 51] or spermidine and spermine [18] administration 1–24 h, after dosing. The preferential accumulation and persistence of radioactive spermidine and spermine in virtually all cellular layers of the mouse brain, after administration of trace amounts of labeled putrescine, has been documented [54]; however, a study is missing on the distribution and metabolism of the relatively large quantities of exogenous polyamines which were administered in the pharmacological experiments described in the preceding paragraphs. In view of the metabolic capacities of the brain and the intricate regulation of the polyamines, it does not seem likely that their long-lasting central effects are paralleled by elevated concentrations. A more likely explanation is the presence of lesions produced by the exogenous polyamines.

The formation of brain edema [52] after putrescine administration has already been mentioned. Anderson et al. [44] have reported characteristic patterns of lesions in mice receiving 0.2 μmol spermidine and in rabbits receiving 1.4 μmol spermine, injected into the lateral ventricles. The paralyzed animals regularly exhibited bilateral lesions in the ventral medulla. The affected area included the descending motor tracts. Frequently, lesions were scattered along the cervical cord, situated mainly superficially under the pia mater. The lesions were necrotizing lesions, often with lymphocytic infiltration.

3.3   Central effects on blood glucose

It has been known for many years that spermine produces hyperglycemia in rabbits [55] and man [56]. More recently [57], it was demonstrated that i.c.v. injections of spermidine and spermine in doses of 2 μmol and 1.4 μmol produce an increase of the blood glucose level by 100 %. Normal values were recovered after about 3 h. From the fact that i.v. doses necessary to produce comparable effects with spermidine were 350 μmol $\cdot$ kg^{-1} it was concluded that polyamines exert their hyperglycemic effect centrally. Pretreatment of rabbits for 7 days with 1 mg $\cdot$ kg^{-1} reserpine, or adrenal demedullation of rats, prevented the spermine-induced increase of blood glucose, demonstrating that the release of epinephrine mediates the polyamine effect.
The potential role of polyamines in the regulation of insulin secretion by inhibition of protein kinase C activation in pancreatic islets [58] and a role of transglutaminase in this process, with polyamines acting as substrates [59] are matters of current discussion. However, mM concentrations of the polyamines are needed to inhibit protein kinase C activity and glucose-induced insulin release [58]. A physiological function of the polyamines in the regulation of blood glucose levels is, therefore, at present not evident in spite of high spermidine concentrations in the pancreatic islets.

4   Cardiovascular effects

The first report on hypotensive effects of the polyamines is probably that of Buss [19]. Intravenous administration of 60 μmol $\cdot$ kg^{-1} of putrescine [60], 4 μmol $\cdot$ kg^{-1} of spermidine or 14 μmol $\cdot$ kg^{-1} of spermine [61] produced a significant decrease of the systolic arterial blood pressure in pentobarbital anesthetized dogs between 1 and 10 min after injection. At the same time sinus bradycardia was observed after administration of spermidine and spermine, but tachycardia after putrescine. In animals pretreated with histamine depletors or an antagonist of the histamine H1 receptor, the hypotensive action of the polyamines was not observed. Thus, it was concluded that i.v. injected polyamines exert their cardiovascular effects via histamine release. The release of histamine by polyamines had previously been shown by direct histamine assay in venous blood [17]. The tachycardic effect of putrescine was explained to be due to both histamine release and a reflex stimulation of the carotid sinus baroreceptors [60]. Chideckel et al. [62] also reported a reversible hypotensive effect of spermine and spermidine in anesthetized dogs. However, in the hands of these investigators pretreatment with the histamine H1 and H2 blockers diphenhydramine and cimetidine did not abolish the hypotensive effect of the polyamines. Polyamines relax the isolated aorta of the guinea pig [62] as well as other smooth muscles (see below). The decrease in peripheral vascular resistance was, therefore, considered the reason for polyamine-induced hypotension.

Microinjection of putrescine into the 3rd cerebral ventricle of dogs (1.2 μmol) or into the vertebral artery produced hypotensive responses, but also reduced heart rate without producing significant changes in respiratory rate [60].

Spermidine, if given i.c.v. or into the vertebral artery at a dose of 0.6 μmol or 1.2 μmol, also produced a hypotensive response. At 6 μmol the arterial pressure initially increased, followed by a progressive hypotension. The changes in arterial pressure were accompanied by a transitory reduction of the amplitude of respiration, followed by an increase of both amplitude and rate. Spermine given i.c.v. in doses up to 3 μmol did not change the arterial blood pressure [61]. Cardiovascular effects are an example of a pharmacologic property of the polyamines where spermidine showed a greater effect than spermine.

In dogs pretreated with atropine or in bivagotomized animals the hypotensive and bradycardic effects of the polyamines were reduced. These observations argue in favor of an increase in the parasympathetic output due to polyamine infusion [61].

Both in the isolated rat heart [19] and perfused rat ventricle strips [63] driven at 1 Hz, putrescine, spermidine and spermine produced at 100 μM concentration a rather significant negative inotropic effect. (Spermidine and spermine initially showed a short-lasting increase in contractility).

Koenig and collaborators [20] accumulated evidence in favor of a role of polyamines in Ca^{2+}-influx (see below). In order to test the hypothesis that an intact polyamine metabolism is important for the normal contractility of the heart, rats were treated daily for seven consecutive days with 50 mg · kg^{-1} (i.p.) methylglyoxal-bis(guanylhydrazone) (MGBG), a competitive though not specific inhibitor of AdoMetDC [64], and twice daily with 100 mg · kg^{-1} (i.p.) 2-(difluoromethyl)orni-thine (DFMO, Eflornithine), a selective inactivator of ODC [65]. (The structures of these drugs are shown in Fig. 1). At the end of the treatment period ventricular ODC activity was reduced by more than 60 %, putrescine concentration by 60 % and spermidine content by 40 % [66]. The basal isometric tension developed by ventricle strips was not affected by the treatment, however, the inotropic effects of ouabain (1 μM), noradrenaline (10 μM) and Ca^{2+} (3.6 mM) were significantly reduced. Since an increase of intracellular Ca^{2+} is a common event of many inotropic agents [67] it is tempting to speculate that the observed effects of the polyamine biosynthesis inhibitors were due to the impairment of intracellular Ca^{2+} accumulation. However, owing to the rather numerous side effects of MGBG, among which mitochondrial damage (and with it impairment of bioenergetic functions) [64] may be most important, the results of Bazzani et al. [66] cannot be interpreted unambiguously. In view of the importance of the problem, repetition of this work using more selective methods of polyamine deprivation [27] would be of considerable interest.

5   Actions on isolated muscle preparations

Spermidine and spermine cause relaxation of spontaneous smooth muscle contractions and they antagonize the actions of various spasmogens: rat prostate gland and seminal vesicle preparations [68], guinea pig and rabbit ileum [17, 19, 69–71], rat uterus, rabbit duodenum [17, 71, 72], rat stomach [73], guinea pig respiratory tract smooth muscle [74], guinea pig trachealis [75], frog esophagus [19] and guinea pig aorta [62] are examples. Using guinea pig ileum, relatively high concentrations of spermine (0.2 mM) and spermidine (0.5 M) were needed to antagonize the spasmogenic effects of acetylcholine, histamine and barium chloride. The contractions produced by nicotine were inhibited by 0.014 mM spermine and 0.05 mM spermidine [17] and serotonin-induced guinea pig ileum contractions were also effectively antagonized by the polyamines. Therefore, polyamines were considered as nicotine and serotonin antagonists [69]. On the basis of these and related observations, some investigators believe that circulating polyamines may play a role in the control of the spontaneous motor activity of the gastrointestinal tract [71, 76].

In general, skeletal muscles react less sensitively than smooth muscles, but they are also relaxed after exposure to spermidine and spermine, as has been shown using electrically stimulated frog rectus abdomini and sartorius [19, 70]. Moreover De Meis [70] demonstrated that polyamines relax glycerol-treated myofibrils. This action has been attributed to the inhibition of actomyosin adenosine triphosphatase [77].

Blockade of the neuromuscular junction of skeletal muscles of the cat was achieved at i.v. doses of the polyamines > 0.3 mmol $\cdot$ kg^{-1} [19]. The ganglion-blocking action of the polyamines was demonstrated using the superior cervical ganglion of the cat, which was isolated from the circulation. In order to antagonize the effect of 0.7 μmol acetylcholine, about 17 μmol of spermine and 24 μmol of spermidine were necessary [19]. These observations indicate again a rather weak anticholinergic effect of the polyamines at muscarinic receptors.

6 Inhibition of gastric acid secretion and ulceration

Using bullfrog gastric mucosa, 0.5 mM spermine inhibited the rate of histamine-induced H^+ secretion by 70 %, spermidine by 45 % and putrescine only by 5 %, if added to the secretory side of the membrane [78]. Enhancement of the K^+-concentration antagonized the effects of the polyamines on acid secretion. Unlike H_2-receptor antagonists the polyamines were completely ineffective, when added to the nutrient side. It was assumed that inhibition of gastric acid secretion by the polyamines is due to uncoupling of the gastric H^+/K^+-exchange pump in the secretory membrane in such a way that the vectorial transport of H^+ ceases, although K^+-transport and recycling remain unaltered.

Aihara et al. [79] studied the effects of polyamines on gastric acid secretion and ulceration, based on the observation that the synthesis of the prostaglandins PGE_2 and 6-keto-$PGF_{1\alpha}$ was inhibited by spermine due to its interaction with phospholipids [80]. Assuming that polyamines may substitute some of the functions of PGE_2 or PGI_2, and since PGE_2 has an anti-ulcerogenic action [81], stress-induced gastric ulceration, ulceration and gastric acid secretion after pylorus ligation as well as histamine-induced acid secretion and ulceration were used as models. Spermine if given orally or if administered in s.c. doses of 50 mg $\cdot$ kg^{-1} produced significant protective effects against ulceration and gastric acid secretion was reduced by about 80 %. Spermidine was somewhat less effective. Spermine also inhibited the formation of acetic acid-induced ulcers. The anti-ulcerogenic effect of spermine was assumed to be due to inhibition of gastric acid secretion and due to the stimulation of the formation of glycosaminoglycans and glycoproteins, which are known to have antisecretory and cytoprotective properties.

Still another hypothesis concerning the mechanism by which polyamines prevent gastric ulceration was put forward by Mizui et al. [82]. After the appearance of lesions produced by 150 mM HCl in ethanol, lipid peroxides accumulated in the gastric mucosa. Pretreatment with polyamines not only antagonized the formation of ulcers [82] but also lipid peroxidation. These and related observations [83] suggest that the cytoprotective action of the polyamines may be based on their radical scavenging properties.

7   Anti-inflammatory effects

The polyamines have a number of effects which interrelate them with glucocorticoid actions. For example milk protein synthesis by cultured mammary epithelium is enhanced by hydrocortisone, which can be replaced by spermidine [84]. Bartholeyns et al. [85] showed that inhibition of carrageenan paw edema by dexamethasone requires active de novo synthesis of putrescine. Since serotonin-induced paw edema of mice was inhibited by glucocorticoids, but not by indomethacin, polyamines were considered as potential anti-inflammatory compounds in this model [86], especially since Bird et al. [87] had identified putrescine as the active anti-inflammatory component of sponge exudates.

If given s.c. 3 h before 2.3 μg serotonin, 33 μmol $\cdot$ kg^{-1} spermidine, 80 μmol $\cdot$ kg^{-1} spermine and 340 μmol $\cdot$ kg^{-1} putrescine reduced paw edema formation by 30 percent. Local injection of the polyamines into the paws was ineffective. Carrageenan-induced edema was also antagonized by comparable doses. In order to achieve the same effects after oral administration about four times higher doses had to be administered. Since a certain lag period is required before the polyamines exert an anti-inflammatory effect, it was suggested that they may be mediators of glucocorticoids for the synthesis of the vascular permeability inhibitory protein, or of phospholipase A$_2$ inhibitory proteins [86].

8   Polyamines and ion movements

The effects of polyamines on membrane functions have recently been reviewed [88]. Influence on ion movements is one of the major aspects of the presumed functional roles of the polyamines at membrane sites in all parts of the vertebrate organism, even though at present conclusive results are rather the exception than the rule.

8.1   Ion and water transport in rat jejunum

Intestinal ion and water movements are affected by sympathomimetic and cholinomimetic agents. Their effect can easily be measured by determination of the transmural potential difference [89]. (The lumen of small intestines is electronegative compared with the serosa. Changes in the potential difference are due to active ion transport [90]. Injections of acetylcholine or serotonin into the jugular vein in amounts of 0.1–1 μg cause a dose-dependent increase of the transmural potential difference of the jejunum, which is due to the stimulation of Cl⁻-secretion from the serosa into the lumen. Spermine (70 μmol · kg⁻¹) or spermidine (140 μmol · kg⁻¹) competitively antagonized the effects of both serotonin and acetylcholine and they antagonized also the inhibitory effect of bethanechol (a cholinomimetic) on the water transport in the jejunum of rats [91]. From the fact that increasing external Ca^{2+} concentrations antagonized the effect of spermine on the contraction of rat uterus and since spermine competitively inhibited Ca^{2+}-induced contractions of the uterus [72], it was concluded that the antagonism of spermine against serotonin and acetylcholine in the jejunum is due to prevention of Ca^{2+} entry into the epithelial cells [91].

8.2   Polyamine effects on neuronal ion movements

Ionophoretic application of spermidine to brain stem [92] or cortical neurons [93] decreased the spontaneous firing rate in about 30 % of the neuronal population. Excitatory effects were only seen in 10 % of the neurons while 60 % showed no effect. For reasons which are unclear, spermine seemed to be ineffective in all cortical neurons, but effective in brain stem neurons.

Ionophoretic injections of spermine into neurons reduced amplitudes of action potentials and removed the hump in their falling phase, indicating that intracellular spermine affected several membrane currents underlying action potentials [94]. More detailed studies of pacemaker neurons from the abdominal ganglion of *Aplysia californica* demonstrated a dose-dependent blockade of the Ca^{2+} inward current and of the delayed K^+ outward current [95, 96]. Reduction of the outward K^+ flux by the natural polyamines was also observed [19] in single fiber preparations of the N. tibialis of the frog, using an experimental design [97] which allowed the determination of ion movements across Ranvier nodes.

Millimolar concentrations of spermine inhibit the purified plasma membrane-bound Ca^{2+}-transport ATPase by interacting with associated polyphosphoinositides [98]. Polyphosphoinositides are primary polyamine binding sites in membranes [99]. It is, therefore, not unlikely that polyamines prevent Ca^{2+}-transport by inhibition of the Ca^{2+}-membrane pump, especially if intracellular polyamine concentrations are increased.

Another potential site of polyamine action on ion fluxes is a subtype of a glutamate receptor macrocomplex.

8.3   Is the N-methyl-D-aspartate receptor complex allosterically regulated by spermidine and spermine?

In the central nervous system inhibitory GABAergic and excitatory glutamatergic systems are in delicate balance. Subtypes of glutamate receptors have been characterized by the selective agonists quisqualic acid, kainic acid, N-methyl-D-aspartic acid (NMDA) and 2-amino-4-phosphonobutyrate [100]. The NMDA receptor has been investigated the most, and it became clear that like the $GABA_A$/benzodiazepine/Cl^--channel macrocomplex, the NMDA receptor is also a complex of macromolecules. It is associated with a cation-selective ion channel that gates Na^+ and Ca^{2+} [101]. In addition to the NMDA (i.e. glutamate) binding site separate recognition sites for the following molecules have been identified: glycine ("strychnine insensitive GlyB receptor"), phencyclidine (and other drugs), Mg^{2+} [102, 103], spermidine and spermine [21].

Phencyclidine, ketamine, MK 801 ([+]-5-methyl-10,11-dihydro-5H-dibenzo-[a, d],-cyclohepten-5,10-imine), TCP (N-[1-[thienyl]cyclohexyl] piperidine) and some other drugs which are NMDA receptor antagonists appear to inhibit NMDA responses by binding preferentially to an agonist-activated state of the receptor-ion channel complex [104]. Glycine is a positive modulator of NMDA-activated channels. In cultured neurons it increases the frequency of channel openings in response to NMDA [105]. Both extracellular [106, 107] and intracellular [108] Mg^{2+} block the NMDA-activated ion channel in a voltage-dependent manner.

Allosteric regulation of enzymes by interaction of the polyamines with anionic binding sites of the protein is a known fact. The first well-explored example is the modulation of membrane-bound and solubilized acetylcholine esterase by μM concentrations of spermine and spermidine [109]. The modulation of NMDA-receptors is presumably another example for conformational changes of proteins induced by interaction of the polyamines with anionic binding sites. It is assumed that in the case of the NMDA receptor the polyamines interact with receptor proteins, although interaction with membrane phospholipids cannot be excluded at present as a mechanism underlying the effects of the polyamines on NMDA receptor activity.

If well-washed preparations of rat cortical membranes are exposed to μM concentrations of spermidine or spermine, binding of [^{3}H]MK 801 [21, 110] and [^{3}H]TCP [111] is enhanced. At the same time spermine (but not spermidine or putrescine) increases the affinity of glycine for the strychnine-insensitive binding site [112]. The enhancement of the affinity of TCP to its binding site due to allosteric modulation of the NMDA receptor by polyamines has not only been shown by determination of the dissociation equilibrium, but also by kinetic data: 100 μM spermidine increased the association rate of TCP with the NMDA receptor and decreased the dissociation rate significantly [111]. These findings suggest that polyamines may enhance the activitation of the NMDA receptor or decrease its desensitization.

In addition to the natural polyamines some homologs enhance the affinity of MK 801 and TCP for their binding sites. With an $EC_{50} = 0.78$ μM N,N'-bis(3-aminopropyl)-1,3-propanediamine [111] is the most potent modulator of the NMDA receptor at the polyamine binding site. It is nearly 8 times more potent than spermine ($EC_{50} = 5.9$ μM). Among a homologous series of α, ω-diamines only 1,3-propanediamine affected MK 801 [110] and TCP [111] binding significantly. N-(3-aminopropyl)-1,3-propanediamine and spermidine (N-[3-aminopropyl]-1,4-butanediamine) were about equipotent [110]. These observations suggest that positive charges separated by a C_3-carbon chain are optimal for binding to the NMDA receptor.

Spermidine [111] like glutamate and glycine [113] converted the stimulatory effects of low Mg^{2+} concentrations into inhibitory effects. One
interpretation of these observations is that the stimulatory effects of
Mg^{2+} and spermidine are mediated by the same site and that spermidine at 10 μM masks the stimulatory effect of Mg^{2+} and reveals its inhibitory action. Because putrescine and Mg^{2+} non-competitively
inhibited spermidine-induced binding of TCP [111] it may be assumed
that putrescine and Mg^{2+} share the same inhibitory site. In apparent
agreement with this assumption is the fact that arcaine (1,4-diguanid-
inobutane) inhibited [³H]MK 801 binding with an $IC_{50} = 1.5\ \mu M$ in
the presence of 100 μM glutamate and 30 μM glycine. Agmatine
(1-amino-4-guanidinobutane) was about 10 times less potent than arcaine [114]. (Whether arcaine indeed binds to the Mg^{2+}-site or to the
polyamine site of the NMDA receptor remains to be established).
There are neuropathological conditions which are assumed to be related to overstimulation of NMDA receptors: focal ischemia and
stroke [115], epilepsy [116] and possibly some neurodegenerative disorders [117]. The massive influx of Ca^{2+} into neurons after excessive
release of glutamate (or of other endogenous excitatory amino acids)
is considered of considerable pathogenetic importance [118–120].
Some drugs with cytoprotective activity (Ifenprodil and S.L. 82.0715
(α-[4-chlorophenyl]-4-[[4-fluorophenyl]methyl]-1-piperidine ethanol),
which are non-competitive antagonists of the NMDA receptor [121]
did not bind to the glutamate or glycine recognition site, nor were they
ion channel blockers, such as phencyclidine, TCP or MK 801. Recently, it could be demonstrated that [³H]ifenprodil binds with high affinity (K_D 37 nM) to the polyamine binding site of the NMDA receptor. Likewise SL 82.0715 is a ligand of the same binding site [122–124].
Thus, it is evident now that the polyamine binding site is a suitable target for cytoprotective drugs.
Phencyclidine is bound by both sigma receptors and the NMDA-receptor coupled cation channels [125]. Since polyamines are modulating ligand binding at the NMDA receptor-coupled ion channels,
it was of considerable interest to know whether sigma receptors are
also modulated by polyamines. (+)-3-(3-Hydroxyphenyl)-N-(1-pro-
pyl)-piperidine (R[+]3-PPP) is a selective ligand of sigma receptors,
with only a low affinity for NMDA-coupled phencylidine binding
sites [125, 126]. Spermine ($IC_{50} = 9\ \mu M$) and spermidine
($IC_{50} = 70\ \mu M$) inhibited R(+)3-PPP binding in membrane prepara-

tions from rat forebrain and with lower affinity in preparations from guinea-pig brain and adrenal medulla. Putrescine was a rather weak antagonist (IC_{50} = 411 μM) [127]. These data indicate that sigma receptors may also be allosterically modulated by the polyamines.

In view of the impressive in vitro data on the interaction of the polyamines with the NMDA-ion channel macrocomplex, it is of considerable interest to know whether the polyamines have a physiological role in the regulation of NMDA receptor activity. The concentrations of the polyamines in the extracellular space of the brain are presently not known. In human cerebrospinal fluid the following concentrations have been reported [128].

Putrescine   184 ± 54 nM
Spermidine   150 ± 48 nM
Spermine   below detection limit

Plasma polyamine concentrations are of the same order of magnitude [129]. Spermine is considered to be an intracellular compound, released only from dying cells [130]. Thus it is unlikely that extracellular polyamines interact with NMDA receptors. However, the possibility remains that the polyamine binding site of the NMDA receptor resides on the cytoplasmic domain of the macrocomplex.

At present evidence for a role of the polyamines in the physiologic regulation of NMDA receptor activity is scarce. It has previously been demonstrated that levels of cGMP in the cerebellum are enhanced by excitatory amino acids [131] and the glycine agonist D-serine [132], and that they are negatively modulated by NMDA antagonists [132, 133]. Now it was demonstrated that intracerebellar injections of 0.8 μmol spermidine or 0.6 μmol spermine reversed the effects of D-serine, quisqualic acid and harmaline on cerebellar cGMP levels. No changes of basal cGMP concentrations were observed after administration of the polyamines alone [134]. These results may be interpreted in various ways. In addition to direct interaction with the NMDA receptor, effects of the polyamines on intracellular Ca^{2+} concentrations may be considered.

The blockade of polyamine biosynthesis in primary cultures of cortical neurons of mice, using 5 mM DFMO, prevented completely NMDA-induced cellular loss, whereas exposure of the cells to 100 μM NMDA for 5 days in the absence of DFMO resulted in almost complete loss of the neurons. Phencyclidine (100 μM) had the same protective effect as DFMO [135]. Again, the interpretation of these rather impressive results is not unequivocal: either the decrease of in-tracellular polyamines due to DFMO [136] and the consequent NMDA-receptor inactivation, or the role of the polyamines in NMDA-mediated Ca^{2+} fluxes [137] (see also below) may be consid-ered as potential explanations for the observed cytoprotective effect of DFMO.

More insights into potential regulatory functions of the polyamines at NMDA receptor sites can be expected in the near future, due to a con-siderable current interest in this research area. It is not unlikely that the new targets which were revealed in the course of the exploration of NMDA-polyamine interactions will result in a new generation of drugs.

8.4   Polyamines and Ca^{2+}-fluxes

The role of Ca^{2+} as a universal cellular messenger is now generally ac-cepted [138]. Disregarding the mentioned potential regulation of NMDA receptors, polyamines have been implicated mainly in two Ca^{2+} related processes:
a) Regulation of cellular Ca^{2+}-homeostasis
b) Regulation of Ca^{2+}-fluxes in signal transduction.

8.4.1   Polyamines and Ca^{2+} homeostasis

Cells limit the exchange of Ca^{2+} with the extracellular space and con-trol it with great care. Oscillations of free Ca^{2+} are transient. The en-doplasmic reticulum is assumed to fine-tune cytosolic free Ca^{2+} down to resting levels [139]. In this regard it is of interest that μM concentra-tions of spermidine and spermine were found to prevent the inositol triphosphate independent Ca^{2+} efflux from fractions of the endoplas-mic reticulum by Ca^{2+}-releasing antibiotics (neomycin, streptomycin) [140]. It appears from this work that polyamines, in contrast to cal-modulin, might be able to modulate endoplasmic reticulum channel activity even when cytoplasmic free Ca^{2+} is low.

Mitochondria seem to play a minor role in the control cytosolic Ca^{2+} under physiological conditions. However, mitochondria have an im-pressive capacity for Ca^{2+} accumulation and storage by deposits of hydroxyapatite. Thus, when noxious agents interfere with the Ca^{2+} permeability barrier of the plasma membrane, and permit cytosolic

Ca^{2+} to rise, mitochondria will store away the excess Ca^{2+} [138, 139]. It is, therefore, of considerable importance that the polyamines activate mitochondrial Ca^{2+}-uptake [141–144]. Thorough studies demonstrated that the activation of mitochondrial Ca^{2+}-uptake by the polyamines involves the allosteric modulation of the Ca^{2+}-transporting protein, resulting in an increased affinity of Ca^{2+} for the uniporter [145–149]. Polyamines may also affect Ca^{2+} efflux from mitochondria by decreasing the apparent Km for efflux [142].

8.4.2 Ca^{2+}-signaling and the polyamines

According to a rather generally accepted theory [150–155] external signals (hormones, neurotransmitters, drugs, etc.) which are detected by cell surface receptors are transmitted to a limited number of intracellular second messengers. Among these inositol-1,4,5-triphosphate and diacylglycerol are most eminent. An inositol-containing lipid within the plasma membrane is the precursor used by the receptor mechanism to release inositol-1,4,5-triphosphate to the cytosol, leaving diacylglycerol within the membrane. The primary function of inositol-1,4,5-triphosphate is to mobilize Ca^{2+} from intracellular stores. The other limb of the signalling pathway is controlled by diacylglycerol. The activation of protein kinase C is a key step in this pathway. For small cells (with a large surface/volume ratio) the entry of Ca^{2+} across the plasma membrane (usually through voltage-dependent Ca^{2+} channels) is sufficient for cell activation. The initial response to stimulation by Ca^{2+}-mobilizing agonists is a release of intracellular Ca^{2+} from stores (Phase I) which is soon followed by entry of Ca^{2+} across the plasma membrane (via receptor operated channels) (Phase II). Much of the Ca^{2+} released from internal stores is pumped out of the cell and the intracellular Ca^{2+} content declines by as much as 50 % [151]. In order to answer the question, how Ca^{2+}-entry during Phase II is controlled, and how intracellular Ca^{2+} is mobilized, a number of hypotheses have been proposed. A role of the polyamines in these processes was not considered [151, 154], in spite of a considerable number of observations suggesting a potential function of the polyamines in the control of Ca^{2+}-transport, inositol polyphosphate metabolism and protein kinase activation.
In Table 3 observations which suggest polyamine dependence of Ca^{2+}-fluxes are summarized. In nearly all the work quoted in this

Table 3
Observations suggesting a role of the polyamines in voltage-dependent and receptor-mediated signal transduction and Ca^{2+} mobilization

Stimulus	Organ or tissue preparation	Biological effect	Reference
Testosterone	Mouse kidney cortex slices	Enhancement of endocytosis, enhancement of transport of α-aminoisobutyric acid and deoxyglucose	[156]
		Enhancement of influx and efflux of $^{45}Ca^{2+}$ and release of mitochondrial $^{45}Ca^{2+}$ into the cytosol	[157]
	Rat heart	Acute positive inotropic and chronotropic effect	[158]
Isoproterenol and other β-adrenergic agonists	Rat heart	Acute positive inotropic and chronotropic effect	[159] [160]
	Cardiac myocytes	Enhancement of endocytosis and of hexose and amino acid transport, decrease of free cytosolic Ca^{2+}	[161] [162]
	Mouse kidney cortex slices	Enhancement of endocytosis and of hexose and amino acid transport; mobilization of mitochondrial Ca^{2+}	[163]
Insulin	Mouse kidney cortex slices	Enhancement of endocytosis and of hexose and amino acid transport, enhancement of Ca^{2+}-fluxes	[164]
		Stimulation of pyruvate dehydrogenase activity	[165]
	Mouse liver, bovine aorta myocytes	Stimulation of pyruvate dehydrogenase activity	[20]
	Rat heart	Enhancement of acute contractility	[166]
Thyroid hormone (triiodothyronine)	Mouse and rat kidney cortex slices	Enhancement of Ca^{2+}-fluxes, enhancement of endocytosis, and of amino acid and hexose transport	[167]
	Heart of hypothyroid mice	Enhancement of Ca^{2+}-fluxes, enhancement of endocytosis, and of amino acid and hexose transport	[168]
	Heart of hypothyroid rats	Acute positive inotropic and chronotropic effect	[166]
	Neocortical slices of hypothyroid mice	Enhancement of Ca^{2+}-fluxes, enhancement of endocytosis, and of amino acid and hexose transport in nerve endings	[169]
Depolarization by K^+	Synaptosomes from rat cerebral cortex	Enhancement of $^{45}Ca^{2+}$-influx and efflux	[170]
		Enhanced release of GABA and norepinephrine	[170]

Stimulus	Organ or tissue preparation	Biological effect	Reference
Putrescine	Synaptosomes	Enhanced release of aspartate	[171]
		Elevation of free cytosolic Ca^{2+}	[172]
Intracarotid mannitol infusion	Rat brain	Hyperosmolal opening of the blood brain barrier	[173]
Hyperosmolal mannitol (1.6 M)	Rat cerebral capillaries	Enhancement of $^{45}Ca^{2+}$-fluxes, enhancement of endocytosis, and of hexose and amino acid transport	[174]
Ca^{2+}-free Krebs-Henseleit solution	Rat heart	Loss of contractility, release of cyto-solic enzymes, structural lesions	[175]

table the same cascade of events was reported to take place [20]. After the stimulus (hormone, depolarization, etc.) ODC activity increased, with a peak activity between 1 and 2 min, and returned to basal levels within less than 60 min. Putrescine, spermidine and spermine concentrations increased to maximum concentrations within 5 min; the rate of spermine enhancement was usually somewhat greater than that of spermidine and putrescine. Polyamine concentrations were at least twice the basal levels and remained high for at least 15 min. Addition of DFMO (5 mM) to the incubation medium of tissue slices or cells, or to the perfusion medium in the case of Langendorff heart preparations, abolished the stimulus-coupled biological effects. If, however, in addition to 5 mM DFMO 0.5 mM putrescine was present in the media, the effects of DMFO were nullified.

DFMO is a selective inactivator of ODC. Numerous growth inhibitory effects of DFMO are known to be prevented in the presence of putrescine [2–4, 7, 9, 10]. Therefore, the suppression of the stimulus-coupled effects by DFMO appears to be a rather strong argument in favor of the notion that active ODC is required to induce Ca^{2+}-fluxes by voltage-dependent and receptor-mediated pathways. Mechanisms which allow the rapid activation of latent ODC, or the de novo synthesis of the enzyme within less than one minute are presently not known, nor is clear how spermidine and especially spermine could be formed within one minute in such amounts as to allow doubling of the basal levels. But these questions will be solved in the future, once the role of the polyamines in signal transduction has been unambiguously proven. In view of the importance of the problem it is astounding that nearly no attempt was made to reproduce the rather provocative ob-

servations of H. Koenig and his collaborators [20]. Instead their existence has been widely ignored.

8.5   Polyamines, polyphosphoinositides and protein kinase C

Biochemical evidence for potential roles of the polyamines in signal
transduction is necessarily indirect. In vitro effects on enzymes are
difficult to validate in terms of physiological relevance. Nevertheless,
some examples of interactions of polyamines with enzymes involved
in the signal transduction pathways are mentioned in the following.
Plasma membrane Ca^{2+}-transport ATPase has a major function in the
control of intracellular Ca^{2+} [151, 154]. Its inhibition by polyamines
[98] has already been mentioned.
In view of the role of inositol phosphates in the mobilization of Ca^{2+}
from stores, effects of polyamines on polyphosphoinositide metabolism should be of special importance. Spermine has been shown to
bind tightly to phosphatidylinositol-4,5-diphosphate [99, 176, 177],
even in the presence of physiological concentrations of Mg^{2+} [178]. At
least in vitro this interaction leads to a decrease in the turnover of
polyphosphoinositides: spermine and spermidine inhibit at μM concentrations the hydrolysis of phosphatidylinositol by Ca^{2+}-dependent
phosphatidylinositol phosphodiesterase [179]. Higher concentrations
of the polyamines activate this enzyme [180], suggesting that by changing the Ca^{2+}/polyamine ratio a subtle regulation of the activity of
phosphatidylinositol phosphodiesterase is possible. In line with this
idea is the observation [181] that spermine is able to block Ca^{2+}-sig-
nals in electrically stimulated muscle fibers, by interfering with the
formation of inositol-1,4,5-triphosphate.
Inositol-1,4,5-triphosphate 5-phosphatase terminates the action of the
second messenger. This Mg^{2+}-activated enzyme is also inhibited by
spermine [182] at mM concentrations. This interaction is another potential point of regulation of signaling. The activation of phosphatidyl-
inositol-4-kinase and of phosphatidylinositol-4-phosphate 5-kinase
[183, 194, 195] by the polyamines should contribute to the enhanced
replenishment of the phosphatidylinositol phosphate pools.
Diacylglycerol has been mentioned to be the key regulatory molecule
of the second limb in Ca^{2+}-dependent signal transduction [151]. It ac-
tivates the membrane bound form of (Ca^{2+}/phospholipid-dependent)
protein kinase C. The docking of the enzyme is believed to occur on a

cluster formed by phosphatidyl serine and Ca^{2+}. The binding of diacylglycerol to this complex causes a decrease of the Ca^{2+}-require-
ment for enzyme activation [186, 187]. Protein kinase C is inhibited by
spermine competitively with respect to Ca^{2+} and phosphatidylserine
[188]. Likewise, the activation of protein kinase C in pancreatic islets
by a phorbol ester was inhibited by spermine and spermidine [58].
(This effect was correlated with a decreased insulin secretion, as has
been mentioned above). It is conceivable that spermine competes with
Ca^{2+}-binding sites and interferes with the association of protein kinase C with the plasma membrane and thus modulates its ability to respond to activation by diacylglycerol [189]. But spermine may also interact directly with the catalytic domain of protein kinase C [190].

9   Are the polyamines modulators of mesolimbic dopaminergic neurons?

From the presently available information it is not possible to conclude
that polyamines have a neurotransmitter function [191–193] even
though spontaneous and evoked release of spermine from brain slices
has been demonstrated [194]. The fact that diphenylhydantoin inhibited K^+-stimulated release of spermine suggests that polyamine release
is also Ca^{2+}-dependent, as is mandatory for neurotransmitter release:
Diphenylhydantoin inhibits Ca^{2+} influx into synaptosomes [195] and
inhibits noradrenaline release from K^+-depolarized brain slices [196].
In order to test the potential role of polyamines as neuromodulators,
Law et al. [197] studied the effects of the natural polyamines and of
some α, ω-diamines on the uptake of adenosine, glycine, GABA, glutamate, dopamine and choline into synaptosomes from the forebrain
of rats. None of the natural polyamines inhibited the uptake of adenosine, glutamate and glycine even at 10 mM concentration. Choline
($IC_{50} = 0.22$ mM) and dopamine ($IC_{50} = 2.7$ mM) uptake was significantly inhibited by spermine, less effectively by spermidine and putrescine. GABA uptake was only slightly inhibited by the polyamines
at a concentration of 10 mM.
Richardson-Andrews [198, 199] postulated functional (and structural)
similarities between neuroleptic drugs, some antimalarial drugs and
the polyamines. As the clinical effects of the neuroleptics are believed
to be due to their ability to inhibit mesolimbic dopaminergic activity,
the effects of spermidine and spermine on indices of dopamine-medi-

ated behavior in rats and mice were tested [200]. Spontaneous climbing and wheel running of mice were inhibited dose-dependently by i.p. doses of 15–115 μmol · kg^{-1} spermine. Given at the same doses to rats spermine failed to cause catalepsy or to antagonize the stereotyped behavior induced by apomorphine. Since limbic dopamine systems are involved in the expression of climbing and wheel running behavior [201], it was concluded that polyamines may modulate limbic dopamine functions. In support of this idea were the following observations: 15–60 nmol spermine or 20–80 nmol spermidine injected bilaterally into the nucleus accumbens of rats inhibited amphetamine-induced hyperactivity. The same doses of the polyamines injected unilaterally into the corpus striatum did not initiate any asymmetry or circling. Thus it appears that exogenous polyamines have a selective action on mesolimbic dopamine function. It remains to be clarified whether modulation of endogenous polyamine concentrations is causing specific dopamine-linked behavioral changes, or changes of behavior that is associated with the modulation of the activity of other neuronal systems.

10   Polyamine metabolism as a target for chemotherapy
10.1   Polyamines and growth

Ever since putrescine was suggested as growth factor of mammalian cells [202] effects of exogenous polyamines on growth, regeneration and related processes have been reported. In Table 4, examples are summarized. These and related effects of exogenous polyamines may become an important research topic in the future, should it be possible to substitute the natural polyamines by non-metabolizable, non-toxic analogs.

In the past the recognition of a role of the polyamines in the enhancement of cell cycle traverse by tumor cells, or more generally the enhancement of polyamine biosynthesis in tumor tissue [129] found much attraction. It was this focus of interest on growth-related processes which induced the development of inhibitors for all enzymes of the polyamine biosynthetic pathway and led to the synthesis of polyamine analogs with antitumoral properties [3, 7, 10].

Table 4
Effects of treatment with polyamines in growth and regeneration processes

Polyamine	Biological effect	Reference
Putrescine	Growth factor for a mammalian cell line	[202]
Putrescine	Requirement for growth of neural cells	[203]
Spermine	Enhancement of motor function recovery after axotomy	[204]
Putrescine, spermidine, spermine	Enhancement of survival of sympathetic neurons after postnatal axonal injury	[205, 206]
Putrescine, spermidine, spermine	Increase in the number of sympathetic neurons in early development	[207, 208]
Putrescine, spermidine, spermine	Precocious development of rats	[209]
Spermidine, spermine	Induction of intestinal maturation	[210]
Putrescine, spermidine, spermine	Enhanced repair of duodenal mucosa after stress-induced damage	[211]
Putrescine	Enhanced healing in D-galactosamine-induced hepatitis	[212, 213]
Putrescine, spermidine, spermine	Prevention of the excitotoxic effect of glutamate in neurons	[214]
Putrescine, spermidine, spermine	Protection against acetaminophen hepatotoxicity	[215]

10.2   Polyamine biosynthesis inhibitors in anticancer therapy

As polyamines had been recognized to be indispensable for cell proliferation, the limitation of the access of tumors to polyamines by inhibition of enzymes of their biosynthetic pathway was the logical step towards a new strategy of anticancer therapy. It appeared that ODC, AdoMetDC and spermidine and spermine synthase were suitable targets. Inhibitors of these enzymes are presently available [3, 4, 10], but among the many compounds, which were synthesized in the course of the last decade [3, 10, 216–220] only two gained therapeutic significance: the ODC inactivator 2-(difluoromethyl)ornithine (DFMO, Eflornithine) [65] and methylglyoxal-bis(guanylhydrazone) (MGBG) [221] (The structures of these compounds are shown in Fig. 1. Their structural analogy to ornithine and spermidine, respectively, is evident in this Figure).

10.2.1   Methylglyoxal-bis(guanylhydrazone) (MGBG)

MGBG is apparently not metabolized in the mammalian organism [222]. As has been mentioned before it is a competitive inhibitor of

AdoMetDC ($K_i < 1 \mu M$) [64]. The closely related ethylglyoxal-bis(guanylhydrazone) is even more potent than MGBG. Another structural analog, 1,1'-([methylethanediylidene]dinitrilo)bis(3-amino-guanidine), is an irreversible inhibitor [223]. Presumably it forms a hy-drazone with the terminal pyruvoyl group of AdoMetDC.

It has been mentioned briefly that MGBG is not specific: It inhibits diamine oxidase and other Cu^{2+}-containing amine oxidases and it in-duces cSAT [64]. These effects, but especially injury to mitochondria [64] makes it difficult to assign effects of MGBG on DNA replication and cell division exclusively to polyamine depletion. However, the following observations suggest that antitumor actions of MGBG might be polyamine-related: MGBG added to cell culture media caused a decline in intracellular spermidine and spermine concentra-tions, as is expected from the metabolic scheme (Fig. 2) and an in-crease of ODC activity and of putrescine formation [10, 64] due to de-repression of the ODC gene [2, 4]. In animals MGBG administration blocks incorporation of labeled putrescine into spermidine and sper-mine in various tissues [226] and likewise in many types of normal and tumor cells in culture. Administration of spermidine to L1210 leu-kemia-bearing mice counteracted the inhibition of tumor growth by MGBG, as well as gastrointestinal toxicity, lymphoid depression, bone marrow depression and immunosuppression, but not its hepato-toxic, cardiotoxic, nephrotoxic and hypoglycemic effects [220, 227]. Recent experiments with a selective inactivator of AdoMetDC with structural features of decarboxylated AdoMet, challenge the idea that MGBG is antitumoral exclusively by inhibition of spermidine and spermine formation. The new AdoMetDC inhibitor [228] depletes profoundly spermine and somewhat less spermidine concentrations in the tumor and induces putrescine formation [229], as has been de-scribed for MGBG, but it has only weak antitumoral effects. In view of the structural similarity between spermidine and MGBG (Fig. 1) it is likely that MGBG can occupy intracellular spermidine and sper-mine binding sites and may prevent in this way physiological func-tions of the polyamines. The fact that the more potent ethylglyoxal-bis(guanylhydrazone) is less antitumoral than MGBG is additional in-direct support to this suggestion. Competition of MGBG with spermi-dine at the level of ribosomal protein synthesis is a likely site of its an-titumoral action: it is known that MGBG interferes with spermidine stimulation of polyphenylalanine and globin synthesis directed by appropriate mRNAs [230]. A decrease in protein synthesis rate is the first defect in macromolecular syntheses of cells which are gradually deprived of spermidine [231].

After having been abandoned by clinicians for almost 15 years, MGBG resurged owing to the discovery of less toxic dose schedules that have demonstrated significant antitumor activity [232]. The development of analytical methods which allowed to determine the pharmacokinetic properties of MGBG and to follow therapeutic regimen was also of considerable clinical importance [233].

The major application of MGBG as a single agent was in patients with acute leukemias, with a 30 % response rate in acute myeloblastic leukemia. But a number of solid tumors (malignant lymphoma and tumors of the esophagus, breast, head and neck, among others), showed also significant response rates [234, 235]. Nevertheless, the usefulness of MGBG is limited by a rather narrow therapeutic window. More recently MGBG has been used in combination with DMFO with variable success (see below).

10.2.2   2-(Difluoromethylornithine) (Eflornithine; DFMO)

DFMO was designed as an enzyme-activated irreversible inhibitor of ODC [65]. It inactivates ODC irreversibly by binding to the enzyme protein. The postulated reactions involved in the inactivation of ODC are shown in Fig. 5. The scheme implies that DFMO undergoes the normal reactions which are involved in the decarboxylation of ornithine. Since, however, F$^-$ is released in the course of the decarboxylation reaction, a chemically reactive species is formed from the inert DFMO, which may react with a nucleophilic residue of the enzyme protein. For more details of mechanistic aspects of ODC inactivation, see [217]. DFMO has a Ki = 39 μM ($\tau_{1/2}$ = 3.1 min) which suggests that the rate of inactivation of ODC by DFMO is relatively slow. In view of the short half-life and the inducibility of the enzyme, this is a considerable disadvantage. Over the years numerous structural analogs of DFMO and also structural analogs of putrescine have been synthesized, some of which are considerably more potent inhibitors of ODC than DFMO [217]. With one of these compounds (R)-α-ethynyl-(R)-δ-methyl-1,4-butanediamine (MAP) (Ki = 3 μM; $\tau_{1/2}$ = 1.7 min) a phase I study was carried out [236]. However, owing to lacking toxicity and a high selectivity, DFMO has remained the most important ODC inhibitor up to date.

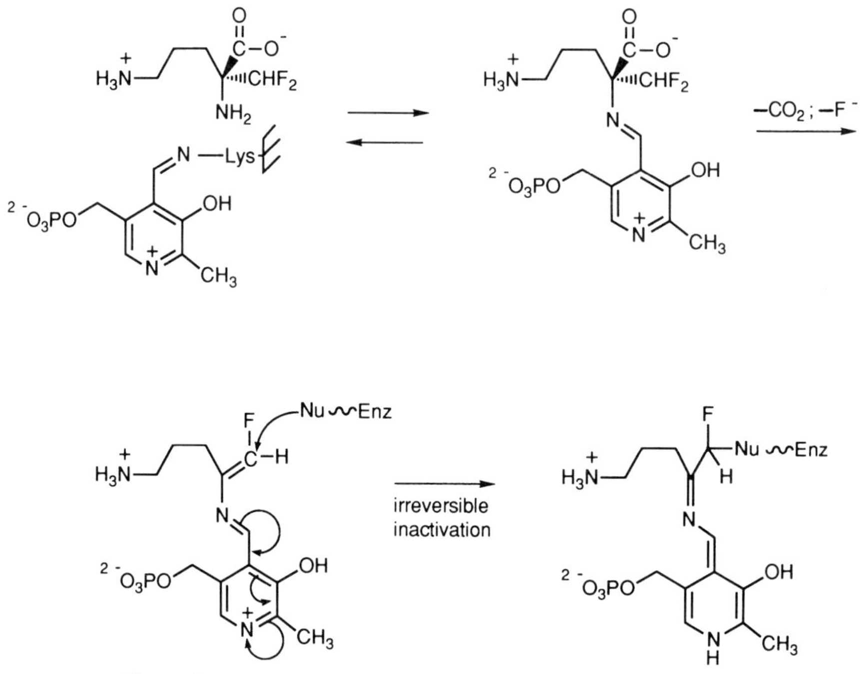

Figure 5
Proposed mechanism for the inactivation of ornithine decarboxylase by 2-(difluoro-methyl)ornithine (DFMO).

Exposure of cells to 1–10 mM DFMO causes a gradual depletion of putrescine and spermidine, whereas spermine concentrations increase somewhat due to the induction of AdoMetDC [237]. Numerous studies have demonstrated that cells stop growing, once the spermidine concentration has reached a critical level. With few exceptions, e.g. small cell lung carcinoma, which are losing viability [238, 239] the growth effects of DFMO are reversed by polyamines. The behavior of different cells with regard to cell cycle traverse varies, but most cells arrest in G0 or early G1 phase if spermidine is depleted [240].

When administered either systemically or with the drinking water in doses of 3–5 g · kg^{-1} per day, some animal tumors, such as EMT6 mouse mammary sarcoma [241, 242], B16 melanotic melanoma in mice [243] and human small cell lung carcinoma [239, 244] responded rather well; however, other tumors (L1210 leukemia, Lewis lung carcinoma) showed little growth inhibition, if treatment started when the tumor was established [245]. Growth processes related to hypertrophy and regeneration processes are likewise only marginally affected by administration of DFMO and other ODC inhibitors, even though ODC activity is considerably reduced by the treatment [246]. Under the mentioned premises it is not astonishing that DFMO used as single agent had only marginal effects in human malignancies [247]: About 500 patients with a variety of advanced malignancies receiving $2–4 \text{ g} \cdot \text{m}^{-2}$ DFMO every 8 h were studied. Stabilization of disease progression occurred in some patients and there were few complete responses, but no general pattern of response to the treatment was evident. Similarly treatment with DFMO of psoriasis, a nonmalignant skin disease, had no effect on the clinical status of the skin, despite polyamine depletion in the psoriatic plaques [248]. Even in the case of patients with small cell lung carcinoma, which responded so well to administration of DFMO in an animal model [239], the results were not encouraging.

In recent experiments with several tumor models, which are weak responders to treatment with DFMO (L1210 leukemia [27, 249]), Lewis lung carcinoma [27, 250] U-251 human glioblastoma [251] it was unambiguously demonstrated that intracellularly synthesized polyamines are not the only polyamine source for tumor growth. Circulating polyamines can be utilized by the tumor, inspite of their low concentration. Circulating polyamines may be of exogenous origin (gastrointestinal tract) or they may derive from various tissues either by physiological release, or pathologically by release from dying cells.

If access to gastrointestinal polyamines is reduced by decontamination, using non-absorbable antibiotics and polyamine-free diet, the antitumoral effect of DFMO can be considerably improved. Polyamine interconversion is another source of polyamines, which can be blocked by inhibition of PAO [252]. If N,N'-bis-(2,3-butadienyl)-1,4-butanediamine (MDL 72527), a selective inactivator of PAO [253] is administered together with polyamine deficient diet, antibiotics and DFMO, a near-to-complete blockade of the growth of the above-mentioned tumors could be achieved, the formation of metastases from Lewis lung carcinoma almost completely prevented and the life-time of L1210 leukemia-bearing mice considerably prolonged. These observations not only suggest the significance of three major polyamine sources for tumor growth, but also that polyamine deprivation may be a general approach to limit the growth rate of rapidly growing tumors. However, even the complete blockade of tumor growth by polyamine deprivation will normally not result in remission of the malignancy, unless an active cellular immune system or a suitable cytotoxic drug finishes with the tumor. Obviously, the clinical use of DFMO as a single agent was inappropriate since no care was taken in the past to exclude alternative polyamine sources. The same is true for all clinically used drug combinations with DFMO.

10.2.3   Combination therapy with DFMO and MGBG

One of the consequences of the structural similarity between spermidine and MGBG is the fact that MGBG shares the polyamine uptake system. MGBG is effectively concentrated from the extracellular space into the cells interior [254, 255]. The fact that MGBG competes with extracellular polyamines for uptake may be a further factor that contributes to its antiproliferative effect, in addition to those mentioned in the previous section, a feature which is not shared by AdoMetDC inhibitors with a structure unrelated to that of the polyamines.

It is well established [26] that depletion of intracellular polyamine stores enhances the uptake of exogenous polyamines. Since inhibition of ODC causes the preferential depletion of putrescine and spermidine in tissues with a high de novo polyamine synthesis rate, i.e. of rapidly growing tumors, but also in intestinal mucosa and other tissues with a high cell proliferation rate and in prostate, it was expected to enhance relatively selectively MGBG concentrations in tumors by pretreatment with DFMO. Early studies were in support of a selective enhancement of the uptake of MGBG into tumor cells by DFMO [233]. However, this principle seems not generally applicable [256]. This may be one reason for the limited clinical success of DFMO-MGBG combinations.

Clinical trials with combined use of DFMO and MGBG started as early as 1981 in childhood leukemia [257]. This early study produced impressive clinical results, but attempts to reproduce them have only occasionally been successful. In general, it was found that priming with DFMO prior MGBG administration enhanced equally antitumor and toxic effects [235, 258–260]. Most significant are, however, the findings of Levin et al. [261] who used combinations of DFMO and MGBG in the treatment of brain tumors (e.g. astrocytomas). This group found sustained response or stable disease in more than 50 % of the patients, and even a total remission was observed. Some complete responses in patients with metastatic thyroid carcinoma and lymphoma with intermittent dosing schedules were also reported [262].

10.2.4   Combination of DMFO with other therapies

The amplification of the antitumoral effect of α-interferon in the case of mouse melanoma [263] stimulated clinical trials with patients suffering from malignant melanoma [264, 265]. DFMO was also combined with standard chemotherapy and radiotherapy in the treatment of patients with a wide selection of malignant tumors [247], but no unequivocal benefit of DFMO was established.

10.2.5   Preventive therapy with DFMO

Irrespective of the insufficient knowledge of the role of ODC in cancerogenesis, DFMO with its low toxicity and known mechanism of action may be of potential value as a chemopreventive agent. This is, at least, suggested by animal studies. Administration of DFMO (by repeated injections or orally with the drinking water) prevented or at least reduced the incidence of tumor formation in several models, such as promotion of skin tumors by 12-0-tetra-decanoylphorbol-13-acetate [266, 267], colonic tumors by 1,2-dimethylhydrazine, colorectal cancer by tumor promotors [268, 269], bladder cancer induced by N-methyl,N-nitrosourea [270] and mammary tumors induced by 7,12-dimethylbenz(α)anthracene [271] or N-methyl,N-nitrosourea [272]. However, Kamatani et al. [273] reported that polyamine depletion by DFMO increased the spontaneous mutation frequency in basophilic leukemia cells treated with N-nitroso,N-nitro,N'-nitrosoguanidine. Human studies on the chemopreventive effect of DMFO are not available at present.

10.2.6   DFMO and parasitic diseases

For reasons which are not entirely clear [274] certain parasites are rather sensitive to treatment with DFMO. Mice infected with *Trypanosama b. brucei* [275], *T.b. gambiense* [276] and *T. congolense* [277] were cured when given a 2–4 % solution of DFMO for several days. This effect of DFMO is certainly polyamine dependent, since administration of putrescine, spermidine or spermine concomitant with

DFMO prevented the curative effect of the ODC inhibitor [278]. DFMO is only partially effective or ineffective [279] against the more virulent. *T.b. rhodesiense* strains (the cause of East African sleeping sickness).

Based on these observations clinical trials with patients suffering from *T.b. gambiense* (West African sleeping sickness) started in 1981. Among 380 evaluable patients all were positively responding to treatment with DFMO, i.e. trypanosomes disappeared from body fluids and the characteristic symptoms of the sleeping sickness ameliorated. Since the reported cases [280] include also patients refractory to treatment with arsenicals, it appears that DFMO is a safe and effective new treatment for human gambiense trypanosomiasis.

DFMO has no effect on *Trypanosoma cruzi,* the parasite causing American trypanosomiasis (Chagas disease) [281]. *T. cruzi* replication is, however, markedly inhibited by 2-(difluoromethyl)arginine, an inactivator of arginine decarboxylase. This suggests that *T. cruzi* uses a putrescine-forming pathway which is absent in the mammalian organism. Thus it is not excluded that an inactivator of arginine decarboxylase could become an effective drug against the now incurable Chagas disease.

Pneumocystis carinii is a common cause of death in AIDS patients. The growth of *P. carinii* can be inhibited by DFMO [282, 283]. In clinical studies [284] DFMO showed some efficacy. DFMO is, therefore, used by some investigators in the therapy of AIDS patients. DFMO has also some potentials in the treatment of *Leishmania infantum* [285].

10.3   Current developments in polyamine-related anticancer
          therapy

Even though clinical success was modest, the work of the past decade nevertheless has demonstrated that polyamine metabolism is a suitable target for new drugs against malignancies and protozoan infections. Based on a more intimate knowledge of the principles of polyamine regulation and function, current efforts are concentrated on the following aspects:
a) Development of improved inhibitors of the biosynthetic enzymes
b) Exploration of combinations of polyamine-directed drugs with (usually cytotoxic) agents not directly related to polyamine metabolism

c) Development of structural analogs of the polyamines with antitumor properties

New inhibitors of ODC and AdoMetDC necessarily have to be irreversible inactivators with a rapid inactivation rate. Owing to the short
half-life of ODC and AdoMetDC and due to their rapid induction
and overproduction due to gene amplification, competitive inhibitors
are not capable of preventing putrescine respectively dAdoMet formation to a sufficient extent over a long time. Favorable pharmacokinetic properties, i.e. uptake into cells and slow elimination are further important properties of a new generation of polyamine biosynthesis inhibitors.

Most probably inhibitors of AdoMetDC and of spermidine and spermine synthase will have to be used in combination with an ODC inhibitor, since depletion of spermidine and spermine causes the compensatory induction of ODC with a consequent enhancement of putrescine formation, as has already been mentioned. The development of
methylglyoxal-bis-(butylamidinohydrazone) and related compounds
[286] which inhibit ODC, AdoMetDC and spermidine synthase have,
therefore, interesting therapeutic potentials.

Based on the assumption that depletion of intracellular polyamines
might increase the accessibility of the DNA to alkylating or cross-linking agents, Marton and his collaborators studied a number of known
cytotoxic drugs in combination with DFMO [287] and found especially with alkylating nitrosoureas a potentiation of the cytotoxic effect by polyamine depletion. In contrast, cross-linking drugs, such as
cis-diammine dichloroplatinum (II) (cisplatin) showed decreased
cytotoxicity against spermidine-depleted cells.

The more complete spermidine depletion by systematic polyamine deprivation and depletion of spermidine and spermine concentrations
by inhibitors of AdoMetDC or spermidine and spermine synthase inhibitors, may have even more favorable effects on the therapeutic efficacy of certain cytotoxic agents.

A current promising development are structural analogs of the natural
polyamines. The following characteristics, are ideally combined in
these compounds:

1) They share the polyamine uptake system and thus act as competitive uptake inhibitors.
2) They bind to polyamine binding sites and displace the natural
   polyamines, preventing their functions especially their growth-

related functions. This implies that the analogs do not support polyamine-dependent reactions essential for growth and cell proliferation.

3) The analogs act as polyamines with respect to their regulatory functions in the biosynthetic pathway and repress biosynthetic enzymes (ODC, AdoMetDC) and induce cSAT, thus causing the depletion of intracellular polyamines.

4) They do not share the toxic effects of the natural polyamines.

Porter, Bergeron and their colleagues found that N^1,N^8-bis(ethyl) spermidine and N^1,N^{12}-bis(ethyl)spermine combine some of the above-postulated properties [10, 288–290] and a considerable number of analogs of the natural polyamines with antitumoral properties were reported by Edwards et al. [291]. The therapeutic potentials of these polyamine analogs are under current investigation. N^1,N^{12}-bis(ethyl)spermine has recently been found to be less toxic than spermine and it inhibited gastric ulceration [292] similarly to spermine [79, 82]. Since research in this field is rather active, more new analogs can be expected in the near future and with them perhaps a new type of anticancer drug.

11   Conclusions

Examples of drug-like actions of the natural polyamines as well as attempts to introduce polyamines as potential therapeutic agents have been demonstrated on the preceding pages. The major thrust of the pharmacological exploration was the elucidation of functions of the natural polyamines in the major organs of the vertebrate organism, admittedly with modest success. There are several reasons for the fact that the pharmacology of the polyamines has not yet passed a preliminary, essentially descriptive stage. One is that during the period between 1950–1980 polyamine catabolism was not well understood. Therefore, metabolic transformations of polyamines were generally not taken into consideration as potential influence on the observed phenomena. Catabolism of exogenous polyamines may or may not be important, however, the lack of pertinent information is a considerable obstacle in the interpretation of reported results.

A second, even more obstructive factor in the exploration of the polyamines was the lack of specific and potent inhibitors of polyamine metabolism. DFMO, the first and still most important tool, became generally available only during the last decade. But even with this and more recent specific enzyme inhibitors [3] in our hands, it is still rather difficult to manipulate intracellular polyamine concentrations in an intact animal, owing to their careful control by multiple regulatory circuits [2, 4]. Long-term depletion of putrescine and partial depletion of spermidine by polyamine deprivation is now possible: after treatment with DMFO, the PAO inhibitor MDL 72527 and polyamine deficient diet containing neomycin and metronidazole, spermidine concentrations in mice are decreased by 40–65 %, depending on the organ, total polyamine concentrations only by 15–33 %, owing to the compensatory increase of spermine [27].

This method should allow us to explore organ functions in a state of chronic spermidine deficiency. From the available (unpublished) observations it appears, however, that disregarding weight loss (respectively retarded weight gain in young animals) no gross behavioral or other changes were observed. Clinical trials with DFMO are in agreement with the animal studies: daily DFMO doses up to 20 g did not cause any changes in muscle tone, blood pressure or heart rate [247], indicating that at least the partial depletion of endogenous polyamines does not produce effects which might occur if Ca^{2+}-fluxes are significantly impaired, as is expected from the work of Koenig and his colleagues [20].

There are several potential explanations for the apparent lack of pharmacologic effects under the treatment conditions. The most likely ones are the relatively small extent of polyamine depletion and the activation of compensatory mechanisms.

Long-term enhancement of endogenous polyamine concentrations by administration of polyamines is not possible, due to the activation of the interconversion pathway and of oxidative deaminations (see section 2).

Inhibition of ornithine transamination (the major degradative reaction of ornithine) causes an enormous accumulation of this amino acid in various tissues, including the brain. As a consequence, the enhancement of endogenous putrescine levels is observed. However, the increase of the spermidine concentration is small, again due to the induction of cSAT, so that as a net result the turnover of spermidine is enhanced. Unusual behavior was not observed under these conditions [293].

It may be possible in the future to substitute the natural polyamines by analogs which are stable against degradative reactions but capable of fulfilling physiologic functions. This type of compound would allow us to pinpoint physiologic or pathophysiologic reactions in the presence of excessive polyamines, and they might be useful in enhancing regenerative processes in situations of limited access to polyamines.

Even though the therapeutic success, at least in hyperproliferative diseases, was modest in the past, the inhibitors of polyamine biosynthetis were nevertheless of great scientific importance. They had a key role in the elucidation of the various aspects of polyamine regulation and opened views into the molecular mechanisms involved therein, as well as into growth-related functions of the polyamines. It seems not too daring to speculate that with our better understanding, the chances for polyamine-related drugs in cancer chemotherapy have considerably increased, especially since the role of exogenous polyamines in tumor growth is now evident. A direct consequence of this knowledge is that the development of polyamine uptake inhibitors will be a prime target in the coming years.

With the description of the polyamine binding site at the NMDA macrocomplex [21], functional aspects of the polyamines not related to growth have been brought to general attention. Since this finding implies a potential regulatory role of the polyamines in major excitatory neuronal systems, a strong stimulatory effect on pharmacologic research can be expected from this observation. It may indeed initiate a new active period of polyamine pharmacology, and we may expect our rather preliminary knowledge of the functions of the polyamines in the central nervous system [191–193] to especially profit from this shift of interest. Perhaps even the puzzling situation concerning the participation or non-participation of the polyamines in Ca^{2+}-signaling may be brought closer to clarification.

References

1   C. W. Tabor and H. Tabor: Microbiol. Rev. 49, 81 (1985).
2   A. E. Pegg: Biochem. J. 234, 249 (1986).
3   A. E. Pegg: Cancer Res. 48, 759 (1989).
4   N. Seiler and O. Heby: Acta Biochim. Biophys. Hung. 23: 1 (1988).
5   S. S. Cohen: Introduction to the Polyamines. Englewood Cliffs, Prentice-Hall, 1971.
6   L. Selmeci, M. E. Brosnan, N. Seiler (eds.): Recent Progress in Polyamine Research. Budapest, Akademiai Kiado, 1985.

7 P. P. McCann, A. E. Pegg and A. Sjoerdsma (eds.): Inhibition of Polyamine Metabolism. Orlando, Academic Press, 1987.

8 V. Zappia and A. E. Pegg (eds.): Progress in Polyamine Research. New York, Plenum Press, 1988.

9 U. Bachrach and Y. M. Heimer (eds.): The Physiology of Polyamines, 2 volumes. Boca Raton, CRC Press, 1989.

10 C. W. Porter and Sufrin: Anticancer Res. 6, 525 (1986).

11 F. G. Fischer and H. Bohn: Ann. Chem. 603, 232 (1957).

12 H. Jackson and P. N. R. Usherwood: TINS 11, 278 (1988).

13 W. S. Skinner, P. A. Dennis, A. Lui, R. L. Carney and G. B. Quistad: Toxicon 28, 541 (1990).

14 P. J. A. Davies, E. A. Chiocca, J. P. Basilion, S. Poddar, J. P. Stein, in: Progress in Polyamine Research (V. Zappia and A. E. Pegg, eds.), p. 391, New York, Plenum Press.

15 S. M. Rosenthal, E. R. Fischer and E. F. Stohlman: Proc. Soc. Exp. Biol. N.Y. 80, 432 (1952).

16 H. Tabor and C. W. Tabor: Pharmacol. Rev. 16, 245 (1963).

17 G. G. Shaw: Arch. Intern. Pharmacodyn. Therap. 198, 36 (1972).

18 T. Sakurada, K. Onodera, T. Tadano and K. Kisara: Japan J. Pharmacol. 25, 653 (1975).

19 J. Buss, M. D. Thesis, Institute of Pharmacology, Faculty of Medicine, Freie Universität, Berlin, 1963.

20 H. Koenig, A. D. Goldstone, C. Y. Lu, Z. Iqbal and C. C. Fan, in: The Physiology of Polyamines (U. Bachrach and Y. M. Heimer, eds.), vol. 1, p. 57, CRC Press, Boca Raton, 1989.

21 R. W. Ransom and N. L. Stec: J. Neurochem. 51, 830 (1988).

22 L. Persson, J. E. Seely and A. E. Pegg: Biochemistry 23: 3777 (1984).

23 T. Kameji and A. E. Pegg: Biochem. J. 243, 285 (1987).

24 F. Dezeure, F. Gerhart and N. Seiler: Int. J. Biochem. 21, 889 (1989).

25 E. S. Canellakis, D. A. Kyriakidis, C. A. Rinehart, S. C. Huang, C. Panagiotidis and W. F. Fong: Biosci. Rep. 5, 189 (1985).

26 N. Seiler and F. Dezeure: Int. J. Biochem. 22, 211 (1990).

27 S. Sarhan, B. Knödgen and N. Seiler: Anticancer Res. 9, 215 (1989).

28 G. A. van den Berg, G. T. Nagel and F. A. J. Muskiet: J. Chromatogr. 339, 223 (1985).

29 S. M. Janes, D. Mu, D. Wemmer, A. J. Smith, S. Kaur, D. Maltby, A. L. Burlingame and J. P. Klinman: Science 248, 981 (1990).

30 R. E. Shaff and M. A. Beaven: Biochem. Pharmacol. 25, 1057 (1976).

31 N. Seiler, F. N. Bolkenius and B. Knödgen: Biochem. J. 225, 219 (1985).

32 J. Kusche, R. Mennigen and J. R. Izbicki: Diamine oxidase, the regulator of intestinal mucosa proliferation, in: Recent Progress in Polyamine Research (L. Selmeci, M. E. Brosnan and N. Seiler, eds.), p. 329, Academic Press, Orlando, 1987.

33 M. Piacentini, C. Sartori, S. Beninati, M. Bargagli, M. P. Cerû-Argento: Biochem. J. 234, 435 (1986).

34 N. Seiler, in: Inhibition of Polyamine Metabolism (P. P. McCann, A. E. Pegg and A. Sjoerdsma, eds.), p. 49, Academic Press, Orlando, 1987.

35 N. Seiler: Physiol. Chem. Phys. 12, 411 (1980).

36 N. Seiler, B. Knödgen, M. W. Gittos, W.-Y. Chan, G. Griesmann and O. M. Rennert: Biochem. J. 200, 123 (1981).

37 G. A. van den Berg, H. Elzinga, G. T. Nagel, A. W. Kingma and F. A. J. Muskiet: Biochim. Biophys. Acta 802, 175 (1984).

38 N. Seiler, B. Knödgen, G. Bink, S. Sarhan and F. N. Bolkenius: Adv. Polyamine Res. 4, 135 (1983).

39 N. Seiler, B. Knödgen and K. Haegele: Biochem. J. 208, 189 (1982).

40 F. Wrede: Hoppe Seyler's Z. Physiol. Chem. 153, 291 (1926).

41   L. C. Rodichok and A. H. Friedman: Life Sci. 23, 2137 (1978).
42   C. W. Tabor and S. M. Rosenthal: J. Pharmacol. Exp. Ther. 116, 133 (1956).
43   R. Teradaira, K. Fujita and H. Takahashi: Pharmacometrics 25, 489 (1983).
44   D. J. Anderson, J. Crossland and G. G. Shaw: Neuropharmacology 14, 571 (1975).
45   T. Sakurada, H. Kohno, T. Tadano and K. Kisara: Japan J. Pharmacol. 27, 453 (1977).
46   W.-W. Shin, W. F. Fong, S.-F. Pang and C.-L. Wong: J. Neurochem. 44, 1056 (1985).
47   R. M. Di Giorgio, G. De Luca, G. Nistico and R. Ientile: J. Neurochem. 45, 739 (1985).
48   S. Genedani, M. Bernardi, S. Tagliavini and A. Bertolini: Life Sci. 38, 1293 (1986).
49   G. B. De Sarro, C. Ascioti, G. Bagetta, V. Libri and G. Nistico, in: Neurotransmitters, Seizures and Epilepsy (G. Nistico, P. L. Morselli, K. G. Lloyd, R. G. Fariello and J. Engel, eds.) p. 423, Raven Press, New York, 1986.
50   G. Nistico, R. Ientile, D. Rotiroti and R. M. Di Giorgio. Biochem. Pharmacol. 29, 954 (1980).
51   S. Genedani, G. Piccinini and A. Bertolini. Life Sci. 34, 2407 (1984).
52   S. Genedani, M. Bernardi, S. Tagliavini, A. Botticelli and A. Bertolini. Pharmacol. Toxicol. 61, 224 (1987).
53   E. T. Wei: Fed. Proc. 40, 1491 (1981).
54   H. A. Fischer, H. Korr, N. Seiler, G. Werner: Brain Res. 39, 197 (1972).
55   E. A. Evans, E. Vennesland and J. J. Schneider: Proc. Soc. Exp. Biol. Med. 41, 467 (1939).
56   U. Risetti and G. Mancini: Acta Neurol. 9, 391 (1954).
57   J. Anderson and G. G. Shaw: Br. J. Pharmacol. 52, 205 (1974).
58   P. Thams, K. Capito and C. J. Hedeskov: Biochem. J. 237, 131 (1986).
59   P. J. Bungay and M. Griffin: Biochem. Soc. Transactions 13, 353 (1985).
60   F. Rossi, G. Nistico, G. De Marco, L. Berrino, C. Matera, G. Bile and E. Marmo: Res. Commun. Chem. Pathol. Pharmacol. 46, 43 (1984).
61   E. Marmo, L. Berrino, M. Cazzola, A. Filippelli, G. Cafaggi, N. Persico, R. Spadaro and G. Nistico: Biomed. Biochim. Acta 43, 509 (1984).
62   E. W. Chideckel, H. H. Dedhia, J. S. Fedan, L. Teba and A. Jain. Cardiovasc. Res. 20, 931 (1986).
63   C. Bazzani, S. Genedani and A. Bertolini: Pharmacol. Res. Commun. 18, 503 (1986).
64   H. G. Williams-Ashman and J. Seidenfeld: Biochem. Pharmacol. 35, 1217 (1986).
65   P. Bey, in: Enzyme-Activated Irreversible Inhibitors (N. Seiler, M. J. Jung and J. Koch-Weser, eds.), p. 27, Elsevier-North Holland Biomedical Press, Amsterdam, 1978.
66   C. Bazzani, S. Genedani, S. Tagliavini, G. Piccinini and A. Bertolini. Pharmacol. Res. Commun. 20, 23 (1988).
67   M. C. Schaub, J. G. Watterson and P. G. Waser: TIPS 4, 116 (1983).
68   T. Martins and J. Velle: Compt. Rend. Soc. Biol. 129, 1129 (1938).
69   K. Onodera, T. Unemoto, K. Miyaki and M. Hayashi: Arch. Int. Pharmacodyn. Therap. 174, 491 (1968).
70   L. De Meis: Amer. J. Physiol. 212, 92 (1967).
71   M. F. Tansy, J. S. Martin, W. E. Laudin, F. M. Kendall and S. Melamed: Surg. Gynecol. Obstet. 154, 74 (1982).
72   H. Hashimoto, J. Unemoto and M. Hayashi: Amer. J. Physiol. 225, 743 (1973).

73   E. J. Belair, G. R. Carlson, S. Melamed, J. N. Moss and M. F. Tansy: J. Pharm. Sci. 70, 347 (1981).
74   E. W. Chideckel, J. S. Fedan and P. Mike: Eur. J. Pharmacol. 116, 187 (1985).
75   E. W. Chideckel, J. S. Fedan and P. Mike: Br. J. Pharmacol. 89, 27 (1986).
76   J. S. Martin and M. F. Tansy: Clin. Exp. Pharmacol. Physiol. 13, 87 (1986).
77   L. De Meis and M. J. De Paula: Arch. Biochem. Biophys. 119, 16 (1967).
78   T. K. Ray, J. Nandi, N. Pidhorodeckyj and Z. Meng-Ai: Proc. Natl. Acad. Sci. USA 79, 1448 (1982).
79   H. Aihara, S. Otomo, Y. Isobe, M. Ohzeki, K. Igarashi and S. Hirose: Biochem. Pharmacol. 32, 1733 (1983).
80   K. Igarashi, R. Houma, H. Tokuno, M. Kitada, H. Kitagawa and S. Hirose: Biochem. Biophys. Res. Commun. 103, 659 (1981).
81   T. P. Dousa and R. R. Dozois: Gastroenterology 73, 904 (1977).
82   T. Mizui, N. Shimono and M. Doteuchi: Japan J. Pharmacol. 44, 43 (1987).
83   S. Ohmori, T. Misaizu, M. Kitada, H. Kitagawa, K. Igarashi, S. Hirose and Y. Kanakubo: Res. Commun. Chem. Pathol. Pharmacol. 62, 235 (1988).
84   T. Oka and J. W. Perry: J. Biol. Chem. 249, 7647 (1974).
85   J. Bartholeyns, J. R. Fozard and N. J. Prakash: Br. J. Pharmacol. 64, 182 P (1981).
86   Y. Oyanagui: Agents and Actions 14, 228 (1984).
87   J. Bird, S. Mohd-Hidiv and D. A. Lewis: Agents and Actions 13, 342 (1983).
88   F. Schuber: Biochem. J. 260, 1 (1989).
89   K. A. Hubel: Amer. J. Physiol. 231, 252 (1976).
90   R. A. Frizzel and S. G. Schultz: J. Gen. Physiol. 59, 318 (1972).
91   T. Yajima: Japan J. Pharmacol. 33, 261 (1983).
92   M. A. Wedgwood and J. H. Wolstencroft: Neuropharmacol. 16, 445 (1977).
93   M. N. Perkins and T. W. Stone: Mol. Physiol. 1, 311 (1981).
94   A. L. F. Gorman and A. Hermann: J. Physiol. (Lond.) 333, 681 (1982).
95   H. Drouin and A. Hermann: Ann. N. Y. Acad. Sci. USA 435, 534 (1984).
96   H. Drouin and A. Hermann, in: Water and Ions in Biomolecular Systems (D. Vasilescu, J. Jaz, L. Packer and B. Pullman, eds.), p. 213, Birkhäuser, Basel, 1990.
97   R. Stämpfli: Ergeb. Physiol. 47, 71 (1952).
98   L. Messiaen, F. Wuytack, L. Raeymaekers, H. De Smedt and R. Casteels: Biochem. J. 261, 1055 (1989).
99   B. Tadolini and E. Varani: Biochem. Biophys. Res. Commun. 135, 58 (1986).
100 D. T. Monaghan, R. J. Bridges and C. W. Cotman: Ann. Rev. Pharmacol. Toxicol. 29, 365 (1989).
101 M. L. Mayer and G. L. Westbrook: Prog. Neurobiol. 28, 197 (1987).
102 G. L. Collingridge and R. A. J. Lester: Pharmacol. Rev. 41, 143 (1989).
103 P. L. Wood, T. S. Rao, S. Iyengar, T. Lanthorn, J. Monahan, A. Cordi, E. Sun, M. Vazquez, N. Gray and P. Contreras: Neurochem. Res. 15, 217 (1990).
104 J. A. Kemp, A. C. Foster and E. H. Wong: TIPS 10, 294 (1987).
105 J. W. Johnson and P. Ascher: Nature 325, 529 (1987).
106 M. L. Mayer, G. L. Westbrook and P. B. Guthrie: Nature 309, 261 (1984).
107 L. Nowak, P. Bregestrovski, P. Ascher, H. Herbet and A. Prochiantz: Nature 307, 462 (1984).
108 J. W. Johnson and P. Ascher: Biophys. J. 57, 1085 (1990).
109 A. Kossorotow, H. U. Wolf and N. Seiler: Biochem. J. 144, 21 (1974).
110 K. Williams, C. Romano and P. B. Molinoff: Mol. Pharmacol. 36, 575 (1989).
111 A. I. Sacaan and K. M. Johnson: Mol. Pharmacol. 37, 572 (1990).

112   A. I. Sacaan and K. M. Johnson: Mol. Pharmacol. 36, 836 (1989).
113   K. M. Johnson, L. D. Snell, A. I. Sacaan and S. Jones: Drug Dev. Res. 17, 281 (1989).
114   I. J. Reynolds: Eur. J. Pharmacol. 177, 215 (1990).
115   S. M. Rothman and J. W. Olney: TINS 10, 299 (1987).
116   M. J. Croucher, J. F. Collins and B. S. Meldrum: Science 216, 899 (1982).
117   D. W. Ellison, M. F. Beal, M. F. Mazurek, J. R. Malloy, E. D. Bird and J. B. Martin: Brain 110, 1657 (1987).
118   G. Garthwhite and J. Garthwhite: Neurosci. 18, 437 (1986).
119   D. W. Choi: J. Neurosci. 7, 369 (1987).
120   B. K. Siesjo and I. Bengtsson: J. Cereb. Blood Flow Metab. 9, 127 (1989).
121   J. Benavides, B. Gotti, A. Dubois, E. T. MacKenzie, B. Scatton and M. Theraulaz: J. Cereb. Blood Flow Metab. 9 (Suppl. 1), S 748 (1989).
122   C. Carter, J. P. Rivy and B. Scatton: Eur. J. Pharmacol. 164, 611 (1989).
123   I. J. Reynolds and R. J. Miller: Mol. Pharmacol. 36, 758 (1989).
124   H. Schoemaker, J. Allen and S. Z. Langer: Eur. J. Pharmacol. 176, 249 (1990).
125   R. Quirion, R. Chicheportiche, P. C. Contreras, K. M. Johnson, D. Lodge, S. W. Tam, J. H. Woods and S. R. Zukin: TINS 10, 444 (1987).
126   B. K. Koe, C. A. Burkhart and L. A. Lebel: Eur. J. Pharmacol. 161, 263 (1989).
127   I. A. Paul, G. Kuypers, M. Youdim and P. Skolnick: Eur. J. Pharmacol. 184, 203 (1990).
128   L. J. Marton, M. S. Edwards, V. A. Levin, W. P. Lubich and C. B. Wilson: Cancer Res. 39, 993 (1979).
129   J. Jänne, H. Pösö and A. Raina: Biochim. Biophys. Acta 473, 241 (1978).
130   S. Sarhan, V. Quemener, J.-Ph. Moulinoux, B. Knödgen and N. Seiler: Int. J. Biochem. 23, 617 (1991)
131   P. L. Wood, J. W. Richard, C. Pilapil and N. P. V. Nair: Neuropharmacol. 21, 1235 (1982).
132   P. L. Wood, M. R. Emmet, T. S. Rao, S. Mick, J. A. Cler and S. Iyengar: J. Neurochem. 53, 979 (1989).
133   P. L. Wood, D. J. Steel, S. E. McPherson, D. L. Cheney and J. Lehman: Can. J. Physiol. Pharmacol. 65, 1923 (1987).
134   T. S. Rao, J. A. Cler, E. J. Oei, M. R. Emmett, S. J. Mick, S. Iyengar and P. L. Wood: Neurochem. Int. 16, 199 (1990).
135   M. A. K. Markwell, S. P. Berger and S. M. Paul: Eur. J. Pharmacol. 182, 607 (1990).
136   N. Seiler, S. Sarhan and B. F. Roth-Schechter: Neurochem. Res. 9, 871 (1984).
137   F. Siddiqui, Z. Iqbal and H. Koenig: Soc. Neurosci. Abstr. 14, 1048 (1988).
138   H. Rasmussen and P. Q. Barrett: Physiol. Rev. 64, 938 (1984).
139   E. Carafoli: Ann. Rev. Biochem. 56, 395 (1987).
140   P. Palade: J. Biol. Chem. 262, 6149 (1987).
141   K. E. O. Akerman: J. Bioenerg. Biomembranes 9, 65 (1977).
142   C. V. Nicchitta and J. R. Williamson: J. Biol. Chem. 21: 12978 (1984).
143   J. R. Jensen, G. Lynch and M. Baudry: J. Neurochem. 48, 765 (1987).
144   J. G. McCormack: Biochem. J. 264, 167 (1989).
145   S. Lenzen, R. Hickethier and U. Panten: J. Biol. Chem. 261, 16478 (1986).
146   H. Kroner: Arch. Biochem. Biophys. 267, 205 (1988).
147   H. Rottenberg and M. Marbach: Biochim. Biophys. Acta 1016, 77 (1990).
148   J. R. Jensen, G. R. Lynch and M. Baudry: J. Neurochem. 53, 1182 (1989).
149   J. R. Jensen, G. R. Lynch and M. Baudry: J. Neurochem. 53, 1173 (1989).
150   M. J. Berridge: Biochem. J. 220, 345 (1984).
151   M. J. Berridge: Ann. Rev. Biochem. 56 159 (1987).

152   C. P. Downes and R. H. Michell, in: Molecular Mechanisms of Transmembrane Signalling, p. 3, Elsevier, New York, 1985.
153   S. R. Nahorski, D. A. Kendall, I. Batty: Biochem. Pharmacol. 35, 244 (1986).
154   J. R. Williamson and J. R. Monck: Environ. Health Perspect. 84, 121 (1990).
155   M. J. Berridge and R. F. Irvine: Nature 341, 197 (1989).
156   H. Koenig, A. Goldstone and C. Y. Lu: Biochem. Biophys. Res. Commun. 106, 346 (1982).
157   A. Goldstone, H. Koenig and C. Y. Lu: Biochim. Biophys. Acta 762, 366 (1983).
158   C. Y. Lu, H. Koenig, A. D. Goldstone and C. C. Fan: Fed. Proc. Fed. Am. Soc. Exp. Biol. 44, 830 (1985).
159   H. Koenig, C. C. Fan, C. Y. Lu and A. Goldstone: Trans. Am. Soc. Neurochem. 16, 236 (1985).
160   H. Koenig, C. C. Fan, A. D. Goldstone, C. Y. Lu and J. J. Trout: Circ. Res. 64, 415 (1989).
161   H. Koenig, A. D. Goldstone and C. Y. Lu: Biochem. Biophys. Res. Commun. 153, 1179 (1988).
162   C. C. Fan and H. Koenig: J. Mol. Cell. Cardiol. 20, 789 (1988).
163   H. Koenig, A. D. Goldstone and C. Y. Lu: Proc. Natl. Acad. Sci. USA 80, 7210 (1983).
164   A. D. Goldstone, H. Koenig and C. Y. Lu: Fed. Proc. Fed. Am. Soc. Exp. Biol. 44: 1593 (1985).
165   A. D. Goldstone, H. Koenig and C. Y. Lu: Fed. Proc. Fed. Am. Soc. Exp. Biol. 45, 1011 (1986).
166   C. Y. Lu, H. Koenig, A. D. Goldstone, C. C. Fan: Fed. Proc. Fed. Am. Soc. Exp. Biol. 45, 101 (1986).
167   C. Y. Lu, H. Koenig, A. D. Goldstone and J. J. Trout: Fed. Proc. Fed. Am. Soc. Exp. Biol. 43, 735 (1984).
168   H. Koenig, C. C. Fan and Z. Iqbal: Trans. Am. Soc. Neurochem. 15, 220 (1984).
169   Z. Iqbal, H. Koenig and J. J. Trout: Fed. Proc. Fed. Am. Soc. Exp. Biol. 43, 735 (1984).
170   Z. Iqbal and H. Koenig: Biochem. Biophys. Res. Commun. 133, 563 (1985).
171   S. C. Bondy and C. H. Walker: Brain Res. 371, 96 (1986).
172   H. Komulainen and S. C. Bondy: Brain Res. 401, 50 (1987).
173   C. Y. Lu, H. Koenig, A. D. Goldstone and J. J. Trout: Fed. Proc. Fed. Am. Soc. Exp. Biol. 46, 1321 (1987).
174   H. Koenig, A. D. Goldstone, C. Y. Lu and J. J. Trout: J. Neurochem. 52, 1135 (1989).
175   H. Koenig, A. D. Goldstone, J. J. Trout, C. Y. Lu: J. Clin. Invest. 80, 1322 (1987).
176   L. Chung, G. Kaloyanides, R. McDaniel, A. McLaughlin and S. McLaughlin: Biochemistry 24, 442 (1985).
177   P. Meers, K. Hong, J. Bentz and D. Papahadjopoulous: Biochemistry 25, 3109 (1986).
178   M. Toner, G. Vaio, A. McLaughlin and S. McLaughlin: Biochemistry 27, 7435 (1988).
179   J. Eichberg, W. J. Zetusky, M. E. Bell and E. Cavaugh: J. Neurochem. 36, 1868 (1981).
180   N. Sagawa, J. F. Bleasdale and G. C. Di Lorenzo: Biochim. Biophys. Acta 752, 153 (1983).
181   J. Vergara, R. Y. Tsien and M. Delay: Proc. Natl. Acad. Sci. USA 82, 6352 (1985).

182 M. A. Seyfred, L. N. Farell and W. W. Wells: J. Biol. Chem. 259, 13204 (1984).
183 J. Schacht: J. Neurochem. 27, 1119 (1976).
184 G. A. Lundberg, B. Jergil and R. Sundler: Eur. J. Biochem. 161, 257 (1986).
185 C. Cochet and E. M. Chambaz: Biochem. J. 237, 25 (1986).
186 R. M. Bell: Cell 45, 631 (1986).
187 Y. Nishizuka: Science 233, 305 (1986).
188 D. F. Qi, R. C. Schatzmann, G. J. Mazzei, R. S. Turner, R. L. Raynor, S. Liao and J. F. Kuo: Biochem. J. 213, 281 (1983).
189 M. S. Moruzzi, B. Barbiroli, M. G. Monti, B. Tadolini, G. Hakim and G. Mezzetti: Biochem. J. 247, 175 (1987).
190 G. Mezzetti, M. G. Monti and M. S. Moruzzi: Life Sci. 42, 2293 (1988).
191 N. Seiler: Neurochem. Int. 3, 95 (1981).
192 N. Seiler, in: Handbook of Neurochemistry (A. Lajtha, ed.) 2nd ed., vol. 1, p. 223, Plenum Press, New York, 1982.
193 T. A. Slotkin and J. Bartolome: Brain Res. Bull. 17, 307 (1986).
194 R. J. Harmann and G. G. Shaw: Br. J. Pharmacol. 73, 165 (1981).
195 R. S. Sohn and J. A. Ferendelli: J. Pharmacol. Exp. Therap. 185, 272 (1973).
196 J. H. Pincus and S. H. Lee: Neurology 22, 410 (1972).
197 C.-L. Law, P. C. L. Wong and W.-F. Fong: J. Neurochem. 42, 870 (1984).
198 R. C. Richardson-Andrews: Med. Hypotheses 11, 157 (1983).
199 R. C. Richardson-Andrews: Med. Hypotheses 18, 11 (1985).
200 S. R. Hirsch, R. Richardson-Andrews, B. Costall, M.-E. Kelly, J. de Belleroche and R. J. Naylor: Psychopharmacology 93, 101 (1987).
201 B. Costall, J. F. Enioju Kan and R. J. Naylor: Eur. J. Pharmacol. 96, 201 (1983).
202 R. G. Ham: Biochem. Biophys. Res. Commun. 14, 34 (1964).
203 J. E. Bottenstein: Adv. Cell. Neurobiol. 4, 333 (1983).
204 A. Sebille and M. Bondoux-Jahan: Exp. Neurol. 70, 507 (1980).
205 M. Dornay, V. H. Gilad, I. Shiler and G. M. Gilad: Exp. Neurol. 92, 665 (1986).
206 G. M. Gilad and V. H. Gilad: Devl. Brain Res. 38, 175 (1988).
207 G. M. Gilad and V. H. Gilad: Devl. Brain Res. 28, 163 (1986).
208 G. M. Gilad and V. H. Gilad: Brain Res. 348, 363 (1985).
209 G. M. Gilad, M. Dornay and V. H. Gilad: Int. J. Devl. Neurosci. 7, 641 (1989).
210 C. Dufour, G. Dandrifosse, P. Forget, F. Vermesse, N. Romain and P. Lepoint: Gastroenterology 95, 112 (1988).
211 J.-Y. Wang and L. R. Johnson: FASEB J. 4, 1986 (1990).
212 F. Tamada: Med. J. Kobe Univ. 45, 169 (1984).
213 W. Putnam, A. R. Buckley, J. A. Warneke, F. M. Karrer, B. Rhenman and K. Steinbronn: Surgery 96, 214 (1984).
214 G. M. Gilad and V. H. Gilad: Life Sci. 44, 1963 (1989).
215 L. P. Juhasz, W. Dairman and G. K. S. Roberts: Fed. Proc. Fed. Am. Soc. Exp. Biol. 43, 504 (1984).
216 A. E. Pegg, in: The Physiology of Polyamines (U. Bachrach and Y. M. Heimer, eds.), vol. 1, p. 303, CRC Press Boca Raton, 1989.
217 P. Bey, C. Danzin and M. Jung, in: Inhibition of Polyamine Metabolism (P. P. McCann, A. E. Pegg and A. Sjoerdsma, eds.), p. 1, Academic Press, Orlando, 1987.
218 A. E. Pegg and H. G. Williams-Ashman, in: Inhibition of Polyamine Metabolism (P. P. McCann, A. E. Pegg and A. Sjoerdsma, eds.), p. 33, Academic Press, Orlando, 1987.
219 O. Heby and J. Jänne, in: Polyamines in Biology and Medicine (D. R. Morris and L. J. Marton, eds.), p. 243, Marcel Dekker, New York (1981).

220   C. W. Porter, C. Dave and E. Mihic, in: Polyamines in Biology and Medicine (D. R. Morris and L. J. Marton, eds.), p. 406, Marcel Dekker, New York (1981).
221   J. Thiele and E. Dralle: Liebigs Ann. Chemie 302, 275 (1898).
222   M. G. Rosenblum, M. J. Keating, B. S. Yap and T. L. Loo: Cancer Res. 41, 1748 (1981).
223   A. E. Pegg and C. C. Conover: Biochem. Biophys. Res. Commun. 69, 766 (1976).
224   S. N. Pathak, C. W. Porter and C. Dave: Cancer Res. 37, 2246 (1977).
225   F. Mikles-Robertson, B. Feuerstein, C. Dave and C. W. Porter: Cancer Res. 39, 1919 (1979).
226   A. E. Pegg: Biochem. J. 537 (1973).
227   E. Mihic: Cancer Res. 23, 1375 (1963).
228   C. Danzin, P. Marchal and P. Casara: Biochem. Pharmacol. 40, 1499 (1990).
229   N. Seiler, S. Sarhan, P. Mamont, P. Casara and C. Danzin: Progr. of the Symposium on Polyamines: Biological and Clinical Aspects, Albère di Tenna, 1990 (M. A. Grillo, ed.).
230   R. Onishi, R. Nagami, S. Hirose and K. Igarashi: Arch. Biochem. Biophys. 242, 263 (1985).
231   B. B. Rudkin, P. S. Mamont and N. Seiler: Biochem. J. 217, 731 (1984).
232   W. A. Knight III, R. B. Livingston, C. Fabiani and J. Constanzi: Cancer Treat. Rep. 63, 1933 (1979).
233   J. Jänne, E. Höltta, A. Kallio and K. Käpyaho: Special Topics Endocrinol. Metab. 5, 227 (1983).
234   J. Jänne, L. Alhonen-Hongisto, P. Seppänen and M. Siimes: Med. Biol. 59, 448 (1981).
235   R. P. Warrell Jr. and J. H. Burchenal: J. Clin. Oncol. 1, 52 (1983).
236   M. A. Cornbleet, A. Kingsnorth, G. P. Tell, K. D. Haegele, A. M. Joder-Ohlenbusch and J. F. Smyth: Cancer Chemother. Pharmacol. 23, 348 (1989).
237   P. S. Mamont, M.-C. Duchesne, A. M. Joder-Ohlenbusch and J. Grove, in: Enzyme-Activated Irreversible Inhibitors (N. Seiler, M. J. Jung and J. Koch-Weser, eds.), p. 43, Elsevier-North-Holland Biomedical Press, Amsterdam, 1978.
238   G. D. Luk, G. Goodwin, L. J. Marton and S. B. Baylin: Proc. Natl. Acad. Sci. USA 78, 2355 (1981).
239   G. D. Luk, M. D. Abeloff, P. P. McCann, A. Sjoerdsma and S. B. Baylin: Cancer Res. 46, 1849 (1986).
240   P. S. Sunkara, S. B. Baylin and G. D. Luk, in: Inhibition of Polyamine Metabolism (P. P. McCann, A. E. Pegg and A. S. Sjoerdsma, eds.), p. 121, Academic Press, Orlando, 1987.
241   N. Seiler, C. Danzin, N. J. Prakash and J. Koch-Weser, in: Enzyme-Activated Irreversible Inhibitors (N. Seiler, M. J. Jung and J. Koch-Weser, eds.), p. 55, Elsevier-North Holland Biomedical Press, Amsterdam, 1978.
242   N. J. Prakash, P. J. Schechter, P. S. Mamont, J. Grove, J. Koch-Weser and A. Sjoerdsma: Life Sci. 26, 181 (1980).
243   P. S. Sunkara, N. J. Prakash, G. D. Mayer and A. Sjoerdsma: Science 219, 851 (1983).
244   G. D. Luk and S. B. Baylin: Cancer Res. 46, 1844 (1986).
245   N. Claverie and P. S. Mamont: Cancer Res. 49, 4466 (1989).
246   C. Danzin and P. S. Mamont, in: Inhibition of Polyamine Metabolism (P. P. McCann, A. E. Pegg and A. Sjoerdsma, eds.), p. 141, Academic Press, Orlando, 1987.
247   P. J. Schechter, J. L. R. Barlow and A. Sjoerdsma, in: Inhibition of Polyamine Metabolism (P. P. McCann, A. E. Pegg and A. Sjoerdsma, eds.), p. 345, Academic Press, Orlando, 1987.

248 H. M. Juillard, G. Tell, P. J. S. Schechter, J. Grove, J. Koch-Weser and E. Grosshans: Br. J. Dermatol. 105 (Suppl. 20), 33 (1981).
249 J. Hessels, A. W. Kingma, H. Keij, G. A. van den Berg and F. A. J. Muskiet: Int. J. Cancer 43, 1155 (1989).
250 N. Seiler, S. Sarhan, C. Grauffel, R. Jones, B. Knödgen and J. P. Moulinoux: Cancer Res. 50, 5077 (1990).
251 J. P. Moulinoux, F. Darcel, V. Quemener, R. Havouis and N. Seiler: Anticancer Res. 11, 175 (1991).
252 N. Seiler, in: Progress in Polyamine Research (V. Zappia and A. E. Pegg, eds.), p. 127, Plenum Press, New York (1988).
253 P. Bey, F. N. Bolkenius, N. Seiler and P. Casara: J. Med. Chem. 28 (1985).
254 M. Field, J. B. Block, V. T. Oliverio and D. P. Rall: Cancer Res. 24, 1939 (1964).
255 J. B. Block, M. Field and V. T. Oliverio: Cancer Res. 24, 1947 (1964).
256 D. L. Kramer, B. Paul and C. W. Porter: Cancer Res. 45, 2512 (1985).
257 M. Siimes, P. Seppänen, L. Alhonen-Hongisto and J. Jänne: Int. J. Cancer 28, 567 (1981).
258 R. P. Warrell, C. J. Coorley and J. H. Burchenal: Cancer Chemother. Pharmacol. 11, 134 (1983).
259 T. A. W. Splinter and J. C. Romijn: Eur. J. Cancer Clin. Oncol. 22, 61 (1986).
260 H. W. Herr, R. P. Warrel and J. H. Burchenal: Urology 28, 508 (1986).
261 V. A. Levin, M. C. Chamberlain, M. D. Prados, A. K. Choucair, M. S. Berger, P. Silver, M. Seager, P. H. Gutin, R. L. Davis and C. B. Wilson: Cancer Treat. Rep. 71, 459 (1987).
262 R. B. Natale, K. Meyer and A. Forastiere: Proc. Am. Soc. Clin. Oncol. 4, 137 (1985).
263 P. S. Sunkara, N. J. Prakash, G. D. Mayer and A. Sjoerdsma: Science 219, 851 (1983).
264 M. Talpaz, K. Plager, J. Quesada, R. Benjamin, H. Kantarjian and J. Gutterman: Eur. J. Clin. Oncol. 22, 685 (1986).
265 E. T. Creagan, D. L. Ashmann, H. J. Long and D. J. Schaid: Amer. J. Clin. Oncol. 13, P218 (1990).
266 M. Takigawa, A. K. Verma, R. C. Simsian and R. K. Boutwell: Biochem. Biophys. Res. Commun. 105, 969 (1982).
267 C. E. Weeks, A. L. Herman, F. R. Nelson and T. J. Slaga: Proc. Natl. Acad. Sci. USA 79, 6028 (1982).
268 A. N. Kingsnorth, W. W. King, K. A. Diekema, P. P. McCann, J. S. Ross and A. R. Malt: Cancer Res. 43, 2545 (1983).
269 J. Rozhin, P. S. Wilson, A. W. Bull and N. D. Nigro: Cancer Res. 44, 3226 (1984).
270 Y. Homma, S. Ozono, I. Numata, J. Seidenfeld and R. Oyasu: Cancer Res. 45, 648 (1985).
271 J. R. Fozard and N. J. Prakash: Arch. Pharmacol. 28, 1 (1982).
272 H. J. Thompson, Z. D. Meeker, E. J. Herbst, A. M. Ronan and R. Minocha: Cancer Res. 45, 1170 (1985).
273 N. Kanatani, K. Nishioka, T. Morita, Y. Morita, F. Takeuchi, K. Matsuta, Y. Nishida and T. Miyamoto: Cancer Res. 44, 4262 (1984).
274 C. J. Bacchi and P. P. McCann, in: Inhibition of Polyamine Metabolism (P. P. McCann, A. E. Pegg and A. Sjoerdsma, eds.), p. 317, Academic Press, Orlando, 1987.
275 C. J. Bacchi, H. C. Nathan, S. H. Hutner, P. P. McCann and A. Sjoerdsma: Science 210, 332 (1980).
276 P. P. McCann, C. J. Bacchi, A. B. Clarkson Jr., J. R. Seed, H. C. Nathan, B. O. Amole, S. H. Hutner and A. Sjoerdsma: Med. Biol. 59, 434 (1981).

277   E. Karbe, M. Böttger, P. P. McCann, A. Sjoerdsma and E. K. Freitas: Tro-
      penmed. Parasitol. 33, 161 (1982).
278   H. C. Nathan, C. J. Bacchi, S. H. Hutner, D. Rescigno, P. P. McCann and
      A. Sjoerdsma: Biochem. Pharmacol. 30, 3010 (1981).
279   C. J. Bacchi, T. Livingston, M. Saric, A. R. Njogu, H. C. Nathan, G. Valla-
      dares, P. D. Sayer and A. B. Clarkson: Antimicrob. Agents Chemother. 34,
      1183 (1990).
280   P. J. Schechter and A. Sjoerdsma, in: Enzymes as Targets for Drug Design
      (M. G. Palfreyman, P. P. McCann, W. Lovenberg, J. G. Temple, Jr., and A.
      Sjoerdsma, eds.), p. 201, Academic Press, Orlando, 1989.
281   F. Kierszenbaum, J. J. Wirth, P. P. McCann and A. Sjoerdsma: Proc. Natl.
      Acad. Sci. USA 84, 4278 (1987).
282   M. T. Cushion, D. Stanforth, M. J. Linke, P. D. Walzer: Antimicrob.
      Agents Chemother. 28, 796 (1985).
283   A. B. Clarkson Jr., D. E. Williams and C. Rosenberg: Antimicrob. Agents
      Chemother. 32, 1158 (1988).
284   A. Sjoerdsma, in: Proceedings of the 10th International Congress of
      Pharmacology (M. J. Rand and C. Raper, eds.), p. 643, Elsevier, Amster-
      dam, 1987.
285   L. Gradoni, M. Gramiccia, M. A. Iorio and S. Orsini: Farmaco (Pavia) 44,
      1157 (1989).
286   K. Nakashima, H. Hibasami, T. Tsukada and S. Maekawa: Eur. J. Med.
      Chem. 22, 553 (1987).
287   L. Marton: Pharmac. Therap. 32, 183 (1987).
288   C. W. Porter and R. J. Bergeron, in: Progress in Polyamine Research (V.
      Zappia and A. E. Pegg, eds.), p. 677, Plenum Press, New York, 1988.
289   C. W. Porter, B. Ganis, T. Vinson, L. J. Marton, D. L. Kramer and R. J.
      Bergeron: Cancer Res. 46, 6279 (1986).
290   C. W. Porter, J. McManis, R. A. Casero and R. J. Bergeron: Cancer Res. 47,
      2821 (1987).
291   M. L. Edwards, N. J. Prakash, D. M. Stemerick, S. P. Sunkara, A. J. Bitonti,
      G. F. Davis, J. A. Dumont and P. Bey: J. Med. Chem. 33, 1369 (1990).
292   K. Igarashi, K. Kashigawi, J. Fukuchi, Y. Isobe, S. Otomo and A. Shira-
      hata: Biochem. Biophys. Res. Commun. 172, 715 (1990).
293   N. Seiler, G. Daune, F. N. Bolkenius and B. Knödgen: Int. J. Biochem. 21,
      425 (1989).

Potassium channel openers: Airway pharmacology and clinical possibilities in asthma

By David Raeburn and Jan-Anders Karlsson

Rhône-Poulenc Rorer Ltd., Dagenham Research Centre, Dagenham, Essex RM10 7XS, England

1   Introduction

Asthma is a common disease worldwide, generally affecting 5–10% of the population, and its incidence is, unfortunately, still on the increase. This is despite intensive research into its pathophysiology and the development of several new therapeutic agents. The clinical symptoms of asthma are very obvious and distressing yet we still have only a rudimentary picture of the pathophysiological mechanisms involved. Airway inflammation and hyperreactivity are characteristic features and, since they seem to correlate with the severity of the disease, asthma is now widely regarded as an inflammatory disease [1–3]. Consequently, research into the physiology and pharmacology of airway smooth muscle and the role of bronchodilator drugs has attracted comparatively less interest in recent years. However, the importance of controlling airway smooth muscle contractility to improve airflow and so provide immediate, symptomatic relief for the asthmatic patient is still vital and indeed the bronchodilators remain the first line therapy [3].

Bronchodilators widely used in clinical practice belong to one of three groups: β_2-adrenoceptor agonists (salbutamol, terbutaline), methylxanthines (theophylline) or muscarinic cholinoceptor antagonists (ipratropium bromide). Compounds modifying airway smooth muscle contractility via novel mechanisms of action and with distinct advantages over currently used drugs are now being sought. Possibly the most encouraging approach to date has been with the development of agents which modify plasmalemmal potassium ion (K^+) channel function. Cromakalim and related K^+ channel openers (KCOs) act to increase K^+ conductance [4, 5], the consequence of this being a reduction in smooth muscle contractility.

Akasaka *et al.* [6] demonstrated that asthmatic airways exhibit considerable electrical excitability compared with normal airways *in vivo* and subsequently it has been suggested [7] that the airway hyperreactivity associated with asthma may be a consequence of a partial blockade of K^+ channels in the smooth muscle plasmalemma. The possibility thus exists that compounds which open K^+ channels (and hence reduce cell excitability) may act not only as bronchodilators but also to reduce airway hyperreactivity and inflammation. This chapter will review the pharmacology of compounds acting via modulation of K^+

channel function at various targets in the respiratory tract and discuss their potential as novel anti-asthma drugs.

2   Potassium channels in airway smooth muscle

In electrical terms, airway smooth muscle cells are relatively quiescent and spontaneous or depolarization-induced action potential discharge is not commonly seen. This electrical stability of the tissue is thought to be the result of membrane rectifying behaviour where membrane *depolarization* (produced by the inward Ca^{2+} current) is limited by the activation of an outward, *hyperpolarizing,* current carried by K^+ through specific K^+ channels in the plasmalemma. In the presence of agents such as tetraethylammonium (TEA) to prevent K^+ channel opening and thus block the rectifying K^+ current, it becomes possible to demonstrate action potential discharge and contraction in airway smooth muscle – see review by Kotlikoff [8].
In smooth muscle and other tissues several distinct K^+ channel types have been identified by their relative conductance, Ca^{2+}-dependence, voltage-dependence and the effects of "specific" channel blockers (4,5,8,8a]. In airway smooth muscle at least four types of K^+ channels so far have been implicated in regulating smooth muscle contractility:

a) delayed rectifier (K_V), conductance 5–60 pS, activated by membrane depolarization (above -45mV), inhibited by TEA and aminopyridines

b) large conductance, Ca^{2+}-activated (BK_{Ca}), conductance 100–250 pS, activated by membrane depolarization, inhibited by charybdotoxin, cromakalim (high $conc^n$), TEA, phenothiazines

c) small conductance, Ca^{2+}-activated (SK_{Ca}), conductance 6–14 pS, activated when $[Ca^{2+}]_i > 0.05 \mu M$, inhibited by apamin and methylene blue

d) ATP-sensitive (K_{ATP}), conductance 135 pS, activated by KCOs (cromakalim, RP 49356, pinacidil), inhibited by elevated $[ATP]_i$, sulphonylureas, phentolamine.

Of the above-mentioned channels the K_{ATP} channel is proving, at present, to be the most interesting and feasable target for pharmacological manipulation. The pharmacology of the compounds acting at this channel will now be discussed in more detail.

3   **ATP-sensitive potassium channels and potassium channel openers (KCOs)**

3.1   Basic pharmacology

A group of K^+ channels (K_{ATP}) with a novel pharmacological profile recently has been described [4,5,9]. The conductance of these channels is thought to be regulated by changes in the intracellular concentration of adenosine triphosphate (ATP), increased concentration of the nucleotide producing closure. K_{ATP} channels were first described in pancreatic B cells where they are involved in regulating insulin secretion. Subsequently, a similar type of channel has been demonstrated in many cell types including smooth muscle where activation (opening) of the channel leads to a relaxant response. Although nicorandil (which also possesses nitro vasodilator properties) was the first compound demonstrated to act on the K_{ATP} [9], cromakalim (BRL 34915) is generally regarded as the archetypal KCO. There is now a variety of compounds with differing chemical structures (Fig. 1) which relax smooth muscle by opening a purported K_{ATP} channel. It must, however, be emphasized that definitive proof of K_{ATP} homology

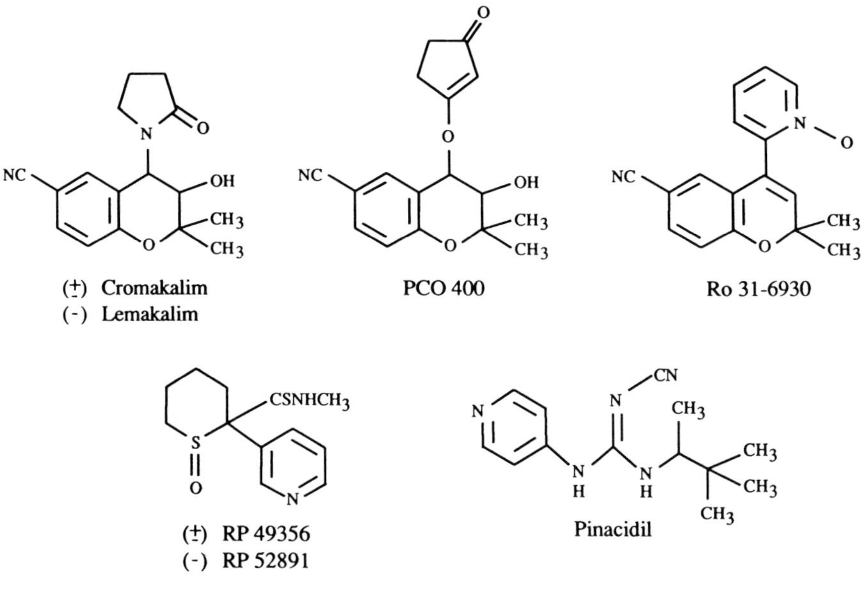

Figure 1
Structural diversity of some compounds which act by opening the K_{ATP} channel in airway preparations *in vitro* and *in vivo*.

between pancreatic B cells and smooth muscle cells is still lacking, especially electrophysiological studies and ATP sensitivity, and classification has been based largely on pharmacological sensitivity to the sulphonylureas (see below).

The precise mechanism by which KCOs relax smooth muscle is not clear. Initially it was proposed that opening the K_{ATP} channel hyperpolarized the smooth muscle plasmalemma towards the K^+ equilibrium potential to limit further depolarization and reduce the probability of opening of voltage-gated Ca^{2+} channels (VOCs). This in turn would prevent depolarization-induced Ca^{2+} entry and inhibit contraction. Evidence supporting this idea came from electrophysiological and ion flux studies demonstrating an increased K^+ conductance and efflux of $^{86}Rb^+$ (a marker of K^+ loss). However, it has since been shown that KCOs can relax electrically "silent" smooth muscle (where Ca^{2+} influx through VOCs plays only a minor role in regulating contraction) and that spontaneous mechanical activity in some vascular smooth muscle is suppressed at concentrations of KCOs which produce only very small hyperpolarizations and do not stimulate $^{86}Rb^+$ efflux [4,5]. Hence, an additional, intracellular action of KCOs to prevent Ca^{2+} release from and/or to inhibit refilling of intracellular Ca^{2+} stores after discharge of their contents has to be considered [4,5]. This may be particularly important in airway smooth muscle where influx of Ca^{2+} through VOCs may only play a minor role in producing contraction (see review by Fedan *et al.* [10]).

3.2   Possible sites/mechanisms of action of KCOs
          in the airways

There is now much evidence to demonstrate that K_{ATP} can regulate airway smooth muscle contractility. The principal determinant for inhibition or reversal of smooth muscle contraction is a reduction in the free cytosolic Ca^{2+} concentration ($[Ca^{2+}]_i$) below a threshold value of approximately 0.1 μM [11]. This generally is achieved by inhibiting Ca^{2+} influx and/or stimulating Ca^{2+} removal by promoting intracellular sequestration or efflux. Several mechanisms are available to the cell to achieve this objective [11,12]. The question is at which cellular locus or loci do the KCOs act?

The standard criteria applied to identify a compound as a K_{ATP}-sensitive KCO is its ability to relax smooth muscle contracted with low

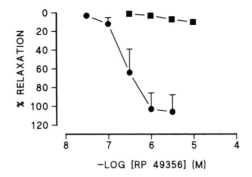

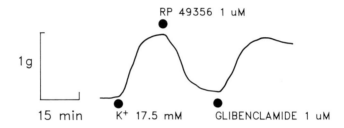

Figure 2
a. Reversal by RP 49356 of spasm induced by low (17.5 mM, ●) but not high (40 mM, ■) K⁺ in guinea-pig isolated trachealis (n = 7);
b. Representative trace showing the effect of glibenclamide on relaxation of K⁺ (17.5 mM)-induced tone by RP 49356.

(< 20 mM) but not with high (> 40 mM) concentrations of K^+ and the inhibition or reversal of this relaxation by a sulphonylurea such as glibenclamide or glipizide. An example of these effects in guinea-pig isolated trachealis is shown in Fig. 2 a, b). In airway smooth muscle *in vitro,* the relaxant actions of KCOs have been shown to be accompanied by an increase in negativity of the resting membrane potential (hyperpolarization) towards the calculated K^+ equilibrium potential and by a reduction in spontaneous slow wave activity [7, 13, 14]. The KCO-induced electrical changes also are inhibited by the sulphonylureas [13, 14]. Unlike TEA which, by blocking K^+ conductance at the K_V and BK_{Ca} channels, can produce action potential discharge, membrane depolarization, Ca^{2+} influx and contraction of airway smooth muscle, glibenclamide alone does not produce any significant changes in resting membrane potential or in contractility. This suggests that the K_{ATP}

may be closed under basal conditions [13,15]. It is likely, based on these findings, that K_{ATP} does not play a role in regulating electrical events in resting airway smooth muscle cells.

In radiolabelled ion flux studies in guinea-pig and bovine isolated trachealis cromakalim and pinacidil (bovine only) have been shown to promote $^{86}Rb^+$ and/or $^{42}K^+$ efflux [7,16–18] which can be inhibited by glibenclamide [17,18]. This lends further support to a role for K_{ATP} channel opening in the relaxant actions of these compounds.

In airway smooth muscle relaxant responses to cromakalim are unaffected by apamin [7] suggesting no involvement of the SK_{Ca} channel. Berry *et al.* [14] failed to demonstrate BK_{Ca} opening with cromakalim (but see section 5.3) or RP 49356. Additionally, the BK_{Ca} channel inhibitor charybdotoxin did not significantly inhibit responses to cromakalim or pinacidil [19]. Indeed, if anything, charybdotoxin augmented the relaxation seen with cromakalim. These findings argue against opening of Ca^{2+}-activated K^+ channels in the smooth muscle relaxant actions of cromakalim and other, similar, KCOs.

KCOs do not appear to produce airway smooth muscle relaxation by increasing the cyclic nucleotide content within the cell. No increase in cAMP or cGMP was seen in airway preparations following treatment with cromakalim or RP 49356 and neither compound was able to potentiate the effects of forskolin [14, 20, 21]. Pinacidil and cromakalim do not appear to be inhibitors of phosphodiesterase activity [14,22]. Experiments using "skinned" trachealis muscle indicate that cromakalim has no direct effect on the contractile proteins [7]. KCOs do not appear to act directly with VOCs since no effect on Ca^{2+}-induced contractions in depolarized tissues was seen [23].

While there is strong evidence to support the claims that the KCOs are acting at an airway smooth muscle plasmalemmal K_{ATP}, this mechanism does not explain all their smooth muscle relaxant actions in the airways. A notable example being their ability *in vivo* to prevent initiation of contraction (see section 5.1) which presumably involves an action against the mobilization of intracellular Ca^{2+} and which would not be expected to be affected by a hyperpolarization-induced reduction in voltage-dependent Ca^{2+} influx. Lemakalim (BRL 38227, the active $(-)$ enantiomer of cromakalim) has been shown to inhibit the release of Ca^{2+} from intracellular stores in rabbit airway smooth muscle cells in culture [24]. Some preliminary evidence also exists to suggest that RP 49356 but not cromakalim may additionally stimulate

Na$^+$/K$^+$ ATPase (which also produces hyperpolarization) [23] to relax airway smooth muscle.

4   KCOs and airway function *in vitro*
4.1   Smooth muscle relaxation; pre- and post-junctional actions

In animal airway preparations *in vitro,* several KCOs including cromakalim [7,13,15,20,21,25,26], RP 49356 [15,21,23,26], Ro 31–6930 [27], pinacidil [28] and PCO 400 [29] have been shown to have airway smooth muscle relaxant properties. As previously indicated, the KCOs generally are able to relax tissues under basal tone and reverse spasm induced by low concentrations of many different spasmogens and the effects are concentration-dependent. The degree of smooth muscle relaxation produced approximates to that seen with the β-adrenoceptor agonists but at approximately 30-fold higher concentrations (Fig. 3). The KCOs are notably less potent at reversing spasm induced by high concentrations of spasmogens and are virtually unable to prevent the initiation of the contractile response, i.e. they have spasmolytic but only poor antispasmogenic properties *in vitro*. This, however, is not the case *in vivo* (see section 5.1). Interestingly, the organic Ca^{2+} entry blockers (CEBs, e.g. verapamil, nifedipine), the β-adrenoceptor agonists and the methylxanthines also are considerably more potent at reversing than at inhibiting contractile responses to mediators in the guinea-pig trachea *in vitro* and their efficacy is like-

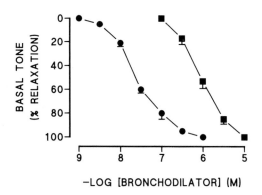

Figure 3
Comparison of potencies of RP 49356 (■) and salbutamol (●) in guinea-pig isolated trachealis (n = 10).

wise dependent on the degree of contraction [10, 30]. The spasmolytic effects of the KCOs can in part be explained by a hyperpolarization-induced inhibition of voltage-dependent Ca^{2+} entry since the maintained phase of the contractile response in airway smooth muscle may involve Ca^{2+} influx (see Raeburn and Brown [15]). However, the channel inhibited seems to be different from the VOCs blocked by the CEBs since the latter group of drugs do not relax tissues under basal tone and are significantly more potent against high K^+ than mediator-induced contractions of the trachea [10, 15, 31].

Pre-junctional effects of KCOs on airway smooth muscle contractility *in vitro* have also been examined. Pre-ganglionic stimulation of vagal nerves produced a cromakalim-sensitive increase in contractility [32]. The effect was considered to reflect a KCO-induced reduction in neurotransmitter release. A complementary study [33] has suggested that cromakalim may inhibit ganglionic transmission without altering post-ganglionic neurotransmitter release. Recently, Good and Hamilton [34] have shown a preferential inhibitory action at a prejunctional site against cholinergic- and noncholinergic-induced contraction of guinea-pig isolated bronchus. The most potent effects were seen with lemakalim. Pinacidil and RP 52891 demonstrated a similar degree of selectivity but were approximately 10-fold less potent. The antagonism of the effects of lemakalim by glibenclamide suggest an action at a K_{ATP} channel.

4.2   Human airway smooth muscle studies

A few studies have now examined the action of KCOs in human airway smooth muscle *in vitro*. Cromakalim, lemakalim and PCO 400 relax human bronchial muscle under basal conditions and after it has been contracted with histamine, carbachol and neurokinin A [29, 35–37]. As was the case in the animal studies, the relaxant effects of lemakalim were antagonized by glibenclamide indicating the involvement of K_{ATP} channels. The relaxation produced was significantly greater than that seen with verapamil and therefore the KCO must be acting at a separate site. In addition to inhibition of inward Ca^{2+} transport across the plasmalemma the KCOs could perhaps act to sequester Ca^{2+} from the cytosol [36, 37]. Human bronchial muscle has a greater sensitivity to KCOs when compared to the guinea-pig trachealis, and this difference is especially marked when considering spasm induced by muscarinic cholinoceptor agonists. These data reinforce the importance of potential species differences.

5   KCOs and airway function *in vivo*
5.1   Smooth muscle relaxation: Pre- and post-junctional effects

In the anaesthetized guinea pig cromakalim, lemakalim, pinacidil, RP 49356, RP 52891, Ro 31–6930 and PCO 400 have been shown to antagonize bronchospasm induced by mediators such as histamine,

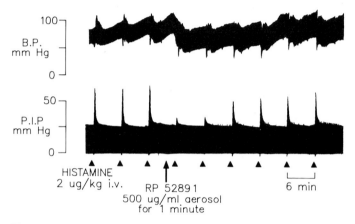

Figure 4
Representative traces showing the effect of RP 52891 on histamine-induced bronchospasm and on mean arterial blood pressure in the anaesthetized guinea pig.

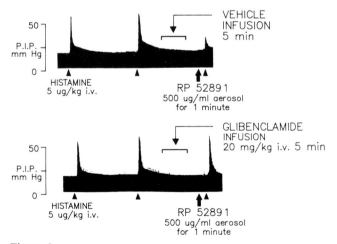

Figure 5
Inhibition by glibenclamide infusion of RP 52891-induced reduction in histamine-induced bronchospasm in the anaesthetized guinea pig.

5-hydroxytryptamine and antigen as well as by cholinergic and non-cholinergic nerve stimulation [22, 25, 27, 29, 35, 38–43]. A typical sample trace with RP 52891 is shown in Fig. 4. The smooth muscle relaxant effects are seen following administration of the KCOs by the oral, intravenous and aerosol routes and are inhibited by glibenclamide [38] and see Fig. 5. KCOs most readily prevent spasm induced by histamine and 5-hydroxytryptamine with little or no effect on responses to acetylcholine or substance P. This mediator-dependency shown by the KCOs was unexpected since it is less evident in guinea-pig or human airway preparations *in vitro*. It remains to be shown whether this property of the KCOs *in vivo* in confined to the guinea pig.

KCOs are potent relaxants of vascular smooth muscle and systemic administration produces a dose-related hypotensive effect which accompanies the inhibition of bronchospasm. However, aerosol administration may separate bronchial and vascular actions and indeed inhaled lemakalim was shown selectively to produce bronchodilation in the guinea pig [38]. A similar separation of airway from vascular events can be seen with RP 52891 (Fig. 6).

In studies in conscious animals [25, 38] cromakalim (2.5 mg/kg orally) and cromakalim and lemakalim (0.125 to 2 mg/ml inhalation) protected against histamine and antigen-induced convulsive cough. Lemakalim was twice as potent as cromakalim. RP 49356 (Raeburn

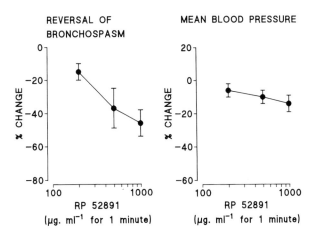

Figure 6
Relative potency of aerosolized RP 52891 on histamine-induced bronchospasm and on mean arterial blood pressure in the anaesthetized guinea pig (n = 5).

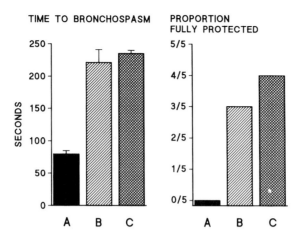

Figure 7
Effect of a single administration (2.5 mg/kg, p. o.) or repeated administration (2.5 mg/ kg, p. o. daily for 7 days) of RP 52891 on histamine-induced dyspnoea in the conscious guinea pig. In the single dose study the KCO was given 60 min before histamine challenge. In the repeated dose study the last dose of KCO was given 60 min before histamine challenge (n = 5). A, vehicle control; B, RP 52891 single dose; C, RP 52891 repeat dose.

unpublished) and RP 52891 [42] confer similar protection to that seen with cromakalim. There is no evidence for the development of tachyphylaxis, animals pretreated with RP 52891 for 7 days showed the same level of protection seen after a single oral dose (Fig. 7).

Taken together, the *in vivo* data clearly demonstrate that KCOs protect against mediator-induced bronchoconstriction. This contrasts with *in vitro* data where the compounds are poorly active if given before the constrictor challenge. β-adrenoceptor agonists and xanthine bronchodilators behave similarly so the implications of these findings remain speculative.

5.2   Anti-inflammatory properties of KCOs:
Neurogenic inflammation and microvascular leakage

It has been proposed [44] that release of peptide mediators (e. g. tachykinins) from capsaicin-senstive sensory nerve endings by an axon reflex may be important in producing airway inflammation in asthma. Changes produced by tachykinins such as substance P and neurokinin A include bronchospasm, increased secretory activity and oedema. These effects may be augmented by the actions of the co-released vasodilator substance calcitonin gene-related peptide. This nervous pathway (the non-adrenergic non-cholinergic system, NANC) is particularly well developed in rodents and studies investigating these NANC effects mostly have been carried out these species.

There is now some convincing evidence that *in vivo* cromakalim [40,41] and RP 49356 and its active (−) enantiomer RP 52891 [40,42] preferentially inhibit bronchospasm induced by cholinergic and excitatory NANC (eNANC) nerve stimulation compared with bronchospasm of a similar magnitude induced by the exogenous application of the respective putative neurotransmitters acetylcholine and substance P. Lemakalim appears to be the most selective of the compounds studied so far being about twenty times more potent as an inhibitor of eNANC neurogenic bronchospasm than of substance P-induced bronchoconstriction (Lewis and Raeburn unpublished). These observations indicate that KCOs may selectively act prejunctionally to inhibit neurotransmitter release.

Another index of inflammatory changes in the lung is the presence of plasma proteins in airway tissues and in the airway lumen (see review by Persson [45]) as a result of plasma leakage from the bronchial blood vessels. Plasma leakage can be induced by many mediators (including antigen) and by vagal nerve stimulation in the guinea pig. Inhaled cromakalim inhibited vagal- but not antigen-induced leakage

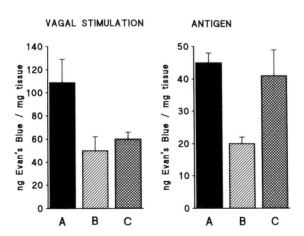

Figure 8
Comparison of the effects of cromakalim and salbutamol on microvascular leakage in intra pleural airways induced by vagal stimulation or antigen (OA)-inhalation in the anaesthetized guinea pig (n = 5,7). A, vehicle control; B, salbutamol (50 μg/ml/1 min inhalation); C, cromakalim (500 μg/ml/1 min inhalation).

(Fig. 8), supporting the view that KCOs selectively inhibit neurotransmitter release. Thus, the selective inhibition of the release of pro-inflammatory transmitters clearly points to potential anti-inflammatory properties in the KCOs. The significance of these actions to asthma in man remain to be established. More studies are required in this area.

5.3   Effects of KCOs in animal models of airway hyperreactivity

As indicated earlier (see Introduction) K^+ channel blockade may be implicated in the development of airway hyperreactivity in experimental animals and in man [6, 7]. While this is an attractive hypothesis no conclusive evidence is available at present. The effects of KCOs have been examined in several models of airway hyperreactivity in animals both *in vitro* and *in vivo*. Lemakalim was able to prevent sephadex bead-induced hyperreactivity to carbachol but not to 5-hydroxy-

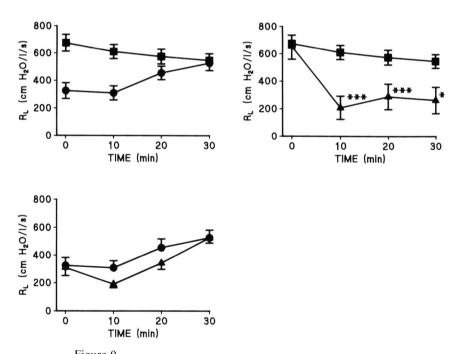

Figure 9
Effect of PCO 400 on responses to histamine (1.8 μg/kg, i. v.) given at 10-min intervals in normoreactive and hyperreactive guinea pigs *in vivo* ●, normoreactive control; ■, hyperreactive control; ▲, PCO 400 (0.1 mg/kg i. v.) redrawn from data from [43].

tryptamine in rat lung parenchymal strips *in vitro* [46]. *In vivo,* cromakalim [43, 47] and PCO 400 [43] have been shown to inhibit and/or reverse hyperreactivity induced by PAF (both compounds), isoprenaline and immune complex (PCO 400) (Fig. 9). The anti-hyperreactive
effects of PCO 400 were obtained at reportedly sub-bronchodilator
doses [43] and were antagonized by glibenclamide. Interestingly,
neither cromakalim nor PCO 400 had an effect on the concomitant
eosinophil accumulation in the lung.

A second type of K^+ channel also may be involved in the development
of airway hyperreactivity in the rat *in vitro*. In this model it has been
demonstrated [48–50] that sub-contractile concentrations of TEA produce airway smooth muscle hyperreactivity to cooling, 5-hydroxy-
tryptamine and acetylcholine. This, presumably, as a result of the
blockade of BK_{Ca} channels.

Chand *et al.* [50] also have reported that in this model cromakalim at
high concentration (100 μM) inhibited TEA-induced hyperreactivity
to cooling and to acetylcholine. At this high concentration it is
claimed that cromakalim is able also to activate the BK_{Ca} channels
(but see [14]), and it is therefore difficult to ascertain its mechanism of
action.

6   Are *β*-adrenoceptor agonists KCOs? Actions at BK_{Ca}

It is now well established that airway smooth muscle relaxation induced by *β*-adrenoceptor agonists is associated with activation of
adenylyl cyclase and an increase in cyclic adenosine 3′,5′ monophosphate (cAMP) content which, in turn, stimulates the activity of the
cAMP-dependent protein kinase (A-kinase). This produces relaxation
as a result of the phosphorylation of a number of target proteins – see
review by Giembycz and Raeburn [51].

Recently, Kume *et al.* [52] have presented electrophysiological evidence in rabbit isolated tracheal myocytes to suggest that opening
a K^+ channel (BK_{Ca}) may be involved in the relaxant actions of the *β*-
adrenoceptor agonist isoprenaline. Extracellular application of isoprenaline at a physiologically relevant concentration (0.2 μM) significantly increased the probability of Ca^{2+}-activated K^+ channel opening. The effect was further enhanced by the application of the protein
phosphatase inhibitor okadaic acid which prevents the inactivation of
A-kinase. The isoprenaline-induced effects were inhibited by pro-

pranolol (suggesting a specific action at β-adrenoceptors) and were dependent on the presence of extracellular Ca^{2+}. Like isoprenaline, application of A-kinase (in the presence of cAMP, ATP) increased the probability of K^+ channel opening and this effect also was augmented by okadaic acid. The authors [52] concluded that activation of a Ca^{2+}-activated K^+ channel may be an important mechanism of action for bronchodilator agents which act via stimulation of A-kinase.

Further evidence implicating the BK_{Ca} channel in the relaxant responses subsequent to activation of A-kinase has recently been published [19]. Relaxant responses to the β-adrenoceptor agonists isoprenaline and salbutamol and to the cAMP analogue di-butyryl-cAMP in guinea-pig trachealis *in vitro* were markedly inhibited by pretreatment of the tissues with the selective BK_{Ca} channel blocker charybdotoxin. These findings add weight to the previous electrophysiological findings [52] and again suggest a role for BK_{Ca} opening in mediating the relaxant responses to agents which act by stimulation of A-kinase. This study additionally demonstrated a similar antagonism by charybdotoxin of responses to sodium nitroprusside implicating an action of G-kinase on the BK_{Ca} channel.

Taken together, these studies [19, 52] suggest that a hitherto unexpected action may, at least partly, explain the mechanism of β-adrenoceptor-induced bronchodilation. Thus, it may not be inappropriate to refer to these important anti-asthma compounds as K^+ channel openers.

7   Clinical pharmacology: Anti-asthma actions of KCOs

To date, very few clinical studies have been performed to determine the therapeutic potential of KCOs as anti-asthma compounds. The studies which have been conducted have examined the effect of cromakalim (usually administered orally) on histamine-induced bronchospasm in non-asthmatic volunteers and on the decline in lung function seen during the early hours of the morning ("morning dipping") which is associated with nocturnal asthma [53].

7.1   Bronchodilator studies

In randomized, double-blind, placebo-controlled, crossover trials, Baird *et al.* [54] and Williams *et al.* [55] demonstrated that cromakalim at a dose of 2 mg p.o., which did not produce bronchodilatation *per se*, provided significant protection against challenge with a provocation concentration of histamine which caused a 40% fall in partial expiratory flow rate (PC_{40}). The effects seen were significantly greater than with placebo and compared favourably with the protective effects of salbutamol (4 mg p.o.). Cromakalim reduced diastolic blood pressure and increased heart rate. However, these cardiovascular effects were similar to those produced by salbutamol [54].

Currently clinical trials with lemakalim and pinacidil are underway but no data is yet available [56, 57].

7.2   Nocturnal asthma

Since the prevention of morning dipping in nocturnal asthma is a highly desirable characteristic of novel anti-asthma drugs, compounds with a long duration of action enabling overnight control of symptoms are of great interest. Cromakalim and lemakalim have a prolonged plasma half-life of about 24 h in man [57–59] and several studies have now examined the potential benefit of KCOs in nocturnal asthma [55, 60–62]. When compared with placebo, a single dose of cromakalim (0.25 to 1.5 mg orally) given at 23.30 h at night significantly and dose-dependently attenuated the predicted fall in FEV_1 measured at 6.30 h the following morning. The maximum effect was seen at a dose of 0.5 mg [60, 61].

7.3   Potential for cardiovascular side effects

KCOs are potent relaxants of vascular smooth muscle *in vitro* and *in vivo* and initially were developed as anti-hypertensive agents. It is therefore important when considering the potential of KCOs in asthma to be aware of their concomitant effects on the cardiovascular system in man which, in this case, is to be considered an unwanted side effect.

In the studies in nocturnal asthma [60, 61] the effect of the KCOs on cardiovascular parameters is not clear. No significant effects of the KCO on blood pressure were reported [60, 61]. Yet, in a review of his earlier study the author states that the highest dose of cromakalim (1.5 mg) used reduced blood pressure and increased heart rate coincident with the improved FEV_1 seen the morning after dosing [63].

While no studies on the anti-asthmatic properties of cromakalim given by the inhaled route have been published so far, a recent report has examined its cardiovascular side effects following nebulized aerosol administration [64]. When inhaled in concentrations of 0.05 to 1 mg, cromakalim was without effect on blood pressure, heart rate, cardiac output or arterial O_2 saturation. While these findings point to a separation between cardiovascular and airway actions, concomitant measurement of lung function is required to establish purported airway selectivity.

The reportedly limited cardiovascular side effects of cromakalim suggests that normotensives are less sensitive than hypertensives to the blood pressure-lowering effects of the KCOs. Administration of the KCOs by the inhaled route may further separate the airway from the cardiovascular effects.

8   Conclusions

KCOs are a chemically diverse group of novel compounds which can relax airway smooth muscle contracted by different types of mediators. Interestingly, these compounds appear to be more potent and less dependent on the spasmogen used in human than in animal tissues. The profile of action of the KCOs differs from those of the β-adrenoceptor agonists, the methylxanthines and the CEBs. KCOs seem to act on the sulphonylurea-sensitive K_{ATP} channel but much remains to be discovered about their exact mechanisms of action. Cromakalim has been shown to inhibit bronchospasm induced by several mediators including histamine and to prevent "morning dipping" in asthmatics. Whether these actions can be explained by its smooth muscle relaxant properties or whether KCOs also possess anti-hyperreactive and anti-inflammatory properties remains to be established. There is no doubt that compounds which act to open the K_{ATP} channel merit further evaluation as anti-asthmatic agents.

References

1   R. Pauwells: Bronchial hyperresponsiveness, Blackwell Scientific Press, San Francisco 1987, p. 315.
2   N. C. Barnes and J. F. Costello: Br. Med. Bull. *43*, 445 (1987).
3   British Thoracic Society, Guidelines for the management of asthma in adults: I – chronic persistent asthma: Br. Med. J. *301*, 651 (1990).

4   N. S. Cook: Trends Pharmacol. Sci. *9*, 21 (1988).
5   U. Quast and N. S. Cook: Trends Pharmacol. Sci. *10*, 431 (1989).
6   K. Akasaka, K. Konno, Y. Ono, S. Mue, C. Abe, M. Kumagai and T. Ise: Tohoku J. Exp. Med. *117*, 55 (1975).
7   S. L. Allen, J. P. Boyle, J. Cortijo, R. W. Foster, G. P. Morgan and R. C. Small: Br. J. Pharmacol. *89*, 395 (1986).
8   M. I. Kotlikoff: Airway smooth muscle in health and disease, Plenum Press, New York 1989, p. 169.
8a F. Dreyer: Rev. Physiol. Biochem. Pharmacol. *115*, 93 (1990).
9   T. C. Hamilton and A. H. Weston: Gen. Pharmacol. *20*, 1 (1989).
10 J. S. Fedan, D. W. P. Hay and D. Raeburn: Current topics in pulmonary Pharmacology and toxicology, Elsevier, New York 1987, p. 53.
11 I. W. Rodger: Asthma: Basic mechanisms and clinical management, Academic Press, London 1988, p. 57.
12 D. Raeburn: Biologist *34*, 16 (1987).
13 M. A. Murray, J. P. Boyle and R. C. Small: Br. J. Pharmacol. *98*, 865 (1989).
14 J. L. Berry, K. R. F. Elliot, R. W, Foster, K. A. Green, M. A. Murray and R. C. Small: Pulm. Pharmacol. (1991) *4*, 91.
15 D. Raeburn and T. J. Brown: J. Pharmacol. Exp. Ther. *256*, 480 (1991).
16 K. A. Foster: Br. J. Pharmacol. *96*, 233P (1989).
17 P. R. Gater: Br. J. Pharmacol *98*, 660P (1989).
18 J. Longmore and A. H. Weston: Br. J. Pharmacol *98*, 804P (1989).
19 T. R. Jones, L. Charette, M. L. Garcia and G. J. Kaczorowski: J. Pharmacol. Exp. Ther. *255*, 697 (1990).
20 J. S. Gillespie and H. Sheng: Br. J. Pharmacol. *94*, 1189 (1988).
21 M. A. Murray, R. W. Foster and R. C. Small: Br. J. Pharmacol. *100*, 367P (1990).
22 P. P. K. Ho, R. D. Towner, M. Esterman and B. Bertsch: Eur. J. Pharmacol. *183*, 2132 (1990).
23 J. Sweetland and D. Raeburn: Br. J. Pharmacol. *98*, 882P (1989).
24 L. C. Chopra, C. H. C. Twort and J. P. T. Ward: Br. J. Pharmacol. *100*, 368P (1990).
25 J. R. S. Arch, D. R. Buckle, J. Bumstead, G. D. Clarke, J. F. Taylor and S. G. Taylor: Br. J. Pharmacol. *95*, 763 (1988).
26 T. J. Brown, J. Sweetland and D. Raeburn: Pflügers Arch. *414 (Suppl. 1)*, S188 (1989).
27 P. M. Paciorek, I. S. Cowlrick, R. S. Perkins and J. C. Taylor: Br. J. Pharmacol. *98*, 720P (1989).
28 J. E. Nielsen-Kudsk, S. Mellemkjaer, C. Siggaard and C. B. Nielsen: Eur. J. Pharmacol. *157*, 221 (1988).
29 I. D. Chapman: Agents Actions Suppl. (1990) in press.
30 J.-A. Karlsson and C. G. A. Persson: Br. J. Pharmacol. *74*, 73 (1981).
31 J. E. Nielsen-Kudsk, J.-A. Karlsson and C. G. A. Persson: Eur. J. Pharmacol. *128*, 33 (1986).
32 A. K. Hall and J. MacLagan: Br. J. Pharmacol. *95*, 792P (1988).
33 D. J. McCaig and B. de Jonckheere: Br. Pharmacol. *98*, 662 (1989).
34 D. M. Good and T. C. Hamilton: Br. J. Pharmacol. (1991) *102*, 336P.
35 S. G. Taylor, J. Bumstead, J. E. J. Morris, D. J. Shaw and J. F. Taylor: Br. J. Pharmacol. *95*, 795P (1988).
36 P. J. Barnes, C. L. Armour, L. Alouan, P. Johnson and J. L. Black: Thorax *45*, 308 (1990).
37 J. L. Black, C. L. Armour, P. R. A. Johnson, L. A. Alouan and P. J. Barnes: Am. Rev. Resp. Dis. *142*, 1384 (1990).
38 N. E. Bowring, J. F. Taylor, G. R. Francis and J. R. Arch: Br. J. Pharmacol. *98*, 805P (1989).

39   R. N. DeSouza, P. R. Gater and V. A. Alabaster: Br. J. Pharmacol. *98*, 803P (1989).

40   S. A. Lewis and D. Raeburn: Br. J. Pharmacol. *100*, 474P (1990).

41   M. Ichinose and P. J. Barnes: J. Pharmacol. Exp. Ther. *252*, 1207 (1990).

42   D. Raeburn: S. L. Underwood and S. A. Lewis: Thorax (1991) *46*, 294P.

43   I. D. Chapman, A. Kristersson, L. Mazzoni, B. Amsler and J. Morley: Br. J. Pharmacol. *102*, 335P (1991).

44   P. J. Barnes PJ: Lancet *i*, 242 (1986).

45   C. G. A. Persson: Lancet *ii*, 1126 (1986).

46   J. S. Ward, B. A. Spicer and S. G. Taylor: Br. J. Pharmacol. *100*, 369P (1990).

47   S. Sanjar, J. Morley, I. Chapman and M. Kings: Am. Rev. Resp. Dis. *139*, A467 (1989).

48   N. Chand, W. Diamantis and R. D. Sofia: Am. Rev. Resp. Dis. *139*, A327 (1989).

49   N. Chand, W. Diamantis and R. D. Sofia: Br. J. Pharmacol. *101*, 541 (1990).

50   N. Chand, R. Jakubicki, W. Diamantis and R. D. Sofia: Am. Rev. Resp. Dis. *141*, A657 (1990).

51   M. A. Giembycz and D. Raeburn: I. Auton. Pharmacol. *11*, 345 (1991).

52   H. Kume, A. Takai, H. Tokuno and T. Tomita: Nature *341*, 152 (1989).

53   P. J. Barnes: Practitioner *231*, 479 (1987).

54   A. Baird, T. C. Hamilton, D. H. Richards, T. Tasker and A. J. Williams: Br. J. Clin. Pharmacol. *25*, 114P (1988).

55   A. J. Williams, T. Vyce, D. J. Richards and T. Lee: NEJ Allergy Proc. *9*, 249 (1988).

56   J. Carlsen: Potassium Channels '90: Structure, modulation and clinical exploitation, I. B. C. Technical Services, London 1990.

57   S. G. Dilley: Potassium channels '90: Structure, modulation and clinical exploitation, I. B. C. Technical Services, London 1990.

58   B. E. Davies, D. Dierdorf, K. M. Eckl, W. H. Greb, G. Mellows and T. Thomsen: Br. J. Clin. Pharmacol. *20*, 136P (1988).

59   J. N. Bullman, T. S. Gill, A. C. Taylor and C. M. Kaye: Br. J. Clin. Pharmacol. (1991) in press.

60   A. J. Williams, A. Hopkirk, E. Lavender, T. Vyse, V. F. Chiew and T. H. Lee: Am. Rev. Resp. Dis. *139*, A140 (1989).

61   A. J. Williams, T. H. Lee, G. M. Cochrane, A. Hopkirk, T. Vyse, F. Chiew, E. Lavender, D. H. Richards, S. Owen, P. Stone, S. Church and A. A. Woodcock: Lancet *336*, 334 (1990).

62   S. Owen, S. Church, P. Stone, B. Bosch, S. Webster, E. Lavender, A. Williams and A. Woodcock: Thorax *44*, 852P (1989).

63   A. J. Williams: Potassium channel modulators: new drugs with novel mechanisms of action, IBC Symposium, London, December 1988.

64   A. J. Williams, P. Verden and E. Lavender: Eur. J. Pharmacol. *183*, 1045 (1990).

Antifungal chemotherapy – Are we winning?

By A. Polak and P. G. Hartman

F. Hoffmann-La Roche Ltd, 4002 Basel, Switzerland

1　Introduction

Medical mycology has always been somewhat overshadowed by bacteriology, and if judged simply by volume will never reach the status of its big sister in the field of infectious diseases. Nevertheless, fungal infections are of growing importance in the medical world of today, and they pose a unique set of problems both in a clinical setting and in the laboratory.

Various aspects of the chemotherapy of fungal diseases have been reviewed recently [1–5] and we shall not attempt to cover the same ground, but rather to identify and highlight the most pressing problems of today and of the next few years, to put them into perspective, and to assess how successfully they are being tackled by recent advances in the field. Finally, we shall look at what we can realistically expect in the future.

Fungal diseases divide themselves naturally into two major classes – dermatomycoses and gynecological infections, and deep mycoses. We have kept to this division, not for microbiological reasons but rather because the problems in the two areas are of a completely different order of magnitude. It can be said that today there are no major problems remaining in the field of dermatomycosis and vaginal candidosis. That is not to say that no difficulties are encountered in the treatment of individual cases, but thanks to the recent development of highly active, fungicidal agents with appropriate pharmacokinetic properties high success rates are obtainable. So we have restricted ourselves to reviewing the most recent innovations and few remaining problems in this area, despite its importance in terms of patient numbers and sales of antimycotics.

In the therapy of deep mycoses, by contrast, we are still struggling to overcome the old problems, while new problems are arriving with disturbing regularity. Progress has been made, but in this indication area one can with justification ask "Are we winning?". Comparison with the antibacterial field, where there is an enormous and steadily increasing choice of effective agents – almost as many as there are pathogens – serves to further underline the dearth of antimycotics.

The problems encountered in antifungal chemotherapy may be regarded as an interactive triangle, or perhaps more picturesquely as a devil's trident:

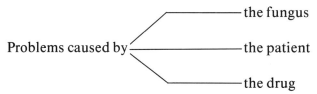

Problems caused by the fungus / the patient / the drug

The difficulty of killing the eukaryotic fungal cell without damaging the host is perhaps more akin to the problems of cancer chemotherapy than those of antibacterial treatment; and the ability of fungi to colonize and infect is awesome. At a recent congress, M. Rinaldi, a leading mycologist, likened human beings to walking Petri dishes, and he believes that there is no fungus left that cannot kill. The list of fungi causing deep mycosis is indeed growing rapidly.

The problem with the patient is that he is seldom only suffering from a fungal infection. The list of predisposing factors is long, and the mycosis is very often set against the complex background of an underlying disease and its treatment. AIDS has served to highlight the problem of immune depression, but there is an increasing number of cancer, leukemia, transplant, surgical and similar patients who are holding their own, only to become victims of opportunistic infection because of their weakened immune status. Indeed, the whole patient population is gradually changing and now requires even greater protection against infection.

The problem with the available antifungal drugs is that they all have problems. The superlative antifungal activity of amphotericin B (Amp B) against the agents of deep mycosis is unfortunately associated with a toxicity that would rule out its use were there a genuine alternative. The narrow spectrum and resistance problems of 5-flucytosine (5-FC) reduce its potential and confine its use to combination therapy, which is only just beginning to gain acceptance. The azoles, despite opening up a new era in antifungal chemotherapy, have not completely fulfilled their early promise. Their lack of fungicidal action, weakness against opportunistic pathogens and the occasional but well-documented occurrence of serious side effects and resistance have all served to dampen the enthusiasm for this class of compounds, and a truly safe across-the-board azole does not yet exist.

"Are we winning?" We hope that the following will provide food for thought and stimulate discussion of the problems that still exist in this field which presents a challenge from the molecular level to the clinic. To quote Dr. Rinaldi again, AIDS has been the eye-opener which has led to the feeling that mycotic infections could be the diseases of the future. Three congresses that have just taken place [6–8] show that the interest, application and ideas are there. These must now be converted into real progress before we can confidently give a positive answer to our question.

2   Dermatomycosis and vaginal candidosis
2.1   Dermatomycosis

The treatment of most forms of dermatomycosis is no longer a problem. Enormous improvement has been achieved since the time when various dyes were used for the treatment of dermatophytic infections. One of the first antibiotics active against dermatophytosis and onychomycosis was introduced in the year 1959 and is still on the market. This drug, griseofulvin, still has a place in the treatment of these diseases, but the era of the azoles has revolutionized the therapy of dermatomycosis. Not only is an enormous palette of topical agents available, there are also numerous galenic forms – tablets, creams, tinctures, sprays, shampoos, nail lacquer. Treatment schedules have become shorter and more acceptable. Once daily treatment has replaced twice or more daily, and the duration of therapy, originally as much as six months or even more, is now often as short as three weeks. There are obviously still difficulties in individual cases, but the only real problem remaining in the dermatomycotic field is that of nail infections, which still need long oral treatment (6–12 months) or surgical removal of the nail together with antifungal therapy. But even in this area there is real hope that two new chemical classes, the allylamines and the morpholine derivatives, will bring new treatment possibilities. We shall take one more look at griseofulvin, the patriarch of antifungal chemotherapy, and then examine the claims of its grandchildren, terbinafine and amorolfine, in connection with the therapy of dermatophytosis.

The imidazole and triazole derivatives will be considered only briefly in this connection, as there is a vast literature on their topical use. This class of antimycotic will be examined more closely in the section on

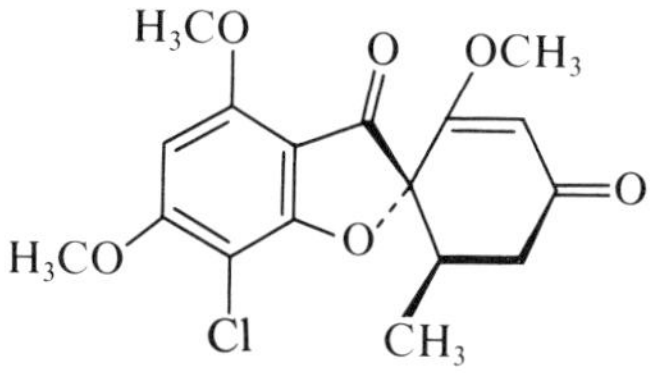

Griseofulvin

deep-seated mycosis, an area where there are still considerable problems to be solved.

Griseofulvin

Griseofulvin is an antibiotic produced by certain species of *penicillium*, particularly *P. griseofulvum*. It is active against various non-pathogenic fungi, but of those pathogenic to humans it inhibits only the dermatophytes (MIC 0.5–5 μg/ml).

The most evident effect of griseofulvin on sensitive fungi is a "curling" phenomenon. Under treatment the cell wall is changed, becoming abnormally soft and rigid at regular intervals. This pronounced distortion of the hyphae is associated with the fungistatic activity of the drug. It is fungicidal due to cell rupture. Griseofulvin has in fact no direct effect on the activity of enzymes synthesizing cell wall constituents, but inhibits microtubular formation in a dose-dependent manner, inducing arrest of mitosis in metaphase.

Griseofulvin interacts with the microtubuli of a variety of mammalian and fungal cells. Its specificity is based on the presence of a particular energy-dependent transport system which is lacking in resistant organisms. Spontaneously resistant strains of dermatophytes can be isolated in the laboratory, there is some primary resistance, and secondary resistance can be selected during therapy [9, 10]. Griseofulvin resistance as a cause for treatment failure or relapses is well established, and comparative studies on MIC values and chemotherapeutic response have shown that there is a sharp division between resistant and sensitive dermatophytes. However, the analysis of griseofulvin resistance is not without problems.

As an example, in one study of 43 cases of *T. rubrum* dermatomycosis of which 20 were treatment successes and 23 were failures, the mean MIC of the successfully treated strains was 1.1 μg/ml (0.1–2 μg/ml) and that of the resistant strains was 4.9 μg/ml (0.5–18 μg/ml) [9, 11].

Although this difference is statistically highly significant, it can only be measured using extremely standardized methods in laboratories with considerable experience in such in vitro testing. Thus although the appearance of resistant strains under therapy was recognized as a potential problem, whether it has had epidemiological consequences is uncertain because of a lack of reliable data. However, in the 30 years of experience with griseofulvin no evidence that the number of resistant strains were increasing has come from authors who routinely performed sensitivity testing [12]. Griseofulvin is still used for treatment of various types of dermatomycosis. If it is less used today, it is not due to an increase in resistance but rather to low efficacy and the incidence of side effects.

Since the introduction of griseofulvin in 1959 a whole host of topically active medicaments for the treatment of dermatophyte infections, as well as some systemically active drugs, has come onto the market. The coming of the azoles, the first of which was clotrimazole, represented a major advance. The advances that have been made since then have been in reducing the frequency and duration of application, which has not only reduced the discomfort of therapy, but has also improved patient compliance. Today the dermatologist can choose from at least 16 compounds from 4 chemical classes.

There are, however, two new classes of antimycotics which may well make an impact even in this crowded field. Although, like the azoles, they are both sterol biosynthesis inhibitors, they each have different targets on the pathway to ergosterol.

Allylamines

Terbinafine and its forerunner naftifine both possess in vitro antimycotic activity against a wide range of pathogen fungi. This activity is exceptionally high against dermatophytes (MIC 0.003–0.2 μg/ml).

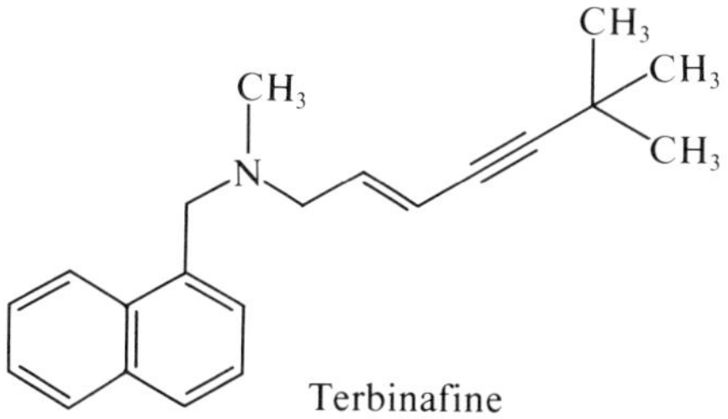

Terbinafine
(Sandoz, SF 86-327)

They are also fungicidal against dermatophytes, although only fungi-static against yeasts. Their primary mode of action is the inhibition of squalene epoxidase, an enzyme in the sterol biosynthesis pathway, leading to depletion of ergosterol and a concomitant accumulation of squalene in sensitive fungal species. There is a clear correlation between growth inhibition and degree of sterol biosynthesis inhibition, and a high specificity for the fungal enzyme. The fungicidal action seems not to be directly related to depletion of ergosterol, but rather to the high intracellular accumulation of squalene [13]. It may also be that the alteration of the sterol content of the membrane leads to a disruption of chitin synthesis. The cell wall of dermatophytes is composed to a greater extent of chitin than that of yeasts, which contain more glucan and mannan. Thus this secondary mode of action may explain the greater sensitivity of dermatophytes to this class of compounds. The mechanism of inhibition of the target enzyme at the molecular level has not yet been established.

Naftifine as a topical ointment and terbinafine applied orally in tablet form are both highly effective in the treatment of a range of dermatophytic infections, and terbinafine has also shown high success rates in the treatment of onychomycosis. The high efficacy of terbinafine may be due to its specific pharmacokinetic properties as it accumulates to high concentration in adipose tissue and skin [14, 15] and is only slowly metabolized and released from these sites with an elimination half-life on the order of 4–7 days. Due to this slow release drug levels are several fold (up to 10 times) higher than the serum levels after repeated dosing. Thus terbinafine has all the desired properties for the treatment of dermatophytosis: – It is fungicidal against dermatophytes and not only fungistatic, it has a high specificity for its target enzyme which leads to a low toxicity, and it is preferentially distributed to the target site of the infecting cells, the skin. Furthermore,

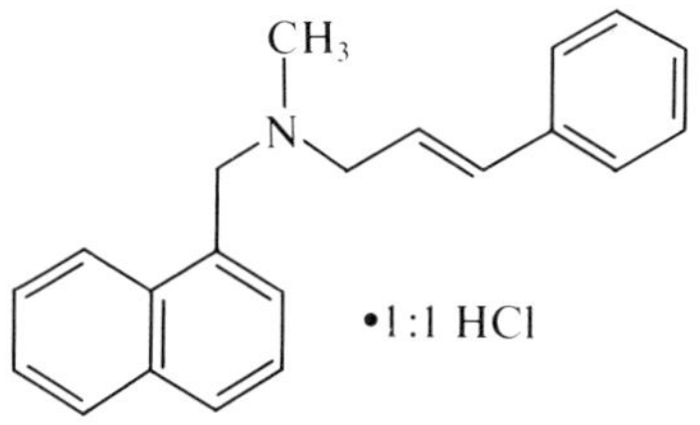

CH₃

•1:1 HCl

Naftitine•HCl

resistant mutants have not yet been described, either in the laboratory or during treatment.

Terbinafine also brings new possibilities to the treatment of onycho-mycosis, which is at the moment still unsatisfactory. 250 mg terbina-fine orally over 6 months for finger nails and for 12 months in the case of toe nails gave a response in clinical trials that was generally excel-lent, with success rates of over 90 % for finger nails and 80 % for toe nails. It was also well tolerated. In addition, terbinafine may give a new alternative for the treatment of nail dystrophy due to dermato-phytic infection [16]. At the recent ICAFC, H. Mieth [17] of Sandoz clearly showed that the fungicidal activity against dermatophytes de-monstrated in vitro has an important impact on therapy in humans. In clinical evaluation it was shown that the onset of mycological cure is very quick and the efficacy both in terms of mycological cure and dis-appearance of symptoms continues even after therapy has stopped.

Amorolfine

Amorolfine is a new morpholine antifungal, a class which is generally active against fungi pathogenic to plants, animals and humans. Amor-olfine has a broad antifungal spectrum including dermatophytes, yeasts, dimorphic fungi, dematiaceae and zygomycetes. It is inactive against *Aspergilli* but active against *Alternaria* and other molds. It is most active against dermatophytes with an MIC of 0.03 μg/ml (0.001–6.2 μg/ml), and is fungicidal against many species [18, 19]. Investigation of its mode of action showed that amorolfine has no in-fluence on the synthesis of RNA, DNA, protein and carbohydrate, but that it interferes with that of lipids, and in particular sterols. In all sensitive species membrane ergosterol is depleted in a time- and con-centration-dependent manner which correlates with growth inhibi-tion, and ignosterol, a Δ14-sterol, is accumulated. At high concentra-tions squalene is also accumulated in some species. Experiments with

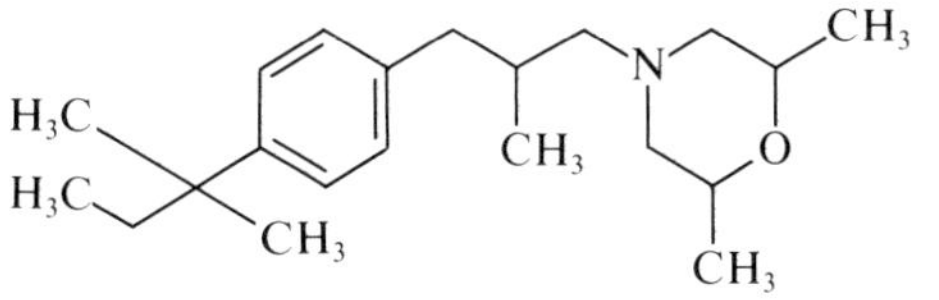

Amorolfine

crude cell extracts from *Saccharomyces cerevisiae* showed that amorolfine inhibits two steps in the pathway of ergosterol biosynthesis, the $\triangle14$-reductase and the $\triangle7$–$\triangle8$-isomerase with IC_{50} values of 2.93 μM and 0.0018 μM, respectively [19, 20].

Whether the inhibition of sterol biosynthesis is solely responsible for the antifungal action of morpholines such as amorolfine has been the subject of discussion. Recent work using fenpropimorph made elegant use of mutants of *S. cerevisiae* not only to provide strong evidence that this is indeed so, but to suggest that it is the lack of ergosterol rather than the accumulation of unusual sterols that causes cessation of growth [314].

However, electron microscopic studies show an abnormal accumulation of chitin in the membrane under amorolfine treatment, indicating that chitin synthesis is also disturbed. The cell wall increases in thickness, electron transparent areas appear in the cytoplasm and extracytoplasmic vesicles are formed and deposited in the cell wall. These are the same observations made in azole-treated cells, but it is not clear to what extent these phenomena are responsible for antifungal activity, or if they are also a result of ergosterol depletion of the membrane [21].

At the molecular level it has been hypothesized that the reactions of both the $\triangle14$-reductase and the $\triangle7$–$\triangle8$-isomerase lead to the formation of a carbonium ion high energy intermediate (at C14 in the reductase and C8 for the isomerase). The morpholinium ion which is present at physiological pH has electronic and structural similarities with this intermediate and may thus have a high affinity for the enzymes [19].

As is the case with terbinafine, it has proved impossible to select amorolfine-resistant mutants under laboratory conditions and none have been observed during clinical trials.

Amorolfine shows great promise as an agent for topical treatment of a variety of dermatomycoses, against which it exerts a fungicidal action. It has shown especially good cure rates in Tinea pedis and Tinea corporis, and is well tolerated. Persistence in the skin for two or three days after application has been measured, but no systemic absorption through the skin was found. Amorolfine also offers an effective topical treatment of onychomycosis. A 5 % nail lacquer applied over 6 months once or twice weekly has shown success rates of around 70 %. Thus amorolfine clearly provides an alternative which avoids the pos-

sible risks associated with oral treatment over the length of time necessary in this indication [22, 23].

It has always been a matter of contention whether one should burden
the system with an oral drug when effective topical treatment is available, and the availability of both amorolfine and terbinafine allows
for a choice of therapy. It would be worth investigating whether a
combination of the two would prove advantageous, especially in difficult cases, and if the duration of therapy could be reduced by such
means.

2.2   Vaginal candidosis

Vaginitis and vaginal discharge have been problems since antiquity.
The earliest report to associate a fungus with this condition was by
Wilkinson in 1849 [24]. Since then there has been a long discussion as
to whether *C. albicans* is a benign commensal in the vagina of normal
women which only under particular circumstances becomes a pathological infection, or whether isolation of *C. albicans* from the vagina is
always a sign of infection even without clinical symptoms of vaginal
thrush [25]. The current opinion is that the presence of *C. albicans* or
other yeast in the vagina is an abnormal state and should always be
treated. Vaginal candidosis is often associated with pregnancy, diabetes or antibiotic therapy (especially with cotrimoxazole). The use of
oral contraceptives may also be a predisposing factor.

There are more pharmaceuticals available for the treatment of vaginal
thrush than for any other type of candida infection. The polyenes amphotericin B, candicidin, hamycin, nystatin and timaricin, and azoles
such as clotrimazole, econazole, miconazole, tioconazole, oxicona-
zole, isoconazole, terconazole, fenticonazole and butoconazole are all
available as cream, lotion, vaginal tablets or ovula. There are also

Clotrimazole

three drugs which can be taken orally, ketoconazole, itraconazole and fluconazole. Even more than in the treatment of dermatomycoses, the improvements in recent years have not been so much in intrinsic efficacy – clotrimazole, the first azole available, achieved cure rates of over 80 % – but in lessening the duration of therapy and thus significantly improving compliance. A 100 % cure rate has, however, never been achieved.

At first sight it would thus seem that therapy for vaginal candidosis is sufficient and there are no further problems in this field. However, there are women who suffer from chronic recurrent vaginal candidosis over periods of months and years, and who have to endure the associated physical and psychological stress. Although this condition has been recognized for a very long time there is even now no suitable therapy, largely because its causes are still unclear. Despite many attempts to investigate predisposing factors there is still no precise knowledge available, and although a variety of metabolic defects are always under discussion, the true pathogenesis of chronic recurrent vaginal candidosis remains obscure.

Some authors have demonstrated the presence of an elevated anticandida IgE titer in the vaginal secretion of affected women, suggesting the occurrence of a localized hypersensitivity. Prostaglandin E2 has also been observed, so it may be that a vaginal allergy induces prostaglandin synthesis which in turn suppresses the cell-mediated immunoresponse, preventing clearance of the infecting yeast cells [26–30]. Witkin et al. have also observed a macrophage defect which could be antagonized by prostaglandin inhibitors [31]. The adherence to vaginal epithelial cells by C. albicans is a known first step in its pathogenicity, but this is not different in normal healthy women and those suffering from recurrent infection.

As therapy, several approaches have been tried, including treatment with transfer factor and immunotherapy with Candida vaccine [32, 33]. Recently, in preliminary phase II studies, an oral vaccine based on C. albicans ribosomes was tested in daily doses of up to nine capsules each containing 0.55 μg active component. Women taking the highest doses had no recurrence during the six months follow-up after vaccination [29].

Another approach to therapy is termed prophylaxis, although it is in fact more of a maintenance therapy. Several treatment schedules are used, but generally the vaginal candidosis is treated, either locally or orally, until the infection disappears, then a "prophylactic" treatment is initiated for a certain period of time, e.g. 3 or 6 months. The drug of choice is given weekly or monthly, locally or orally. A clear reduction in recurrence is always observed, but a proper cure is never achieved. After some time the candidosis reappears, so it would appear that this approach leads to a symptomatic rather than a mycological cure [34–38].

So despite the considerable range of available treatment there is still a pressing problem in the field of gynecological fungal infection. Basic knowledge on the pathology of *C. albicans* and on the predisposing factors for vaginal candidosis is still urgently needed.

3   Systemic mycosis – The problems
3.1   Problems with fungi

Fungi can infect all organs of the body as well as causing fungemia, which is one of the reasons systemic mycoses are so difficult to treat, and it has become clear that each organ is particularly susceptible to a particular pathogen or group of pathogens. For instance, *Candida* often infects the liver, heart valves and kidneys in transplant patients. *Aspergillus* primarily causes lung infections but can also disseminate to the brain. The lungs are also the primary site of infection of *Cryptococcus*, but it mostly progresses to meningitis which is fatal if not treated. However, in severely immune suppressed patients this preference for particular sites disappears and all organs, and also the skin, can be infected.

Agents of deep mycoses can be divided into two groups according to their ability to infect a healthy immunocompetent host. Those that are able to do so are known as primary pathogens, and include *Coccidioides, Histoplasma, Blastomyces* and *Sporotrix*. Opportunistic pathogens, such as *Aspergillus, Candida, Mucor, Rhizopus, Absidia, Trichosporum,* only cause infection under circumstances where the immune defence is not fully functional. Most fungi can be clearly placed in one of the two categories, but occasionally there is uncertainty, as in the case of *Cryptococcus neoformans,* which was for long classified as a primary pathogen but nowadays seems to be regarded as more usually causing opportunistic infections. It is sometimes difficult to classify some of the rarer fungi as true pathogens or opportunists. For instance, dematiaceous fungi can cause chronic subcutaneous infection, but also acute infection of the brain, and no clear correlation between pathogenicity and immunological state has been documented to date.

Primary pathogens cause serious fungal infections even in normal immunocompetent hosts, and there are regular outbreaks in endemic areas. Normal experimental animals are also easily infected and thus the diseases can be studied in animal models. Truly pathogenic fungi are most virulent, but although virulence factors have been tentatively identified for some species they have generally not been well characterized. These species are to a large extent resistant to the defence mechanisms of the host. Their spores overcome the alveolar macrophages, which play an important role in the initial defence against parasites, and in the tissue develop into their invasive form which is also resistant to human neutrophils. This latter is also a property of the heavily capsulated form of *C. neoformans* [39].

The opportunistic pathogen is only a danger if the immune defence has been weakened, and observations of which infections are associated with which form of immune inadequacy have contributed significantly to our understanding of the natural defences against mycoses. Some of the ever-increasing predisposing factors for opportunistic mycoses are discussed in a later section. Which fungi can cause a systemic infection in an immunocompromised host is not something that can be stated with confidence, but as mentioned in the introduction there is a case for saying "any". Ever more fungi which have always been regarded as non-pathogenic and harmless are now causing life-threatening deep mycoses. This tendency brings with it two separate problems, one of which is simply that the appearance of such saprophytic fungi on a culture plate is often not connected with infection, but is assumed to be contamination. And even if the mycosis is recognized as such, many of the less common fungi are simply not sensitive to available antifungal drugs. It is also becoming apparent that fungi that are primary pathogens, but usually cause little actual sickness in a healthy individual, can be devastating in the immune compromised. Cases are also appearing in the literature of people who have travelled in an area where a particular fungus is common and many years later, when their immune system has been weakened by age or sickness, have developed a systemic mycosis caused by this fungus. It is perhaps instructive to look at a few of the "newer" pathogens, as it gives some indication of the problems facing the physician in this area.

Emerging pathogens

There is a case for classifying all opportunistic pathogens under this heading, as they have become significant causes of morbidity and mortality only as the population of patients with reduced immunity has increased. However, mycoses caused by *Candida, Aspergillus* and *Cryptococcus,* for example, are nowadays accepted, indeed expected, to a sufficient extent that they may be considered established pathogens. As mentioned in the introduction, it is becoming difficult to find a fungal species that has not appeared in the literature as having caused a serious infection, but certain fungi are cropping up on a sufficient number of occasions to make themselves noticed.

Among the primary pathogens, *Histoplasma capsulatum* and *Coccidioides imitis* are perhaps those which have appeared more frequently in immune-deficient patients in recent years. *Saccharomyces cerevisiae* would probably be chosen as the least dangerous of fungi, but nevertheless several cases of invasive life-threatening infection have been caused by this common colonizer of human mucosal surfaces [40]. *Blastoschizomyces capitus* has been reported in a number of leukemia patients [41], and *Acremonium* spp., *Fusarium, Cunninghamella, Curvularia, Alternaria* and *Penicillium* in neutropenic and AIDS patients [42–45]. Another unusual pathogen is *Trichosporon beigelii,* which has been reported as a pathogen resistant to Amphotericin B (Amp B) [46], although this does not always appear to be the case [42, 44]. *Candida lusitaniae* infections have also been associated with Amp B resistance, but again this does not seem to be universal. A recent paper [47] reports two cases where infection with this organism was successfully treated. Thus the clinician is faced not only with an increasing battery of pathogens, but also with uncertainty about their sensitivity, with the possible resultant delay in initiating treatment. It is interesting that the authors of this paper [47] specifically state that when this fungus is isolated from an immunocompromised host it should be treated as an opportunistic pathogen and be tested for its sensitivity to antifungal agents. This perhaps illustrates the growing awareness of the possibility of fungal infection afflicting such patients, but the fact that it needs to be said at all suggests that mycoses are not always at the forefront of the physicians mind. The ability of fungi to invade virtually any organ and the plethora of predisposing factors require specialists in every medical area to be aware of their devastating potential.

The question has been asked whether it is not only unusual fungal species that are beginning to be found infecting vulnerable patients, but whether it is particularly virulent strains of the more common pathogens which attack, for instance, AIDS patients. In the case of *H. capsulatum* this appears not to be the case if the indications of a recent investigation by Spitzer et al. [48] are confirmed. Their work suggests that the appearance of a previously unique strain of *H.capsulatum* in three AIDS patients is not the result of an enhanced virulence, but that the strain is common in their particular geographical area where it produces symptoms only in particularly susceptible hosts. A similar conclusion was reached for the case of *Candida albicans* by Whelan et al. [49], who established the similarity between isolates causing infection in 23 AIDS patients and those colonizing 24 healthy subjects. Thus it would seem that it is the immune status of the patient that plays the major role in his vulnerability to a particular fungal strain, rather than any intrinsic property of the fungus itself. As will be mentioned in a later section, it is becoming clear that each particular class of immunosuppressed patient is especially vulnerable to a particular pathogen or group of pathogens. It would contribute to progress in the fight against fungal infection if these trends could be comprehensively documented as an aid to prophylaxis, diagnosis and treatment.

As a final comment to this section it should perhaps be mentioned that a likely problem in the future is the dwindling numbers of those who have the background and training to make a rapid and accurate identification of unusual pathogens, as opportunities for the study of fungal taxonomy are becoming increasingly rare.

Diagnosis

An aspect of medical mycology that causes much concern is that of diagnosis. The figures given vary according to source, but the proportion of deep mycoses first diagnosed or confirmed at post mortem is disturbingly high. Often this results from a failure to consider a fungal infection, which is perhaps due to the lack of emphasis on this area in medical training. But even when the physician thinks of mycosis, his diagnostic problems are just beginning. Absolute proof of fungal infection requires histology and culture growth, but many patients at risk are too ill for invasive approaches, and by the time the cultures have grown in the laboratory it is often simply too late. The need for a swift diagnosis could be filled by serological methods, but in the field of mycoses these have by no means solved all problems. A variety of tests are available for the most common pathogens but not all can be considered satisfactory. Antibody detection methods suffer from the problem of far too high a false negative rate and are of limited use in immunocompromised patients. The detection of circulating antigens gives somewhat better results, but one is still talking of detection rates of little over 70 %, and a further problem is to distinguish between colonization and actual systemic infection. Much effort has gone into attempts to identify antigen structures, up to now with a remarkable dearth of success, and this lack of basic knowledge has held back development of such methods. The one major success is the latex test for *Cryptococcus* antigens.

Progress in this area has been slow, and the prospects for improvement do not appear particularly good. *Candida* infections have received the most attention as this is the commonest opportunistic pathogen. Several commercial diagnostic kits are available, but publications comparing one with another invariably leave the impression that something better is required [50, 51], although various additional tests to identify false positive results [52], for instance, can sometimes improve matters. Even the methods for comparing methods leave much to be desired. The purification and characterization of *Candida* antigens is proceeding, but slowly. The possibility of utilizing antibodies against germ tubes rather than whole cells of *C. albicans* appears to be a promising approach which would attain a higher specificity, and according to recent indications would also be suitable for the immune compromised patient [53]. As with so many other ideas, however, this has not yet reached the stage of practical application.

The situation with aspergillosis is no better. The diagnosis of pulmonary infection is usually difficult to establish as culture of the organism from sputum is most often due to contamination [54]. Clinical diagnosis is no easier, with X-ray images being difficult to interpret, although computer tomography is a new aid that promises considerable help. As with *Candida*, attempts are being made to characterize suitable antigens but these are still at the experimental stage [55]. A new latex agglutination test for *Aspergillus* antigens (Pastorex) does, however, seem promising [55a]. And so it goes on; for some pathogens such as *Cryptococcus* and dermatophytes diagnosis does not cause quite such severe problems, while for the more unusual fungi culture of tissue samples is the only possibility.

What is the outlook? Any mycology congress or meeting contains a good percentage of diagnostics papers, and the theme that binds them all is the real need for new, more effective methods. Most of the contributions, however, tend to be of the type which conclude with words such as "this shows promise for/may be applicable in the diagnosis of invasive fungal infections". One receives the impression that good work is being done by individual laboratories, but that a major coordinated effort in basic research is somehow lacking. Many approaches are reported in the literature and at congresses, but few come to fruition. It has become clear that carbohydrate antigens lack specificity, and several groups are looking at proteins and glycoproteins. The idea of an infection-specific antibody is also under investigation, and this would obviously help rule out colonization. The possibility of monitoring fungal metabolites such as D-arabinitol [56] or β-D-glucan is also under investigation. DNA hybridization and fingerprinting techniques are also being developed, and although they appear at the moment to be more applicable to epidemiological studies than diagnosis this could be the direction from which improvements come.

The absence of rapid and reliable diagnosis is certainly a great hindrance in the battle against deep mycoses. It renders it difficult to decide when, and what, therapy should be initiated, and together with the lack of a genuinely broad spectrum, safe antifungal has led to the situation whereby antimycotics are very often administered only when a "fever of unknown origin" does not respond to antibacterial treatment for several days. For some patients this is too late. This is an area where we are not winning.

3.2   Problems with patients

The major factor in the increase in systemic mycoses is undoubtedly immune deficiency. Be it in the very old or very young, the result of disease, medical treatment or surgical intervention, there is an ever-expanding community of people with a weakened or even nonexistent immune system. Although travel to endemic areas is becoming more common, and diseases caused by primary pathogens such as *Histoplasma capsulatum, Coccidioides immitis, Blastomyces dermatiditis* and *Paracoccidioides brasiliensis* are more often recognized as such, it is the increase in opportunistic infections that has completely changed the significance of antifungal chemotherapy. It has also somewhat blurred the division between primary and opportunistic pathogens, as colonization or asymptomatic infection can flare up into life-threatening disease in a host whose immune system has been weakened years after the endemic area has been left.

Opportunistic fungal infections can be broadly divided into those which take advantage of defects in the non-specific defence based on polymorphonuclear leukocytes, and those which occur when the cell-mediated acquired immunity is lacking. These two groups are often found in distinct clinical settings, but in some cases, for instance granulocytopenic patients who are receiving corticosteroid chemotherapy, broad spectrum antibiotics or other forms of chemotherapy, the danger comes from both categories. We are in constant contact with fungi, we inhale thousands of spores and harbor a large variety of species on our skin and in the gastrointestinal tract, and the majority of us suffer no harm from them. The fungi are not changing, but the factors that turn a saprophyte into a virulent pathogen are becoming more varied and more common.

Although immune suppression as part of medical care, for instance in organ transplant patients, has become more common, it is the AIDS pandemic that dominates the area of defects in cell-mediated immunity, and this field is reviewed regularly [43, 57–59, Dupont in 2]. Common skin pathogens cause much more severe infections in AIDS patients, and also tend to be much more extensive. Practically every tissue and organ can be a target for fungal attack in these patients, but the central nervous system and the upper digestive tract are particularly susceptible. About 50 % of AIDS sufferers have at least one episode of *Candida* infection (some sources put it as high as 80 %) and in most cases it is oral thrush or oesophagitis. In fact, this is often the first sign of the progression of HIV infection to full-blown AIDS. Cryptococcosis is one of the most serious of the fungal infections that commonly affect this patient group, as it usually manifests itself as meningitis and must not only be treated with an effective chemotherapy regime in order to achieve a cure, but also requires some form of maintenance therapy to prevent relapse. It is in these indications that the new triazole antifungals are showing promise. Although these are the two most common, well over 50 fungal species have been documented as causing infections in AIDS patients [43].

In a setting of neutropenia, severe diabetes mellitus, use of broad spectrum antibacterials and certain types of catheters, the main opportunistic infections are caused by *Candida* and *Aspergillus*. Treatment is often ineffective unless the underlying disease can be controlled, and here the triazoles do not offer much hope for improvement. The extent of the problem is illustrated by the fact that 20–30 % of patients with acute leukemia die of *Candida* infection [60]. Risk factors for mycoses have been delineated for various patient groups, and it has become clear that severely ill general medical or surgical patients are at risk as well as those with malignancies [61, 62]. There are still many controversies in the management of fungal diseases in such patients [63], and this situation is likely to remain until more effective and safer drugs become available.

What is gradually becoming clear is that certain organisms have an affinity for particular disease states, i. e. *Candida tropicalis* and *krusei* for leukemic patients, *Candida glabrata* for cancer patients, *Mucor* for diabetes mellitus patients.

More is becoming known about the way the human body defends itself against fungal infection [63, 64], and much information is being gathered about the particular risks of specific groups of patients. Apart from the factors already mentioned these include long hospitalization, alcoholism, radiotherapy, hemodialysis, severe burns, and in many cases there is a combination of predisposing factors in the underlying condition. But there is some way to go before this understanding is sufficient to legitimately be used to guide prophylaxis and treatment in these groups of patients. Again, the sifting and collation of available data is a formidable task, and it is often difficult for a physician to take advantage of the experiences of others simply because of the sheer amount of information available. Until our knowledge of the immunology of fungal diseases becomes more detailed the most important advance will remain an awareness of the possibility of fungal infection in the ever-growing population of the immune compromised.

3.3   Problems with the available drugs

A count of the established drugs for the treatment of systemic mycoses ends at three. Interested parties might add one or two more to the list, and two triazoles are in the process of being introduced onto the market, but at the present time it is still true to say that the large majority of patients are treated with amphotericin B (Amp B), 5-flucytosine

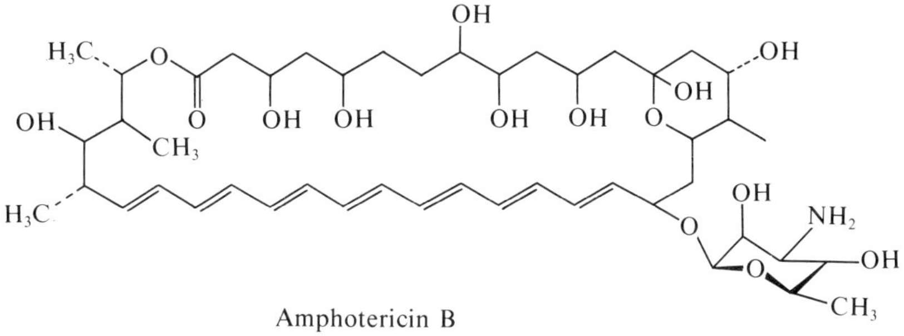

Amphotericin B

(5-FC) or ketoconazole (Keto). Any attempt to judge progress in antifungal chemotherapy must use these drugs as a yardstick, and examine them critically in terms of efficacy and spectrum, resistance and toxicity.

Amphotericin B

Polyene antibiotics are all produced by species of *Streptomyces* and consist of a macrolide ring closed by a lactone. The best known of these, Amphotericin B, has a very broad spectrum of antifungal activity. Most fungal species pathogenic to humans, including *Candida* spp., *Cryptococcus neoformans, Histoplasma capsulatum, Aspergillus fumigatus, Paracoccidioides brasiliensis, Coccidioides immitis* and *Mucoraceae* are inhibited at least fungistatically at concentrations of around 1 μg/ml. Dermatophytes, the dematiaceous fungi and species of *Madurella* are considered resistant with MIC values of > 10 μg/ml. These antibiotics are specifically active against eukaryotic cells, i.e. all cells containing sterols in the cytoplasmic membrane [1, 9].

The mode of action of polyene antibiotics is based on the formation of a complex with the sterols of the cytoplasmic membrane. These complexes are thought to be in the form of long hollow cylinders and arranged perpendicularly to the membrane, forming a non-static aqueous pore, but they may also be simply inserted between the two layers of the membrane. Whatever the details of the polyene/sterol interaction, the result is a disturbance of ergosterol function [10, 65, 66]. The first result in sensitive cells is an increased permeability which leads to a disruption of the proton gradient and leakage of potassium ions. The proton gradient, generated by an ATPase located in the plasma membrane, has a central role in the functioning of this membrane. It energizes the uptake of amino acids and other nutrients and maintains intact the internal pool of potassium ions. Furthermore, it has an important role in the regulation of growth of fungal cells. The fungistatic effect of Amp B is related to efflux of potassium, the fungicidal effect however to an irreversible inhibition of the membrane ATPase.

Amp B has a degree of specificity for ergosterol over cholesterol, the prevalent mammalian sterol, and this is considered the key to the relatively low toxicity of this compound to the human host compared to other polyenes, which have a much greater toxicity [67]. Nevertheless, the major drawback of Amp B is the frequent occurrence of adverse reactions. Amp B also possesses some affinity to lipids other than ergosterol. Its interaction with lipid bilayers has been studied in sensitive cells, liposomal vesicles, black films and artificial membranes. Various models have been proposed to explain how the complex of Amp B and lipids in the membrane is constructed but it is still not clear whether actual pores are formed or merely complexes. The mode of action of Amp B has been extensively reviewed by Polak, Kerridge and Brajtburg [10, 68, 69].

Resistance

It is relatively easy to isolate Amp B-resistant mutants in the laboratory. They are generally distinguished from parent strains by an altered cell membrane lipid composition and are used for studying sterol biosynthesis. But published information on the frequency of the natural appearance of resistance is scarce [9], and despite the ease of obtaining resistant mutants in the laboratory secondary resistance to the drug has remained an extremely rare occurrence despite its extensive use in chemotherapy for more than 30 years. This may be explained by the fact that the very alterations in the membrane that lead to resistance reduce virulence and slow growth rate. Secondary resistance has been described in two cases of *Candida* endocarditis caused by *Candida parapsilosis* [70, 71], two cases of infection due to *C. lusitaniae* [72, 73], and two cases of disseminated infection caused by *C. tropicalis* and one by *C. glabrata* [74, 75]. In most cases the degree of resistance was high (100–500 μg/ml). It is of interest that the most frequent causative agent of candidosis, *Candida albicans,* was not involved in any of these documented cases. Resistant yeast strains in patients prophylactically treated with polyene antibiotics to achieve clearance of the digestive tract is very uncommon, and again no *Candida albicans* strain resistant to Amp B has been reported [9].

It does seem, however, that the observation of Amp B-resistant infection has been increasing in recent years. The first authors to discuss this problem in detail were Dick et al. [76]. They reported the Amp B sensitivity of yeasts isolated from 70 patients in an oncology program undergoing extensive chemotherapy for acute leukemia and bone marrow transplantation. Strict criteria for resistance were used (> $2 \mu g/ml$ for Amp B). 55 isolates (7.4 %) out of 747, originating from 6 patients (8.6 %), were found to be resistant. 27 of the resistant isolates were *C. albicans,* 3 were *C. tropicalis* and 25 *C. glabrata.* All patients had received intravenous Amp B and 5 out of 6 had received oral nystatin. Polyene susceptible isolates of the same yeast species had been obtained from all 6 patients on multiple occasions and all had experienced long periods of neutropenia. By comparison, none of 625 isolates from 238 patients on non-oncology services showed polyene resistance. In 1988 Pouderly et al. made a similar observation. All episodes of bloodstream infection in immunocompromised patients caused by isolates with MIC > 0.8 $\mu g/ml$ were fatal, versus 8 of 17 episodes of similar infection caused by yeasts with MIC < 0.8 $\mu g/ml$. The authors concluded that yeast fungemia in severely immunocompromised patients is often caused by organisms resistant to the usual concentration of Amp B obtainable in vivo, and that this finding was clinically significant.

Apparently, mutants resistant to Amp B chemotherapy may occur in severely ill patients, and such cases are occasionally reported [77–79]. A further source of worry, as mentioned above, is the number of unusual species now causing deep mycoses that are resistant to Amp B.

Toxicity

That Amp B toxicity is a problem in the clinic is well established, although it is sometimes difficult for those not actually in clinical practice to judge how great the problem is. One physician will say that his nurses run a mile when they hear that treatment with this drug is necessary, another will state he has no major problems with it; much is subjective, and patients do not generally publish their experiences in the literature or appear at congresses. It is clear, however, that Amp B can and does induce both acute and chronic side effects that are unpleasant and in many cases dangerous, and the situation has been extensively reviewed [80]. Acute reactions to Amp B, usually fever and chills, are experienced by anything up to half those receiving it. Various strategies have been tried to ameliorate these effects, including the administration of drugs such as meperidine, acetaminophen or hydrocortisone. Some authors suggest that slow infusion rates reduce the discomfort for the patient, but recent studies have tended to come down on the side of infusion times as short as one hour [81–83]. There is a tendency in some hospitals to tailor the time and duration of the infusion to the individual patient, as reactions are so variable. This approach is supported by recent work in animal models which suggests that Amp B toxicity is dependent on circadian biosusceptibility rhythms, which is an interesting result [84]. Chronic toxicity of Amp B is mostly due to renal damage, the mechanism of which has not been defined but which probably involves changes in membrane permeability. Hypokalemia, hypomagnesemia and increased serum creatinine are also common and troublesome, and regular monitoring is essential. Thrombophlebitis and hematological effects are also far from rare.

So what progress has been made in combatting these adverse reactions? As with the duration of the infusion, there is little general agreement on measures to help the situation. Despite a lack of controlled, prospective trials the reversal of sodium depletion by salt loading is gradually gaining acceptance as more reports appear in the literature [80, 85–87]. To date this has been the most successful method of reducing the nephrotoxicity of Amp B. Lack of reliable data on the elimination kinetics of Amp B has always hindered the idea of alternate day dosing, but recent data from Hoeprich [88] supports this method of reducing toxicity and improving the welfare of the patient. An assessment of risk factors for each patient would seem essential, especially in pediatrics [89], and some effort has even been made to quantify this [90]. An example of the diverse sources of toxicity problems is the finding that one particular source of Amp B contained endotoxin in amounts varying according to the batch, which led to induction of Tumor Necrosis Factor and thus to a greater incidence of febrile reaction [91, 92]. This particular trouble has apparently been solved by better product control, but it illustrates the potential for problems when dealing with a drug that is on the limits as far as tolerability is concerned.

Despite its toxic potential, Amp B is still used as therapy of choice for a wide range of systemic mycoses, and for many indications is indis-

putably the "gold standard". Its fungicidal action makes it almost irre-
placable at the present time for the treatment of opportunistic infections in immune suppressed patients, at least as initial therapy. Three
recent reviews of its use are those by Hoeprich [1], Schmitt and Armstrong [93] and Benson and Nahata [94]. It cannot be regarded as satisfactory, however, that after more than 30 years of clinical use there is
no general agreement as to optimal dose, duration of therapy, method
of administration and pharmacokinetics in different patient groups,
and relatively little hard data upon such matters. The lack of a "standard" Amp B therapy also hinders realistic comparison with newer antifungals. Perhaps the greatest progress in this case would be a little
more consensus on how best to use Amp B.

5-Flucytosine

The antifungal spectrum of flucytosine (5-FC) is limited to species of
Candida and *Cryptococcus,* which are highly sensitive (MIC 0.1–2 μg/
ml), and *Aspergillus* and *Dematiaceae,* which are only moderately sensitive (MIC 1–25 μg/ml). After prolonged contact fungicidal activity
is observed against yeasts and *Dematiaceae* but not against *Aspergilli.*
Exposure of sensitive fungi to flucytosine is followed almost immediately by inhibition of the synthesis of DNA and RNA. In yeasts and
dematiaceous fungi appreciable cell growth continues with protein
and carbohydrate overproduction. After prolonged incubation the
cells die due to unbalanced growth – the phrase thymine-less death is
used. In *Aspergilli* the inhibition of nucleic acid synthesis results in an
immediate inhibition of growth, and the lack of overproduction of
proteins and carbohydrates is probably the reason why 5-FC is not
fungicidal in this species. The metabolic pathway of 5-FC in fungi has
been carefully studied using various mutants resistant to its action.
5-FC is taken up actively by a cytosine permease which is normally responsible for the uptake of adenine, guanine, hypoxanthine and cyto-

5-Fluorocytosine

sine [95] and is therefore antigonized by these natural substrates. Inside the cell 5-FC is immediately deaminated to 5-fluorouracil (5-FU), a critical step since it is 5-FU that is the active principle responsible for killing the fungus rather than 5-FC itself. The low toxicity of the drug in human hosts is due to the absence of the cytosine deaminase in mammalian cells. 5-FU acts along two different pathways. It is converted by uridine monophosphate pyrophosphorylase into 5-FUMP which is further phosphorylated and incorporated into RNA (a step which is antagonized by uridine). At the same time it is converted to 5-fluorodeoxyuridine monophosphate, a potent inhibitor of thymidylate synthetase, and this leads to inhibition of DNA synthesis. 5-FU itself cannot be given as an antimycotic drug since its uptake by the fungal cell is poor and its toxicity in mammalian cells precludes systemic use in the quantities necessary for chemotherapy. The details of the pathway and mode of action of 5-FC have recently been reviewed [10]. What is remarkable about the action of 5-FC is that the fungal cell itself produces a fungicidal substance from an inert compound by internal metabolization, and further metabolizes it to cause its own death, a situation unique in medical mycology. However, the length of the metabolic pathways and the several different enzymes involved are also the reason for the frequent appearance of 5-FC-resistant mutants. Every enzyme in this pathway can be altered or deleted in ways which render 5-FC ineffective against the mutant strain [95].

Resistance

There is a certain amount of primary resistance, and secondary resistance appears during chemotherapy or selection in the laboratory. The proportion of primary resistant isolates has been determined as approximately 10 % in a sample of 10,000. A highly significant correlation has been found between the incidence of primary resistance to flucytosine and the serological type in *Candida albicans*. Although representing a minority of isolates in most geographical areas, those of serotype B account for a majority of the instances of primary resistance. This is most pronounced in Europe, where of 583 isolates studied by Drouhet et al. [96], 547 were type A und 36 type B, but only 4 (0.7 %) of type A were 5-FC-resistant compared to 30 (83 %) of type B. The greater proportion of serotype B strains in North America explains at least partially the higher rate of primary resistance to flucytosine found there. In a study by Stiller et al. [97] 196 (49.3 %) of 398 isolates were type B, and of these 29.6 % were resistant to flucytosine. Only 6.9 % of the 202 type A were resistant. Generally, in Europe, Asia, Australia and New Zealand 6 to 9 % of isolates have a primary resistance whereas in the United States and Africa the figure is 20 % or more. Not only type B *Candida albicans* but also other *Candida* species *(C. tropicalis, C. parapsilosis* and *C. pseudotropicalis)* show a high frequency of primary-resistance. *C. glabrata* on the other hand has a similar frequency to *C. albicans* serotype A. *Cryptoccus neoformans* has a low frequency (2.4 % of 280 strains), but *Aspergilli* a high frequency [9].

The resistant isolates are not normally less virulent, although this was observed recently by Fasoli [98] in a 5-FC-resistant mutant lacking the cytosine deaminase and uridine transport system. He concluded that the loss of virulence is the reason why this particular type of resistance is so rarely found during chemotherapy, but it is also true that laboratory selected mutants show a low frequency of cytosine permease and cytosine deaminase activity loss.

Most mutants isolated lack UMP-phosphorylase, and Whelan and Magee [99] observed a clear segregation between highly resistant mutants and partially resistant ones. These were the experiments that demonstrated that *Candida albicans* is a diploid organism, and it appears that the mutation in partially resistant strains is only located in one allele, whereas in totally resistant strains it is in both. In every normally sensitive population of fungi there is a minority which is 5-FC-resistant. The absolute number of resistant cells is species dependent. The lowest resistance frequency is seen in *Candida albicans* (2.7×10^{-7}) followed by *Cryptococcus neoformans* (4×10^{-6}) and the highest is seen in *Aspergilli* (3.5×10^{-5}). In *Dematiaceae* the frequency is in the range of 2×10^{-3} to 1×10^{-7}. During lengthy chemotherapy with 5-FC monotherapy this proportion of resistant cells can so increase such that the population as a whole becomes resistant and therapy fails. The risk of this happening is considered dependent on the number of fungal cells present in the host, the resistance frequency of the particular strain, the degree of resistance of the mutants in question, the duration of treatment before achievement of mycological cure, and inversely proportional to the 5-FC concentration in the body and the state of the host defence mechanism. As there is a clear correlation betweeen therapy failure and the appearance of secondary resistance 5-FC monotherapy is no longer used in long-term chemo-therapy. Since it could be clearly demonstrated in vitro and in animal models [100–102] that a combination of Amp B and 5-FC is not only synergistic but significantly reduces the appearance of secondary resistant isolates, this has become the therapy of choice for a large number of physicians in certain indications. For example, in cryptococcal meningitis 20 to 30 % secondary resistance was observed under 5-FC-monotherapy, whereas only 2 to 3 % with the combination. This topic is dealt with in more detail below and in ref. 9.

Toxicity

The actual clinical relevance of 5-FC toxicity is controversial. Some clinicians emphasize it and speak as if it were a major problem. Others have a different opinion, stating clearly that side effects are uncommon and rarely serious or irreversible [1]. It is assumed that its toxicity is related in some way to the production of 5-fluorouracil by bacteria of the gastrointestinal tract. Indeed, during chemotherapy the level of 5-FU is measurable, but it has no direct relation to the 5-FC level, and is related to the state of the gut flora [103–105]. Toxicity cannot be at all correlated with the level of 5-FU, but is directly correlated with 5-FC concentrations of over 100 mg/l for a sustained period. This has been observed for all patients suffering from side effects during controlled studies, particularly for the subgroup with hepatitis and bone marrow suppression [106–108]. Most importantly, since 5-FC is fully excreted by the kidneys even a minor impairment of renal function by the Amp B-treatment in combination therapy leads to elevated 5-FC levels. Thus it is important to monitor 5-FC levels and adapt the dose to the actual kidney function during combination therapy. Doing so reduces the toxicity of 5-FC to the more acceptable levels reported by many authors [107, 108]. The adverse reactions documented include nausea, vomiting and diarrhea, and liver toxicity, which is more serious but rarely fatal. Of greater concern is the potential for bone marrow depression which occurs, as do the other side effects, in about 5 % of patients, and is not always reversible if not recognized early enough. This aspect of 5-FC toxicity is perhaps overplayed and more careful consideration of the evidence would allay many fears [109]. As with Amp B, exact evaluation of toxicity is complicated by the fact that the patient is almost invariably suffering from an underlying disease that disturbs metabolic functions, and is usually already being treated with a battery of other drugs.

Despite its narrow spectrum and resistance problems, 5-FC finds considerable application in the clinic. This is mostly in combination with Amp B, although recently also with other agents, as its swift onset of action, low acute toxicity and fungicidal action make it an ideal combination partner. The 5-FC/Amp B combination is accepted by many as the therapy of choice for cryptococcosis, and is also frequently used against *Candida* and *Aspergillus* infection.

Ketoconazole

Although it was not the first azole to become available for the treatment of systemic infections, ketoconazole made the breakthrough for this class of compounds and has held its place in the antifungal armament to the present day. Clotrimazole did not really become a serious contender, and questions as to the efficacy and safety of miconazole prevented its acceptance, although the position of this compound is even now contentious.

Ketoconazole is often represented as a broad spectrum antimycotic, although the difference in concentrations required for fungistatic action varies by a factor of a thousand between the most and the least sensitive species; the MIC for the dimorphic fungus *Histoplasma capsulatum* is 0.01 μg/ml, while for *Candida albicans* it is 10 μg/ml [9, 10]. In general ketoconazole performs satisfactorily against true pathogens (except in meningitis) but has not proved itself in opportunistic infections in immune compromised patients, and tends not to be used in critical cases unless Amp B is contraindicated. The lack of fungicidal activity is probably to blame for the more frequent relapses after ketoconazole treatment, and the high doses that are often required. The reduction in absorption in cases of reduced gastric acidity has also

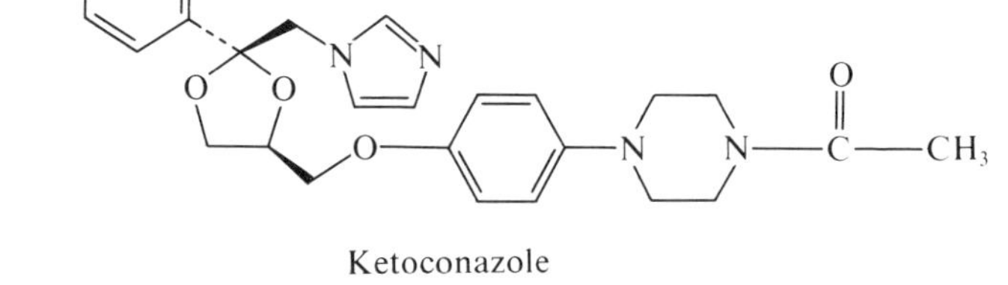

Ketoconazole

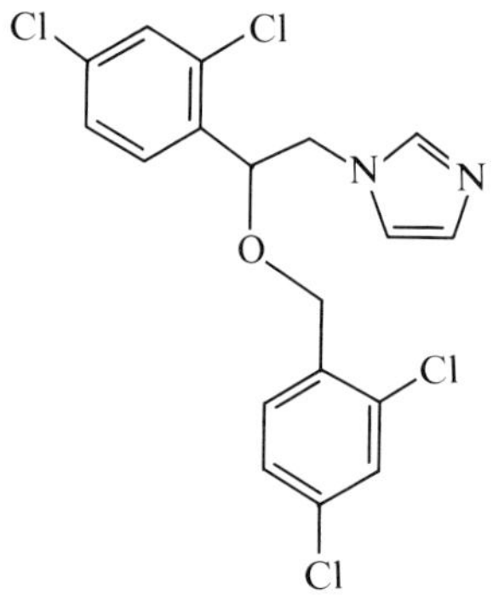

Miconazole

caused problems, but now that this is recognized it can be corrected. Biochemical studies have revealed that azoles disturb the function of the fungal cell membrane by interfering with the cytochrome P450-dependent lanosterol C14-demethylase [vanden Bossche in 7, 9, 10, 68]. The primary mode of action of all azoles and triazoles is related to the inhibition of this enzyme and it is generally agreed that their fungistatic action is due to depletion of ergosterol and accumulation of lanosterol in the membrane. That miconazole and itraconazole are fungicidal is thought to be the result of direct membrane damage leading to the loss of cytoplasmic constituents [vanden Bossche in 110]. The mode of action of azoles has been intensively studied [2] and will be discussed in more detail later.

Resistance

Neither primary resistance nor its appearance during therapy seem to be a great problem with ketoconazole. No increase in resistance rates has been observed in true pathogenic fungi such as *Coccidioides, Histoplasma* etc, but it is of course more difficult to judge resistance in species such as *Candida* where the sensitivity is low to start with. It is possible to obtain resistant strains under laboratory conditions, but few reports have identified clinical problems. This could in part be due to the fact that azole-resistant strains are significantly less virulent than the parent strains. Long-term treatment of chronic mucocutaneous candidosis has led to relapse due to genuine resistance to ketoconazole, but in many cases treatment failure seems to be linked rather to the deteriorating immunological status of the patient [111, 112]. The resistance problem hovers in the background, however, and it remains to be seen how the situation develops with the newer compounds of this class [9].

Toxicity

The necessity of using a high dosage of ketoconazole for various indications has led to significant toxicity problems [113–115] although not of the same order as those associated with the use of Amp B. Gastrointestinal reactions, mostly vomiting, have proved dose limiting for up to 50 % of patients receiving more than 800 mg/day [114]. Endocrinological toxicity due to interference with steroid metabolism is also well documented, but is reversible within a short time after the end of therapy. These effects have in fact been used to advantage in certain cases, as in the treatment of Cushing's syndrome and in patients with prostatic carcinoma [116, 117]. Liver toxicity is also a potential problem, and although its frequency is clouded by the number of patients with underlying diseases involving hepatic function it can be said that its occurrence is most serious although seldom. Drug interactions are also of considerable relevance when assessing the use of ketoconazole. Interaction with alcohol, anticoagulants, rifampicin and barbiturates has been reported. Of particular concern is the interference with the clearance of cyclosporin A, which can cause the serum concentrations of this drug to be sufficiently elevated to be toxic.

The three drugs described above were introduced around 30, 20 and 10 years ago, respectively. They have rendered deep mycoses, previously virtually untreatable, diseases for which effective chemotherapy is available. They are, however, clearly not able to cope with the ever-increasing demands on antifungal drugs. The increasing number of patients requiring treatment who are already desperately ill, their often catastrophic immune status, and the failure of diagnostic methodology to make any real progress has changed the situation considerably over the last decade. Amphotericin B, 5-flucytosine and ketoconazole, although nobody can deny their continuing contribution to antifungal chemotherapy, have simply too many drawbacks to be considered satisfactory. The toxicity of one, the resistance to the other, and the lack of a real efficacy over a wide spectrum of the third leaves the physician constantly hoping for better alternatives. It is clear that what is required is a truly broad spectrum, fungicidal drug that is safe enough to be given prophylactically and over a long period of time to very ill patients and which does not induce resistance. The not altogether surprising failure of such a drug to suddenly appear over the horizon has left the physician looking for less spectacular advances to improve his care of the patient. New treatment methods have been developed to improve the performance of the established drugs, the advantages of newer drugs are being exploited where appropriate, and solutions are being sought outside the range of traditional antifungal chemotherapy.

4   Systemic mycoses – Answers

The present situation in the therapy of deep mycoses can be described as barely satisfactory. These life-threatening infections can be treated, but up to now there has been a limited range of drugs, difficulties in diagnosis in many indications, and significant toxicity problems. And the field is in no way becoming easier. So what are the answers at the present moment?

4.1   Established drugs

Amp B still offers the broadest and most efficacious therapy, regardless of whether the infection is caused by a true or an opportunistic pathogen, and despite having been on the market for more than thirty years its possibilities are clearly not yet exhausted [118]. A great deal of effort is still going into reducing the toxicity of this drug and improving its use. New formulations, derivatives and immunostimulant properties are discussed below. In addition, new galenic forms are coming into use, such as the nasal spray that Meunier [119] has found effective in reducing the incidence of aspergillosis in her cancer patients.

Even with all its drawbacks a good number of clinicians still use Amp B routinely for all types of opportunistic fungal infections where a real fungicidal action is needed. They are not afraid to use it as they are aware of its side effects and have learned how to control them [Armstrong in ref. 63, 118]. An indication area that will probably remain the domain of Amp B, with or without 5-FC, for a long time to come is that of fungal infections in AIDS, particularly against disseminated histoplasmosis, where Amp B remains the drug of choice for initial treatment, although the subsequent maintenance therapy may be better with a triazole [120]. The combination of 5-FC and Amp B will also probably remain the "gold standard" for the therapy of deep candidosis and cryptococcosis for the time being, and has also shown advantages over Amp B monotherapy in aspergillosis in some recent studies [121].

The broad spectrum and the good in vitro activity of the early azoles ketoconazole and miconazole against both true and opportunistic pathogens did not transfer to clinical efficacy as had been hoped. Both drugs are very good against dimorphic fungi such as *Histoplasma,* where keto has replaced Amp B monotherapy outside of AIDS [122] but they have not proved sufficiently effective for systemic candidosis or cryptococcosis in immune-suppressed patients. During a perspective on azoles at the recent ICAFC Congress [7], Hay offered the opinion that miconazole still has a place as therapy of choice for *Pseudoallescheria boydii* infections, but otherwise it is a drug that never really made it, and that keto has established itself as an effective and well-tolerated alternative to Amp B only against mucocutaneous candidosis and madurella feet.

So from where are the new answers coming? Where has progress been made?

4.2   The new triazoles

For a good while all hopes for a higher level of antifungal chemotherapy rested on the new triazole derivatives, represented in the first instance by itraconazole (itra) and fluconazole (flu). But the 1990 ICAAC [8] backed up the Oiso congress [6] in showing that a reexami-

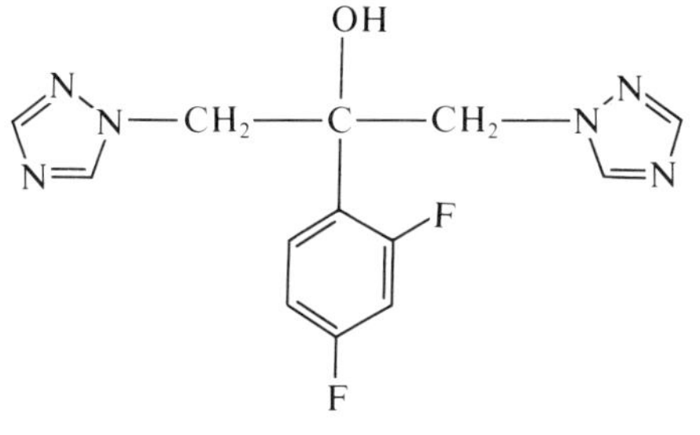

Fluconazole

nation of their role has taken place, even in AIDS where they initially showed such promise. Both drugs have a high specificity for fungal over mammalian cytochrome P450 demethylase and, probably for this reason, have shown significantly less toxicity than the early azoles. However, during their clinical evaluation it became clear that neither could fulfil their promise of reaching the broad efficacy of Amp B. Nevertheless, both are finding their niche, and there are going to be indications where they are more effective, better tolerated and easier to handle than the established drugs. Perhaps this will have to lead to a change of attitude in the field. Up to now one has thought in terms of one drug that is applicable more or less across the board, and has hoped for something similar but better. Very soon there will be three or four drugs which are the best treatment in their own particular indications, and that this greater choice will mean more difficult clinical decisions is something that has already been recognized [123]. It also places pressure on diagnosis, which is not the most satisfactory aspect of the field.

Itraconazole

The place of the triazoles in the therapy of deep mycoses is becoming progressively clear, and has been the subject of several recent reviews [124–127]. Itra has proved superior to keto against several true pathogens, particularly good results being obtained in sporotrichosis where it has now gained the place of first choice therapy [Graybill in 2, 128]. It may also soon replace keto in the treatment of blastomycosis and histoplasmosis in non-AIDS patients, and has also shown convincing efficacy in chromomycosis [Graybill in 2, 129, 130]. *Cladosporium* infections are cured by itra monotherapy, but *Fonsecaea* may require combination with 5-FC for a definite cure. Itra has already become the agent of choice for in South America for sporotrichosis [131].

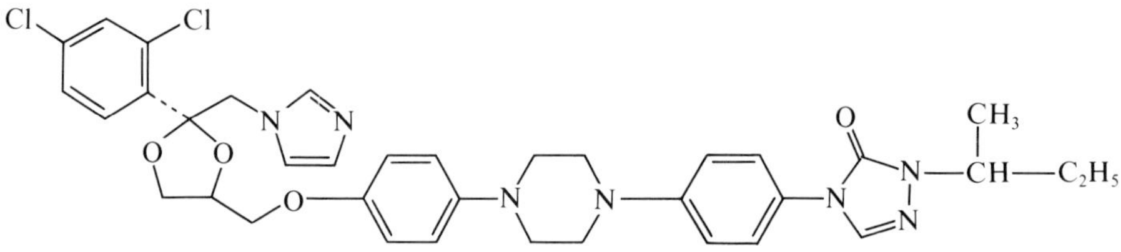

Itraconazole

Thus itra has reached the number one spot against several infections caused by primary pathogens, *Sporotrix schenckii* and dematiaceous fungi, but the situation is rather different in the field of opportunistic pathogens. While too few clinical trials have been carried out to properly place itra in the therapy schedule, what evidence there is suggests that its use will be limited in the treatment of these severe and complicated infections. Nevertheless, several publications [132, 133, A. Restrepo in 110] do show that it is effective in invasive aspergillosis and also against aspergilloma. In the latter indication itra is clearly a breakthrough [134] since up to now no therapy existed, and surgery was the only possibility. Now, surgical intervention can be replaced by therapy in all cases where there is no danger of hemoptysis. More comparative trials are necessary to precisely define the place of itra in invasive aspergillosis, as to date there is no evidence that it is superior to Amp B with or without 5-FC. It may well prove very suitable for the prophylaxis of relapse cases, but here again there is too little clinical data available.

Itraconazole showed good results as initial therapy in cryptococcosis in AIDS patients [132, 135]. As it does not penetrate cerebrospinal fluid, these results are noteworthy and suggest that meningeal and parenchymal penetration are critical [136]. Itra has been widely used as maintenance therapy in cryptococcal meningitis in AIDS patients with results comparable to flu and significantly better than Amp B, and it shares with flu the advantages that an orally available drug brings to long-term therapy [137]. Thus while itra has clearly brought benefit to many patients suffering from chromomycosis, sporotrichosis and aspergilloma, further clinical trials are needed to ascertain if it will find use in other indications.

Fluconazole

Fluconazole has the advantage of being available in two galenic forms for oral and i. v. use, which makes it additionally attractive in an area where many patients are too ill to take drugs orally. Also, the water solubility of flu means that it easily reaches the cerebrospinal fluid, and it was thus regarded as likely to be particularly effective against cryptococcal meningitis in both AIDS and non-AIDS patients. In fact, flu is so much easier to use that one could almost say that a sense of euphoria invaded the treatment of cryptococcal meningitis. At the

ICAAC in 1987 one heard that all AIDS patients with this infection were treated with flu as first choice therapy, and the results seemed satisfactory. In 33 of 46 patients the CSF was cleared [138–140], but these were non-controlled trials. Since then, two controlled trials have been instigated to compare flu with Amp B with and without 5-FC. Some results from these studies have recently been published [141, Mycoses Study Group in 8]. When compared with the Amp B/5-FC combination, clinical failure was reported in 8 of 14 patients receiving flu against none of 7 receiving the combination, and this trial was in fact stopped. In less severe cases the response to flu was better. In a larger trial, conducted by the Mycosis Study Group, flu was compared to Amp B monotherapy. About 50 % of cases showed cerebrospinal fluid culture conversion and the 23 % mortality was evenly divided between the two groups. The different results obtained in this study show that flu is as effective as Amp B monotherapy, but that neither is the optimal treatment. The combination of Amp B and 5-FC is clearly the best therapy in this indication where the real synergy between the two drugs leads to faster conversion to negative cultures and higher cure rates. Based on these results Larsen [141, 120] recommends that for AIDS patients severely ill with cryptococcal meningitis (antigen titer > 1:32) two- to four-week a course of treatment with Amp B plus 5-FC should be followed by flu monotherapy. Only in less severely affected patients with milder symptoms and a titer < 1:32 should initial treatment be with flu.

Although it has failed to replace the "gold standard" for first line treatment, flu has proved excellent for maintenance therapy, which is essential for this patient group. In clinical trials [7, 8, 142, 143] 200 mg per day proved significantly more effective than Amp B as maintenance.

Flu is also a highly active treatment of oropharyngeal and gastrointestinal candidosis [144, 145] and it has become the drug of choice for prevention of recurrence of the former in HIV patients [146]. In practice, many physicians use the less expensive alternatives of clotrimazole troches or Amp B tablets for prophylaxis simply on economic grounds, and resort to flu only if this fails. Flu monotherapy has given some good results in coccidioidal meningitis [147], and although treatment was not without relapses it definitely shows promise in this indication. Success in the treatment of ocular infection has also been reported recently [148].

So flu has certainly found a place in the antifungal armory, even if at present only in the indications mentioned above. Its efficacy in other infections, such as deep candidosis in cancer or other immune suppressed patients, is yet to be properly explored in clinical trials, and it remains to be seen whether flu has already found its niche or will prove to be useful over a broader spectrum in the future.

Resistance

Resistance is not currently a problem as far as the triazoles are concerned, but it is hovering in the background. The number of cases is few, but there are already reports of fluconazole resistance appearing under therapy [149]. The few resistant strains have been intensively studied to understand the mechanisms involved. Some are no longer able to take up or accumulate drug although the target enzyme is still highly sensitive as measured in cell-free extracts. These strains are resistant to all azoles [150, 151]. A *Candida albicans* strain has been isolated in Japan with a lanosterol demethylase that was no longer able to bind drug to its cytochrome P_{450} moiety because of a point mutation [vanden Bossche in 7]. A *Candida glabrata* strain that developed resistance to fluconazole therapy during treatment proved to have significantly more ergosterol in its membrane as well as a higher amount of cytochrome P_{450}. Thus more drug was required to inhibit ergosterol synthesis and even then the cells had a large reserve of ergosterol [vanden Bossche in 7]. So several mechanisms of resistance to this class of compounds have already been identified, and further study in this direction is required to meet the problem as well prepared as possible.

Drug interactions

Although the new triazoles have a far greater specificity for fungal cells than ketoconazole, it is clear that they still react to a certain extent with the human hepatic cytochrome P_{450} system, and they may thus influence the metabolism and clearance of co-administered drugs [125–127, 152, 153]. Such interactions have been reported and represent another problem for the clinician as they must always be taken into account. Cyclosporin A and phenytoin appear to be drugs which require monitoring when used concurrently with flu, and this is an area in which considerable research is required. The interaction of keto with other drugs is well documented, and it would appear that flu is similar in this respect, although less problematic in degree. Itra seems to be less complicated in this matter [154–158].

So the breakthrough hoped for in the treatment of deep mycoses has not really been achieved by the triazoles. They will bring considerable benefit to many patients, and widen the available choice in several areas of the field, but the battle is by no means won.

It is somewhat depressing that a section on new drugs should contain but two. Others are on the way, as we shall see, but even looking further into the future the situation appears somewhat bleak. For these reasons other answers have been sought, in some cases with more than a little success.

4.3   New formulations

The advantages gained from new formulations of established drugs are real, but mostly minimal. In the antifungal field, however, it has long been clear that a liposomal formulation of Amp B could bring tremendous advantages. The physical characteristics of the polyene antibiotics cause intrinsic problems in their application, and the standard form of Amp B contains the detergent deoxycholate as well as active substance and buffer. Although this has been used with great success for many years, its toxicity is well known, and the role of tissue distribution is still controversial [159]. Since the idea of encapsulating Amp B in liposomes was first tested experimentally it has been known that this was a means of lowering the toxicity and increasing the therapeutic index, but bringing this idea from the laboratory to the market place has been a long and painful business despite a great deal of effort [160].

Much work has been done investigating the physical biochemistry of Amp B liposomal complexes, and on the mechanisms by which toxicity is reduced, the details of which are beyond the scope of this review [160–163]. The essentials are that Amp B in any formulation consists of complexed and free substance in equilibrium, and it is only the latter which is active. The greater affinity for ergosterol-containing fungal cells over cholesterol-containing mammalian cells means that a concentration range of free Amp B exists which is sufficient to be toxic only to the fungal cells. The job of the liposomes is to bring the drug into close contact with sterol containing membranes in tissue, where the greater affinity for ergosterol ensures better transfer of active substance to the fungal cells. Less Amp B is delivered to mammalian membranes, and less free substance is around to cause toxicity. There is good evidence that inclusion into liposomes serves to enhance, or simply make the most of, the inherent selectivity of heptaene antibiotics rather than creating structures that are intrinsically more selective [164, 165].

This model of what lies behind the improvements in therapy achieved by liposomal Amp B implies that there is no need for actual inclusion of the polyene molecule into a vesicle, and that simpler complexes with lipids or detergents would bring the same advantages. This has indeed proved to be the case [166–169]. Testing of a variety of formulations in animal models consistently showed efficacy of antifungal action and reduced toxicity, and detailed studies have been made of pharmacokinetics and tissue distribution as well [170–179a]. It has in fact been reported that simultaneously administered liposomes have the effect of lowering the toxicity of Amp B even if no actual complex is formed. A further refinement is the attachment of antibodies to the liposomes [180–182].

Trials in humans started in 1985, and results from small groups of patients have been trickling into the literature ever since [182–188]. They have been universally encouraging, but the step to general availability proved to be greater than was anticipated. The problem of the commercial scale manufacture of uniform, reproducible and stable formulations has been a real stumbling block, and it is only recently that success appears to have been achieved. The Vestar Corporation, formed especially to develop and market a liposomal form of Amp B, seems to have made the breakthrough. They have developed technology for the production of a unilamellar liposome encapsulated formulation of Amp B which is supplied in lyophylized form to be reconstituted with water for use. The problems of reproducibility and stability seem to have been solved, and the product is in the process of being registered in the USA and Europe.

The latest state of affairs in this area was presented at recent congresses in Japan and the USA [6–8]. In a European multicenter study, Ambisome was used in 80 patients who had failed on previous therapy, or had Amp B related toxicity or renal impairment, without signs of renal toxicity despite considerably higher peak serum levels than those obtained with Amp B. The results were very encouraging, especially considering the patient category which was enlisted in the trial, with a particularly good performance in candidosis. Excellent results in pulmonary mycoses were also reported in the USA. This product is sure to find a place in the antifungal armory, and further trials will better define the role it will fulfil.

An Amp B lipid complex with dimyristoylphosphatidyl choline and dimyristoylphosphatidyl glycerol has also shown itself superior to the normal formulation in animal models, and the current evaluation in man by Bristol-Myers Squibb has yielded favorable initial results. An emulsion formulation is also under evaluation in Japan. Detergent preparations are still being looked at, and sucrose monolaurate has given particularly good results, although these have not yet reached the stage of clinical trials [7].

Perhaps the story of liposomal Amp B is in a way typical of antifungal chemotherapy. A good idea, difficult to realize in practice, plenty of research, but perhaps not the commitment from industry because of the feeling that the development costs would not be covered (even the pharmaceutical industry must make a profit to survive). Then the hopes for better drugs are not fulfilled as quickly as anticipated, and an old drug in a new dress proves after all to be a real advance in the field.

4.4   Combination therapy

Chemotherapy with combinations of antimicrobials has always been a contentious subject, and its use perhaps rather more dependent on fashion than on objective considerations of the advantages and disadvantages. Opinions differ between cultures, countries, and even between and within clinics. In the antifungal field the continuing failure of even the much vaunted triazoles to solve the ever-increasing problems has led to a new willingness in many quarters to consider combinations of drugs to broaden antifungal spectrum, attain a fungicidal action, and reduce side effects.

Studies in vitro and particularly in animal models have shown that a real increase in efficacy can be achieved with certain combinations in some indications, but that others should be avoided as they are antagonistic. Based on such results, drug combinations are beginning to be used in clinical situations, and are often able to clear infections significantly faster than monotherapy. The field is rapidly changing, but two recent reviews have covered the subject thoroughly [19, 189]. We shall attempt to illustrate that there is a real possibility for progress if the available evidence is considered and the correct combinations used in the correct indications. As with all other aspects of chemotherapy the steps are clearly defined – in vitro, animal models, clinical use. Although by no means the only factor upon which the effect of a drug combination depends, interactions at the level of the fungal cell do indicate which possibilities are worth further consideration. Looking at the information available, and keeping in mind the great variations in methodologies, the following conclusions can be reached [19, 100, 101, 190]. Amp B plus rifampicin is the most effective synergistic combination. Amp B plus 5-FC also shows good synergy, especially against 5-FC-resistant strains. Amp B and (tri)azoles act antagonistically when added simultaneously, or when the azole is added first, but synergy has been observed in cases where the azole was added to cells that had been pretreated with subinhibitory concentrations of Amp B. Azoles and 5-FC are usually indifferent, occasionally synergistic and never antagonistic.

Combination therapy has been studied in models of a variety of infections in normal and neutropenic mice, rats and rabbits [101, 191–193]. Although other combinations have been studied more recently most work has been done with the combination of Amp B and 5-FC, which has improved activity in cryptococcosis and systemic candidosis. Notably, in neutropenic rabbits only this combination was able to eradicate renal candidosis, which neither fluconazole nor itraconazole was able to achieve [191, 193]. The in vitro synergy of Amp B and rifampicin is confirmed in animal models over a broad range, including aspergillosis and other opportunistic infections, and also against the true pathogens *Histoplasma* and *Blastomyces*. This combination has, however, found only limited clinical use.

The result of combining Amp B and azoles depends on species and strain. Synergy was found with keto, flu and itra in models of cryptococcosis in mice and rabbits, but antagonism in *Candida* and *Aspergillus* infections. The combination of 5-FC with an azole has a beneficial effect in most cases, the degree depending on the nature of the azole, and is never antagonistic. In murine candidosis the synergy is as strong as that of Amp B and 5-FC, but in cryptococcosis it was found to be surprisingly weak for flu. This may be due to the high efficacy of

Table 1
Summary of drug interaction in combined chemotherapy of murine fungal infections

	Candidosis	Cryptococcosis	Aspergillosis	Histoplasmosis Blastomycosis	Chromomycosis Wangiellosis
Amp B + Rif	ADD	–	SYN	SYN	–
Amp B + 5-FC	ADD/SYN	ADD/SYN	INDIFF/SYN	–	SYN
Amp B + Keto	ANT/SYN	SYN	ANT	INDIFF(SYN)	–
Amp B + Itra	INDIFF/ANT	ADD	INDIFF/ANT/SYN		
Amp B + Flu	INDIFF/ANT	ADD	INDIFF/ANT/SYN		
5-FC + Keto	ADD/SYN	INDIFF/SYN	INDIFF	–	INDIFF
5-FC + Itra	ADD/SYN	INDIFF/ADD	SYN/INDIFF	–	–
5-FC + Flu	ADD/SYN	INDIFF/SYN	–	–	SYN

Amp B	Amphotericin B	ANT antagonistic
Rif	Rifampicin	ADD additive
Keto	Ketoconazole	SYN synergistic
Itra	Itraconazole	INDIFF indifferent
5-FC	5-Flucytosine	– not tested
Flu	Fluconazole	

flu on its own in this model, or to pharmacokinetic differences, as 5-FC and itra was an effective combination. Other studies have indeed shown synergy between 5-FC and flu [193 a]. Table 1 summarizes the effect of antifungal drug combinations in murine infections.

Triple combinations have also been investigated, which means addition of an azole derivative to 5-FC plus Amp B. In this respect keto is generally antagonistic, itra indifferent with a tendency to antagonism under certain conditions, but the situation with flu appears more promising as real benefit was observed except at very low concentrations of flu. Again, the best performance of triple combinations was seen in models of cryptococcosis [19].

Thus from animal work it would seem that combination of 5-FC with Amp B, itra or flu may be of benefit in the treatment of systemic mycoses. Whereas Amp B should not be combined with imidazoles or triazoles in candidosis or aspergillosis, this may be of advantage in cryptococcosis and histoplasmosis. Triple combinations should at the moment only be considered for cryptococcosis, especially in AIDS, where fungicidal action can bring particular benefit.

It is of course the clinic that matters, but unfortunately this is where differences in practice and interpretation begin to cloud the issue. It is also far from easy, for both practical and ethical reasons, to perform a proper clinical trial in cases of deep mycoses, which are life-threatening and very often complicated by underlying disease. Up to now a controlled clinical trial has taken place only with one combination in one indication, where the superiority of 5-FC plus Amp B over Amp B monotherapy has been clearly demonstrated [108, 194]. However, there is no lack of what is known as anecdotal information, and this is beginning to suggest that the results in animal models do indeed have a predictive value regarding the potential of combinations of antifungal drugs in human chemotherapy.

The therapy of choice for cryptococcosis in non-AIDS patients is 5-FC plus Amp B, based on the results of the two randomized, prospective studies mentioned above. These authors did, however, note a high incidence of side effects, and this is an illustration of the geographical differences which are noticeable in the field. Examination of the literature reveals that this combination has caused a higher incidence of adverse effects in the USA than in Europe. Likely explanations for this are the readier acceptance in Europe that 5-FC toxicity can be avoided by monitoring serum levels and keeping below

100 mg/l [106], and the non-availability of a parenteral form of flucytosine in the States. The latter is an important factor given the original reluctance to accept that the nephrotoxicity of Amp B can be radically reduced by "salt loading" [195, 196]. This is automatically achieved by an infusion of 5-FC, which contains 9 g of saline, but must be administered additionally when the oral form is used. Despite this problem, the combination has become accepted worldwide as being superior to Amp B monotherapy.

The situation with *Cryptococcus* in AIDS is more confused [197–200]. The illness proceeds differently and is far more difficult to eradicate as reservoirs of infection appear to remain, especially in the prostate, even after therapy has apparently succeeded, and relapse is the rule rather than the exception. Here the variety in treatment is at its greatest. In America Amp B alone was the therapy of choice, and a retrospective study by Chuck and Sande [201] which concluded that the addition of 5-FC did not alter the outcome gave no reason to change. In Europe, especially in France and Italy, the combination was and still is preferred for initial therapy. It is universally agreed that a lifelong maintenance therapy must be given, and this is usually with flu although itra is also used. As stated above, flu monotherapy has been tried but has not proved its worth in this indication. The reluctance to use 5-FC in the USA goes back to the fear of inducing bone marrow toxicity, and also the difficulty in taking oral medication suffered by the many AIDS patients with oropharyngeal candidosis. However, the combination is being used increasingly in the States, and more physicians are being convinced of its benefits. The introduction of a parenteral form of 5-FC there would be an important step in the improvement of care for this patient group.

In Europe flu and itra monotherapy have been used successfully in cryptococcosis, but combination of itra with 5-FC worked better and no bone marrow toxicity was observed [132, 135]. Fluconazole has been used in combination with Amp B and also with 5-FC [202], and results of treatment with the triple combination Amp B/5-FC/flu have also been published recently [203].

This large number of variations that has been used in just one narrow area, cryptococcosis in AIDS, demonstrates clearly that one of the major problems in combination therapy is the sheer number of possibilities. It has become clear that an effective fungicidal treatment followed by maintenance therapy gives the best results, and it is to be hoped that one of the combinations now being tried will prove capable of completely sterilizing the body. It is surely worth persevering to achieve this goal.

Combination therapy has also proved its worth in deep-seated *Candida* infections. In neutropenic patients the need for effective, fungicidal chemotherapy is paramount, and the Amp B/5-FC combination has achieved the best results here [60, 203–206]. Bone marrow recovery is, however, necessary to achieve cure. *Candida* peritonitis is a problem in CAPD patients, and while Cheng et al. have shown that monotherapy without removal of the catheter does not give an acceptable cure rate, various combinations of drugs have given convincing results [207, 208]. Systemic *Candida* infections have also become a significant problem in neonatal intensive care units, where Amp B plus 5-FC is almost exclusively used. This is an area where an alternative is badly needed, since premature infants tolerate Amp B very badly. It is to be hoped that either flu or itra can be proved an effective substitute in the future.

So again it is only the combination of the established drugs 5-FC and Amp B that has really been evaluated to a sufficient extent for conclusions to be reached. It is certainly indicated in all granulocytopenic patients with definite symptoms of CNS candidosis, renal candidosis and hepatosplenic candidosis [209] as well as a diversity of other *Candida* infections. However, there is some hope that one of the new triazoles, although not effective as monotherapy against this opportunistic pathogen, may prove to have the ability to replace Amp B as a combination partner.

Aspergillosis responds so poorly to antifungal chemotherapy that more emphasis is put on prevention than in other indications. For therapy, the Amp B/5-FC combination also seems to be superior here, especially when the dose of Amp B is high [121, 209]. Itra has been used with some success in the clinic, as reported recently by Dupont [209a], and looks promising. Although the author does not comment on this, it is clear from his data that long-term treatment with a combination of Amp B and itra is not effective against invasive aspergillosis, and often leads to treatment failure. This is confirmation of the results of in vitro and animal model experiments [101, table 1]. Although no clinical data are as yet available, its combination with 5-FC is likely to be of value [133, 135, 210]. This has also proved effective in the treatment of chromomycosis [131, 211, 212] and has been successful in treating *Candida* infections with strains resistant to Amp B [Rennie and Hellmann in ref. 8].

New ideas are continually appearing. Combination of Amp B with the new triazole Sch 39304 (genaconazole) in a mouse model of crypto-coccosis has proved better than monotherapy, but the dosage regimen of Amp B is critical [Graybill in ref. 8]. The addition of a monoclonal antibody to Amp B has also improved treatment in another murine model of the same infection [Dromer and Charreire in ref. 8]. The use of immune modulators in combination with antifungal chemotherapy is also something that will become of increasing importance in the years to come, and the role of surgical intervention should also not be forgotten. Thus although the options for the treatment of deep my-coses are perhaps limited, the optimal use of what is available in appropriate combinations can serve to widen the choice available.

4.5   Immune modulators

There is of course more than one way to fight opportunistic fungal infections. The classical approach is chemotherapy with an effective, preferably fungicidal antimycotic. Less conventionally one could, at least in theory, use compounds which influence the virulence of the fungi or the host defences. Knowledge concerning virulence factors is still too scarce to be of practical use in drug design at the present, but the ability to influence the host immune system has become a reality. Knowledge of the host defence against fungal infection is steadily increasing [212a] and research in immunology has characterized much of the body's diverse armament of interleukins, interferons, colony-stimulating factors, tumor-necrosis factor (TNF) etc. as well as developing synthetic immunomodulators such as muramyl peptides. Various cytokines have been isolated and several have been produced using biotechnology methods.

All of these factors have been thoroughly tested in vitro and in animal models to define their capacity to increase the defence against tumor and bacterial cells and protozoic infection. Compared with the intensive study in these fields relatively little has been done to investigate the role of these substances in mycology, but some information is available.

Muramyl peptides increase the natural resistance against fungal infection [6–8, 213], but because of their toxicity they have not been used in human therapy. They are known to induce the production of interleukins in vivo, so the role of these latter has also been studied in neutropenic mice infected with *C. albicans*. Both interleukin 1α and 1β prolonged survival in a lethal *Candida* infection [213, 214].

Histoplasmosis in mice is associated with depression of cellular immune response due to a deficiency in the production of interleukin 2. This cytokine is able to enhance natural killer cell activity through induction of interferon in vitro. However, the cellular immune response of mice with disseminated histoplasmosis could not be modulated by interleukin 2 administration [215]. Interleukin 3 was found to stimulate the phagocytosis of *Candida* cells by peritoneal macrophages, and killing of *Candida pseudotropicalis* (but not of *C. albicans*) was also increased [216]. Interferon γ has been shown to enhance the growth inhibition and even fungicidal activity of macrophages as well as that of polymorphonuclear neutrophils (PMNs). The growth of several fungi including *C. albicans, Histoplasma capsulatum* and *Blastomyces dermatitidis* was significantly more inhibited in the presence of interferon γ-stimulated macrophages and/or PMNs than unstimulated [217]. TNF has a similar effect on PMNs and in fact has shown synergy with interferon γ [218]. Differences in response are observed depending on whether the pulmonary or resident macrophages are studied and which fungal species is involved. For instance, *Blastomyces dermatitidis* is significantly better killed by interferon γ-activated pulmonary macrophages, whereas no stimulation was observed in killing of *C. albicans* [219]. Extracellular killing of *Cryptococcus neoformans,* an encapsulated yeast, is also induced by interferon γ in vitro [220].

In vivo, a stimulation of the killing capacity of macrophages and PMNs after the systemic application of interferon γ has also been observed [221–223]. Treatment with interferon γ also enhances the survival time of mice infected with *H. capsulatum,* but has no effect on *Candida*-infected mice although this might have been expected from the in vitro results (A. Polak, unpublished data). Interferon γ used prophylactically provided significant protection against an extracellular infection with *Aspergillus fumigatus* [224].

These studies show the way in which new treatments may develop, but as far as we are aware no clinical trials have been performed with any of these immune modulators.

The most promising immune modulators for fungal infections appear to be granulocyte- and granulocyte-macrophage-colony stimulating factors (G-CSF and GM-CSF). G-CSF treatment results in significant protection against systemic infections caused by *C. albicans* in neu- tropenic (cyclophosphamide treated) but not in cortisone-treated mice, which have a more complex immunodeficiency. Localized candidosis, however, does not respond. Apparently G-CSF restores the granulocyte-dependent defence mechanism to near normal capac- ity, as the mice only succumb to the same inoculum of infecting agent as normal mice, whereas a hundred-fold lower inoculum is fatal for neutropenic mice [A. Polak, Mycoses in Press 1991, 226]. A recent re- port also demonstrated the beneficial effect of G-CSF in experimental hepatosplenic candidosis in granulocytopenic rabbits [225].

G-CSF has a similar protective effect in mice infected with *Aspergillus fumigatus*. In both models of aspergillosis studied (i. v. and intranasal infection) a life-prolonging effect was observed. Again, cortisone- treated mice did not respond, underlining the high specificity of G- CSF which appears to activate only granulocytes and no other im- mune competent cells. It is interesting that G-CSF affords no protec- tion against cryptococcosis, showing that the main defence against this infection is not granulocyte dependent. The susceptibility of AIDS patients to *Cryptococcus* supports the idea that the T-cell system is the most important in this case [see also 7].

It was clearly of interest to ask whether a synergistic effect exists be- tween G-CSF treatment and conventional antifungal therapy, and in fact this has proved to be the case. The degree of this synergy is de- pendent both on the nature of the antifungal and on its dose; thus it is high with Amp B, 5-FC, ketoconazole and low doses of the triazoles flu and itra, while high doses of flu and itra show such a strong cura- tive effect in neutropenic mice on their own that no synergy with G- CSF could be observed in candidosis. A strong synergy was also ob- served in models of aspergillosis [A. Polak, Mycoses in Press 1991].

GM-CSF broadly exerts similar effects as G-CSF, but there is less data available about its use in models of fungal infections.

The synergy observed between conventional and immune therapy in animal models of fungal infections is mirrored in the bacterial field, and may also begin to play an important role here as well. Thus G- CSF together with various antibacterial agents has been studied in *Pseudomonas aeruginosa* infected mice [227–231], and also in strepto- coccal sepsis in neonatal rats [230]. A similar model, but with

Staphylococcus aureus as the infecting agent, has been used to demonstrate that GM-CSF also induces a protective effect in this field.

There have been as yet no trials of G-CSF in human antifungal therapy, although GM-CSF has been used in combination with Amp B against disseminated mycosis [232]. Survival was improved although the doses of both components were not optimal. An endocarditis due to *Candida parapsilosis* responded well to a GM-CSF combination, although the patient died of bacterial septicemia [233].

Despite this lack of direct evidence, inferences can be made from several clinical trials of the various growth and colony-stimulating factors in cancer and related diseases, and even in AIDS patients. The details of such work are beyond the scope of this chapter, but various aspects have been reviewed recently [234–236]. The success in reducing the rate of infections in immune-suppressed patients has in some cases been remarkable, and awakens real hope for the future. It is becoming abundantly clear that the available knowledge in this extremely complex field barely suffices to use even the substances presently available to the best advantage, but as the most appropriate factors and their correct combination for individual conditions are established more and more patients will benefit from their use. There are still problems with side effects to be solved, but it appears that the more specific factors, such as G-CSF, are less likely to cause trouble.

It would appear, then, that although we are right at the beginning of their development in this field, the augmentation of host defences by immunomodulating agents such as interferons, cytokines and colony-stimulating factors, especially during pharmacological immune suppression, may prevent the development of life-threatening opportunistic fungal infections in immune-compromised patients. These modulators may also become important adjuncts to conventional antifungal therapy of established infections in this setting.

5   Systemic mycosis – Hopes and dreams

Hopes and dreams should perhaps not be dealt with together under one heading, but separation of hopes from dreams is a tricky task and such judgments are bound to be subjective. So we shall look in the direction from which progress is likely to come, starting with drugs that are in full development and progressing to substances and ideas that may come to fruition ever further in the future, and leave the reader to arrive at his own conclusion as to what is hopeful and what is likely to remain a dream.

5.1   New drugs on the way

Genaconazole

As with new drugs on the market, the count of drugs in development for the treatment of deep mycoses just creeps into the plural. Only saperconazole and Sch 39304 have survived to a stage of clinical trials that makes it possible to believe that they will make it onto the market; the few others have fallen at the various hurdles along the way.

Sch 39304, also known as SM 8668, is a triazole under development by Schering-Plough under licence from Sumitomo. It is active orally, parenterally and topically and has been investigated with an impressive intensity. In fact one could almost say that there has been a tendency to go overboard, the literature is so full of animal studies in various species, neutropenic and non-neutropenic, infected with an extensive array of pathogens. The excitement that this new drug has aroused is perhaps some indication of how desperately progress is needed in the field, and its performance to date has indeed been impressive.

Earlier results have been reviewed by Ryley [2], and the information has continued to flood in during 1990. Leaving aside in vitro data which, despite efforts to persuade us otherwise, really do not help much in comparative studies involving azoles, the in vivo news has continued to be good. Sch 39304 compared favorably with Amp B and was much better than fluconazole against *Histoplasma capsulatum* infected normal and neutropenic mice [237]. It was more effective than both itra and flu in a mouse model of coccidioidal meningitis [238],

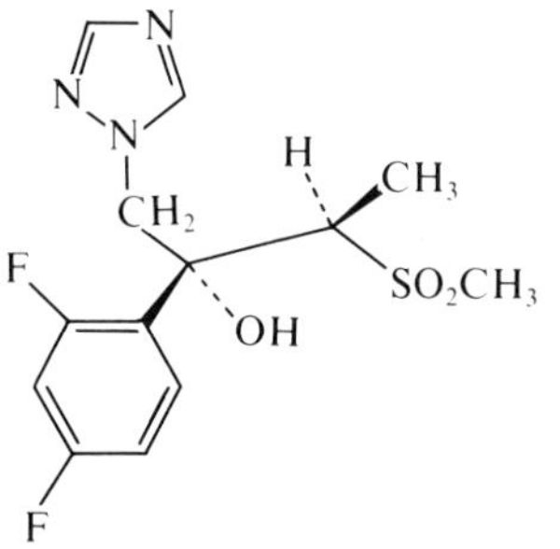

SCH 39304 (SM 8668)

and superior to flu in another study of disseminated coccioidomyco-sis in mice [239]. Two studies confirmed its efficacy in cryptococcal meningitis [240, 241] and good, long-lasting penetration into the cere-brospinal fluid of rhesus monkey was also observed [242]. The drug was also effective in murine blastomycosis [243]. *Candida* infections have received their fair share of attention, and Sch 39304 proved com-parable to flu and Amp B in prevention and early treatment of dissem-inated candidosis in granulocytopenic rabbits, but not as effective as Amp B plus 5-FC once the infection was allowed five days to set in [244]. At the moment this is simply the best azole on the scene.

Sch 39304 is in phase II/III clinical trials in the USA. Initial studies have shown that there is virtually no metabolism, and that renal excre-tion of the unchanged drug accounts for about 80 % of the dose. The serum half-life is very long in humans, averaging 60 hours, which could be a double-edged sword. The possibility of longer intervals be-tween doses is obviously attractive, especially for maintenance ther-apy and prophylaxis, but there could be problems with drug accumu-lation and dosing schedules in severely ill patients, especially those with reduced kidney function. The safety profile also looks good to date. The results of several clinical studies were presented at the 1990 ICAAC [8]. Meunier's group reported efficacy of 50 mg/day in oro-pharyngeal candidosis in cancer patients, and the results in invasive mold infections, again in cancer patients, achieved by Annassie et al. suggested that the drug could significantly improve treatment in this patient group even in the face of profound neutropenia. Pharmaco-kinetic studies showed that it is extremely well absorbed with a high bioavailability, and that the parameters were unchanged in AIDS pa-tients.

One cloud on the horizon is the result of findings presented at the Oiso Congress by scientists from Sumitomo [245]. They have con-firmed that the antifungal activity of SM 8668 depends mostly on the RR-enantiomer (SM 9164). The pure enantiomer apparently has bet-ter activity than the racemate by a factor of about two and is more wa-ter soluble. It is not clear how this will effect the development of the compound, but could lead to considerable delay.

Saperconazole

The other drug which has raised a few hopes is saperconazole, which is under development by Janssen. Its status is, however, difficult to assess for lack of information. A comprehensive review of in vitro and in vivo results appeared at the end of 1989 [246], from which it can be concluded that saperconazole has powerful antifungal activity over a wide spectrum, and is in addition fungicidal. Good activity was reported in disseminated candidosis and cryptococcosis in normal and neutropenic guinea pigs, and the activity against aspergillosis is particularly interesting [247, T. F. Patterson, D. George, R. Ingersoll, P. Minitier, V. T. Andriole in ref. 8]. The drug is lipophilic, but the possibility of an i.v. formulation was opened by animal experiments using β-cylodextrin derivatives. However, we are unaware of any clinical experience with this drug, and will have to await some indication of its progress. Despite the promise of in vitro and in vivo experiments saperconazole seems to be taking a long while to get off the ground and it is to be hoped that it has not run into problems.

5.2   Shattered hopes

It is a fact of life that many of the new drugs that enter development will fall by the wayside on efficacy, toxicological or economic grounds, but nevertheless it is always a disappointment each time it happens. The list of hopes that have foundered is longer than the list of those drugs still in the running.

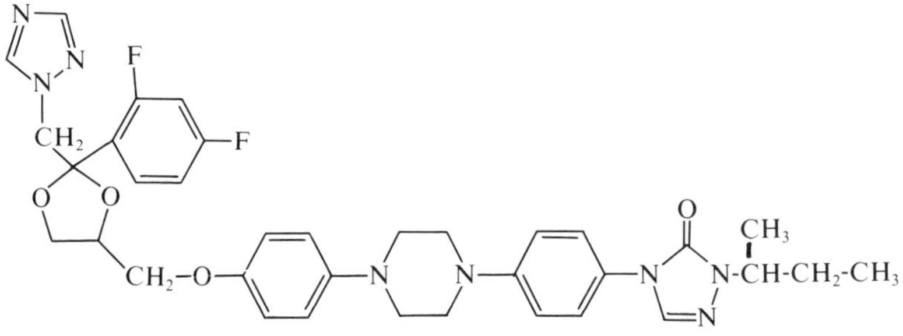

Saperconazole

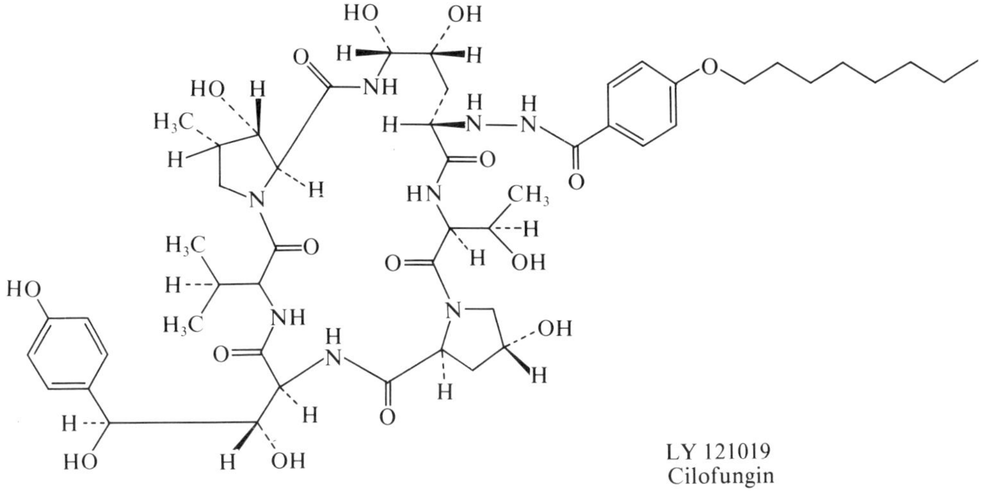

LY 121019
Cilofungin

Cilofungin

It was a brave decision by Lilly to develop a drug with a spectrum re-stricted in practice to *Candida albicans* and *Candida tropicalis*, and which has to be administered four times a day by the i. v. route. A de-ciding factor was no doubt that cilofungin would have been the first drug for many years to have a really novel mode of action [248, 249]. This semisynthetic derivative of echinocandin B is a specific non-competitive inhibitor of the beta-1,3-glucan synthase of *Candida albicans,* and has no effect on the synthesis of chitin, mannan, DNA, RNA or protein [250, U. Taug and T. R. Parr in 8].

Animal studies gave good results in most models studied [251–254], and there were also indications that it could be combined with other antifungals [255]. Preliminary phase II results showed satisfactory

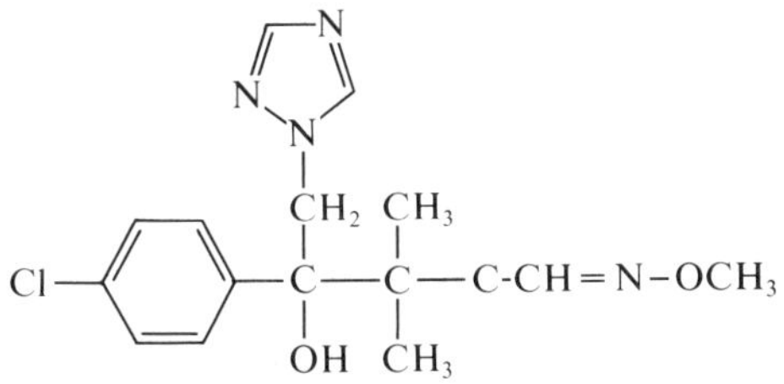

BAY R 3783 (Electrazole)

efficacy in the treatment of *Candida* esophagitis in AIDS patients [C. R. Copley-Merriman, N. J. Ransburg, L. R. Crane, T. M. Kerkering, P. G. Pappas, J. C. Potage, D. L. Hyslop in ref. 8] and disseminated candidosis in non-neutropenic patients [C. R. Copley-Merriman, H. Gallis, J. R. Graybill, B. N. Doebbeling, D. L. Hylop in ref. 8]. Too little information was available to reach any conclusion regarding possible resistance problems, although preliminary work had been done [A. Cassone, L. Angiolettà, C. Bromuro, N. Simonetti in ref. 8]. A somewhat unexpected bonus was that in vivo activity had been found against aspergillosis in a murine model [D. W. Denning, D. A. Stevens in ref. 8]. But cilofungin always seemed to be a marginal case and, although a shame, its demise was not totally unexpected. Toxicity of the vehicle necessary for its administration finally tipped the scales against it and brought an end to this gallant effort to bring something really new onto the market.

Electrazole

A substance that is not from a new chemical class, but nonetheless showed promise, is BAY R 3783 (electrazole – the name never caught on). This triazole has a broad spectrum of in vitro activity [255–258]. A good number of in vivo studies showed BAY R 3783 to be at least as good as the other triazoles in development [259, 260]. However, it was found that this azole was quickly metabolized to several substances. One of these was very persistent and had non-linear kinetics, which lead to the suspension of phase I studies in humans [2].

ICI 195,739

Another azole that fell out of the race at an early stage is the bistriazole ICI 195,739. This compound, identified as a result of an intensive synthesis and screening effort, is extremely active in vitro and in vivo. The efficacy in a range of animal models was reviewed by Ryley. Despite these good results the compound may not be developed [261].

Also ran

And so it goes on. Two compounds from Sandoz, the triazole SDZ 89-485 and the wide spectrum allylamine SDZ 87-469 seem to have

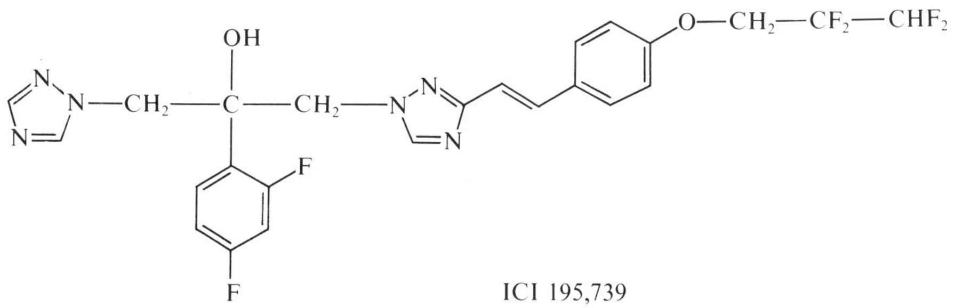

ICI 195,739

submerged, and development of the amino acid derivative RI 331 has also been discontinued by Taisho. The latter was another hope for a product with a novel mode of action, as it interferes with amino acid synthesis at the level of homoserine dehydrogenase, an enzyme lacking in animals. The compound possesses activity against several pathogenic fungi, was shown to be effective against systemic candidosis in animals, and was well tolerated [7]. The properties of another hopeful compound whose development was continued this year suggests that it might also act on the amino acid synthesis pathway. Cispentacin is an amino acid derivative that shows a weak, medium-dependent in vitro activity, but was active in vivo against infections with *Candida albicans* and *Cryptococcus neoformans* [262, 263]. It was also extremely well tolerated in preliminary toxicology. Compound G2, isolated from alfalfa roots, was also around for a long time. It is active in vitro against plant pathogenic fungi, medically important yeasts and dermatophytes [264–267]. A recent paper described in vivo evaluation against experimental dermatophyte infection [268], but its development has now been discontinued.

The chances of a compound that enters phase I trials actually reaching the market are about one in ten, and many never progress beyond

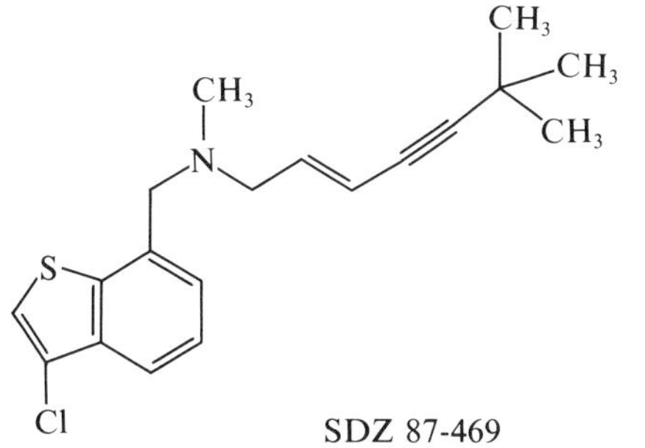

SDZ 87-469 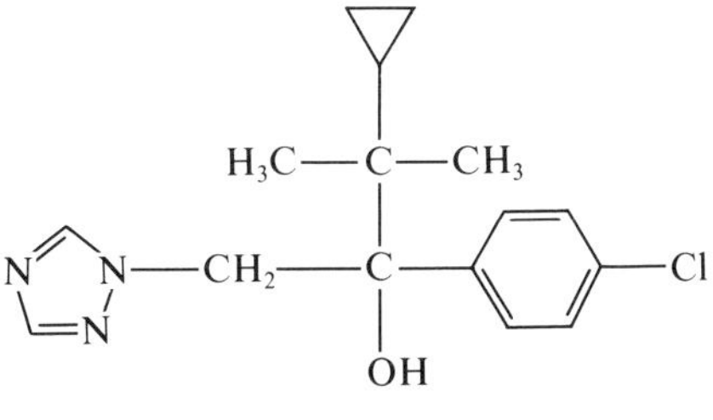   SDZ 89.485

RI 331

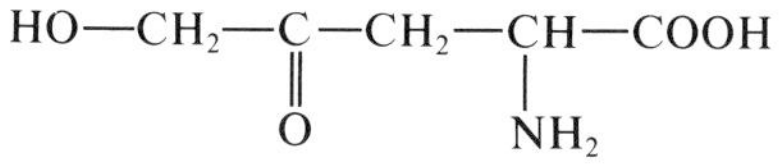

$$HO-CH_2-\overset{\displaystyle C}{\underset{\displaystyle O}{\|}}-CH_2-\overset{\displaystyle CH}{\underset{\displaystyle NH_2}{|}}-COOH$$

(S)-2-amino-5-hydroxy-4-oxopentanoic acid

the preclinical stage, and thus a constant flow of new structures and ideas are required to feed the whole process. So perhaps it is worthwhile examining some of the "dreams", those compounds really still in their infancy from whose ranks the hopes for the future must come.

5.3   Further in the future

The literature is full of new antibiotics, and a good proportion of them are antifungals. Every week one can spend a couple of hours in the library reading of inhibition zones and MIC values of new substances, be they fermentation products or the result of chemical synthesis. Some journals specialize in such reports, which reflects the amount of work being carried out. Some of the substances mentioned stay with us for a while, and one reads of structure determination, activity of derivatives, and structure-function studies. Others are more ephemeral, and after a comment such as ". . . could be useful in the treatment of fungal infections" they are never heard of again. It is encouraging to be constantly reminded of the diversity of active substances that nature presents to us, and it could well be the case that the next significant advance in antifungal chemotherapy has already made its debut in the Journal of Antibiotics.

It is often very difficult to keep up to date with antifungals in the early stages of development, as information tends to be scanty. Indeed, a sudden flood of data on a compound frequently heralds its demise. Some do, however, still seem to be running. The pradimycins are a growing family of antifungal antibiotics produced by *Actinomadura*

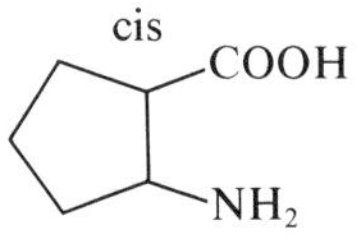

Cispentacin

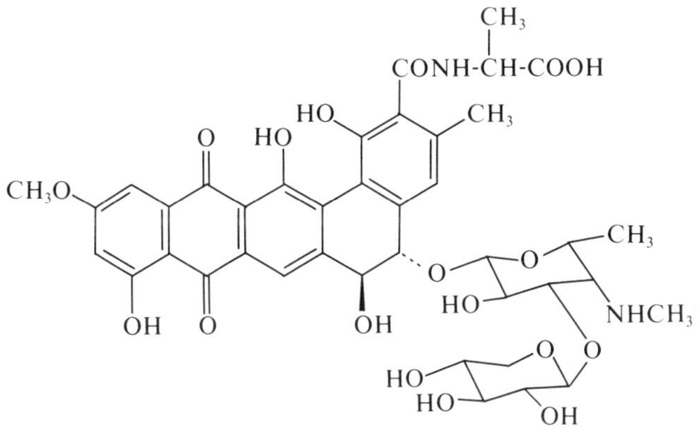

BMY 28567 (Pradimycin)

hibisca, based on a core structure of glycosylated dihydrobenzo(a) naphthacene quinone with a D-amino acid. Pradimicin A and B have been around for three years [269] and have now been supplemented by C, D, E, FA1 and FA2 [270, 271, Y. Sawada et al. in 7] which has allowed some structure-function information to be gleaned. The natural product pradimicin A has a good range of in vitro activity and showed in vivo efficacy against a broad range of fungal infections (candidosis, aspergillosis, cryptococcosis, trichophytosis) [272]. However, the limited solubility made further development difficult, and as a result a chemical program was started at Bristol-Myers Squibb in Japan to identify water soluble derivatives. BMY 28864, the dimethyl analog of pramicidin FA-2 in which the amino acid moiety is D-serine, was chosen for further development, and several reports were to be seen at the ICAAFC in Oiso [7]. It is as active as the parent compound in vitro and in vivo, has superior water solubility and a higher LD_{50} in mice. The mode of action is unique, although not yet defined in detail, and is dependent on the presence of calcium ions [272a]. Under these conditions BMY 28864 binds to sensitive fungi, but not to bacteria, human erythrocytes, cultured mammalian cells or cells of nonsensitive fungi. Electron microscopic studies revealed damage to the cell wall, membrane and nuclei, leakage of cell constituents was noted, and binding to mannan and mannoproteins observed. The reported activity in vivo against *Candida, Cryptococcus* and *Aspergillus* certainly justifies further investigation of this pramicidin derivative.

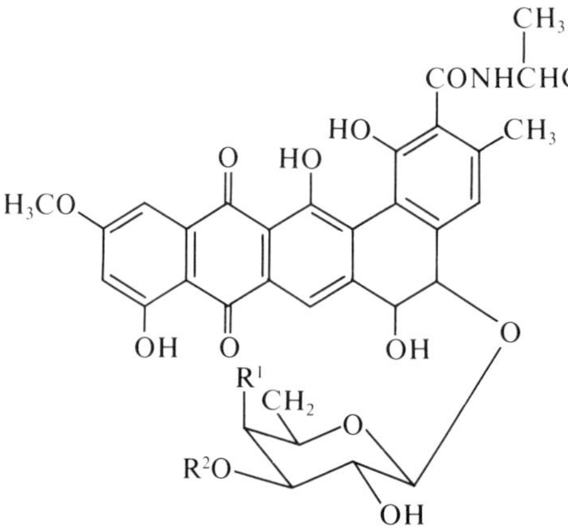

$$CH_3$$
$$CONHCHCOOR^3$$

Benanomycins

Compound	R¹	R²	R³
A	OH	xylosyl	H
B	NH₂	xylosyl	H
A-DX	OH	H	H
B-DX	NH₂	H	H
B-AC	NHCOCH₃	xylosyl	H
B-ME	NH₂	xylosyl	CH₃
B-DXME	NH₂	H	CH₃

A structurally very similar group of antifungal substances, the bena-nomycins, were first reported at more or less the same time. They too have been the subject of derivatization, and appear to have similar ac-tivity to the pramicidins, including fungicidal properties. The mode of action of benanomycin A (ME 1451) has been studied [7, 8] and the results underline the similarity. No significant effect on the synthesis of protein, DNA or RNA was observed, but that of lipid, glucan, and other cell wall polysaccharides was stimulated. Binding to sensitive cells followed by leakage was also observed. It will be interesting to follow the separate development of these very similar antifungals.

Another large family of antifungals, isolated from the fermentation broth of *Aureobasidium pullulans,* are the Aureobasidins A to R, cyclic peptides containing eight amino acids and a hydroxy acid. Aureoba-sidin A is extremely active against a broad range of pathogens includ-ing *Candida* spp., *Cryptococcus* spp., *Blastomyces dermatiditis* and

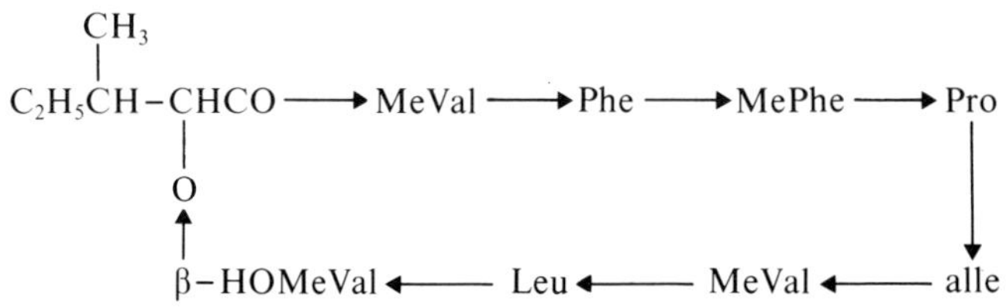

$$CH_3$$
$$C_2H_5CH-CHCO \longrightarrow MeVal \longrightarrow Phe \longrightarrow MePhe \longrightarrow Pro$$

β−HOMeVal ⟵ Leu ⟵ MeVal ⟵ aIle

Aureobasidin A (R 106-I)

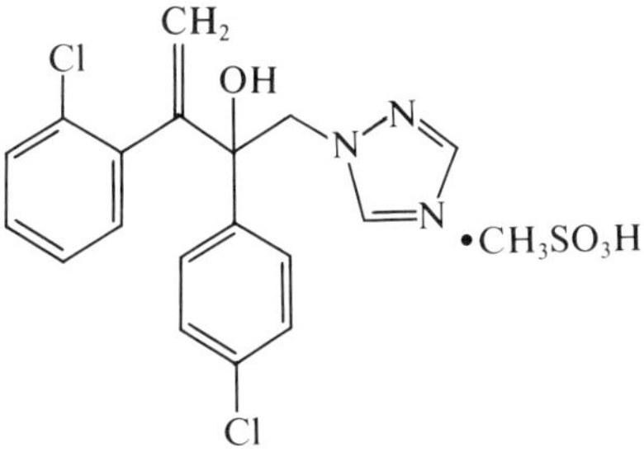

DuP 860

Histoplasma capsulatum. It is more active than Amp B against these organisms, and is fungicidal. Against murine systemic candidosis it was effective at 3.5 mg/kg i. v. for 5 days, and at 14 mg/kg p. o. [6–8]. The *Candida* was almost eradicated by the curative dose, and the acute toxicity is also low. This could also be one to watch.

The seemingly inexhaustable synthetic possibilities of the azoles, akin to the cephalosporins of the antibacterial field, is still potentially capable of producing antifungals with improved performance and DuP 860, an α-styrylcarbinol, is one of the latest to arrive on the scene [8]. The in vitro activity of this compound compares favorably with that of established drugs, especially against *Candida albicans*. Oral efficacy in animal models of systemic and superficial mycoses has been mentioned, but no details given. DuP 860 is the active (S)-(-)-isomer, and two active epoxide metabolites have been identified in the mouse, rat and dog. An azole must be something a bit special to make it nowadays, but the indications are that better structures will be found. Perhaps this one will prove to have that extra something.

Chitin synthase is an enzyme that is considered by many to be one of the most promising targets for the development of novel antifungals,

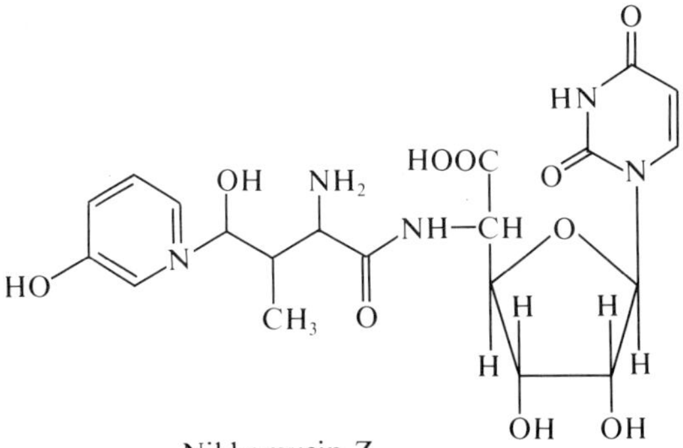

Nikkomycin Z

but its inhibition has up to now not produced any real success. Amongst the most hopeful inhibitors are the nikkomycin group of antifungals. Details of their activity are still appearing [7, 8, 273], and they seem particularly effective against coccidioidomycosis and blastomycosis. Also, combination with cilofungin, another cell wall inhibitor, produced a degree of synergy. Nikkomycin Z is apparently being developed in the USA by the Bayer subsidiary Cutter, and some effort is still being invested in producing analogs by mutasynthesis and chemical modification.

Sometimes there is very little information available, but just enough to whet the appetite. For instance, a recent report indicated that a compound UFC 6401 is undergoing clinical trials against *Trichophyton mentagrophytes, Aspergillus fumigatus,* "etc", but this is the first time that we have heard of this substance. Even more enigmatic was a report in a "popular" scientific journal concerning an antifungal called metapleurin, a substance secreted by ants, which was supposed to be under evaluation as it had shown activity against *Candida albicans* as well as against *Staphylococcus aureus* [274]. A search of the literature and attempts at correspondence failed to uncover any further trace of this compound, but reports such as this serve to keep alive the hope that even if the new antifungals discussed above do not make it into clinical practice, someone, somewhere has got something up their sleeve.

There is no stagnation in the field, the search for new antimycotics is continuing. There is always something new to arouse interest. And there are also a few old ideas that continue to move researchers to further efforts despite many years of disappointing results.

5.4   Still trying

In any field there are a few perennials, lines of research that have not really fulfilled their expectations but have come close enough to make you think that success is just around the corner, or that have proved to be interesting simply for the basic knowledge that they yield. Amp B has such outstanding antifungal activity that it is not surprising that attempts have been made to increase its therapeutic index by derivatization, and this has become one of the perennials of antifungal chemotherapy. The goal of such studies has been to increase solubility and decrease toxicity without losing efficacy.

Amphotericin B derivatives

The names of Borowski and Schaffner are those most often associated with this work, and the latter has reviewed the subject in detail [275]. The first to be investigated were the N-acetyl derivatives [276–278], but these proved not to be truly water soluble, and their decrease in toxicity was matched by a corresponding reduction in activity. Amp B methyl ester (AME) was the next to be considered [279], and this has been the subject of the greatest effort of all Amp B derivatives. Salts of AME are soluble in water, probably existing as micellar aggregates. In vitro results indicated that the toxicity was reduced, but that the activity against fungi was similar to that of Amp B, and in addition a significant antiviral activity had appeared. Inhibition of the human immunodeficiency virus in cell culture was obviously of great interest [280]. A host of studies in animal models of fungal infections did not always produce consistent results [281–284], but pharmacology and toxicology work continued and led to the first clinical trials of AME [285]. The use of higher doses than of Amp B was possible, and results were good. Nephrotoxicity was not a problem, but signs of neurotoxicity became apparent [286]. This toxicity has been extensively investigated, and Schaffner has also reviewed this problem [287]. Recent studies at the molecular level have suggested that AME has in fact less potential for neurotoxicity than Amp B itself on an equimolar basis [288], and strengthened the feeling that one should look at the problem more closely. Indeed a recent review of 53 patients with systemic fungal infections treated with AME concluded that further study of this drug is warranted both for its antifungal potential and its activity against HIV [289].

N-glycosyl [290] and trimethylammonium methyl ester derivatives [291] have also been synthesized but not so thoroughly investigated. More attention has been paid to N-aminoacyl Amp B ester derivatives, and it was concluded that such compounds have potential clinical merit [275, 292]. And so it goes on. The two latest reports from Borowski's group have been on the synthesis of Amp B 2-morpholinoethylamide diaspartate and hydrazide derivatives [293] of polyene antifungals, the latter being currently the subject of pharmacological studies, so there is no sign of interest waning. Indeed, structure-function studies are being actively pursued [6]. A major problem is, of course, that development of a chemotherapeutic agent involves enormous effort and cost, and for a pharmaceutical company to commit itself to such a program the initial results must really show something dramatic. So such expressions as "worthy of further investigation" are in many cases written in vain, although recent patent applications by Beecham show that investigation is in some cases leading to new substances.

Tetaine

Borowski's group have also expended considerable effort to make something of the tetaine group of antibiotics. Tetaine, also known under the names bacilysin and bacillin, is an antibiotic that turns up time and again in the screening of microbial broths. It is active against some bacteria and also against *Candida albicans*. Tetaine is transported into the fungal cell by an oligopeptide transport system and is there cleaved to yield the antibiotic anticapsin, an inhibitor of glutamine-6-phosphate synthetase (more correctly known as L-glutamine: D-fructose-6-phosphate aminotransferase, EC 2.6.1.16). Although they show in vitro and in vivo activity [294, 295] this is somewhat weak, and added to the narrow spectrum is the reason that these compounds have not been further developed. Various derivatives have been synthesized in attempts to improve the spectrum and activity [296–299], but so far none of the substances has really got off the ground. A report of the isolation of a chlorinated analog of tetaine [300] with a somewhat broader spectrum gives hope that further work in this direction would be justified. The target is certainly attractive in theory, as the cell wall synthesis has always been considered of great potential for the design of antifungal drugs. One can only hope that someone is prepared to keep on trying.

Garlic

Something else that shows no sign of fading away is garlic. There is an ever-increasing interest in the antibiotic properties of natural substances, and this is perhaps an area that has not been sufficiently explored in the past. It is undeniable that natural oils and plant extracts have healing properties, but their rationalization – the extraction and characterization of the active principles they contain – has brought little in the way of concrete results. It is beginning to seem that this subject, and the interactions of the substituents of medicinal plants in general, is more complex than the pharmaceutical chemist would wish. Garlic has always been associated with healing properties, and pushing a few cloves into the earth of a pot plant certainly does help to prevent mold [P. Hartman, unpublished], but attempts to develop a useful antifungal from its constituents have so far been without success. This does not prevent continuing efforts, as recent publications and congress reports show. The major flavor product of garlic, allicin, has traditionally been assumed to be responsible for its antimicrobial properties, and recently the target enzyme of this substance has been identified as acetyl-CoA synthetase [301]. A derivative of allicin, ajoene, has been shown to possess activity against *Candida albicans* and *Aspergillus niger* [302], and recently its inhibition of the growth of *Paracoccidioides brasiliensis* has been attributed to damage of the fungal cytoplasmic membrane [6, 7, 303]. The intravenous use of garlic to treat fungal infections in humans has apparently been taking place for many years in the Peoples Republic of China, and a recent paper has investigated the antifungal activity in cerebrospinal fluid during such treatment [304]. It was stated that few side effects were caused by the i. v. administration of commercial *A. sativum* extract, and that these are similar to those encountered after eating fresh garlic, namely "vomiting, diarrhea, nausea, anorexia, flatulence, weight loss or garlicky body odour".

6   Where do we go from here?

There has been a certain amount of progress in the past few years, and further promising drugs are in sight, but which is the way forward from here to ensure that the antimycotics of the future are better than those of today? There are basically three approaches that can be taken:

1. Improve existing drugs
2. Find new compounds for old targets
3. Attack new targets

These are the possibilities to be considered when the rationale is developed, but there is naturally considerable overlap, and any practical approach will inevitably fall somewhere between two of these categories. Derivatization of Amp B clearly comes under heading 1 above, but synthesizing new azoles may be regarded as improvement of old drugs or not, according to point of view. A non-azole inhibitor of the sterol C-14 demethylase would certainly come under heading 2, but are other enzymes of the sterol biosynthesis pathway genuinely new targets? One must also ask whether completely new target areas are one day going to produce effective antifungals despite the lack of success of all efforts up to now. It is perhaps worthwhile looking at the work being carried out in the search for new drugs, and in doing so to see which aspects of basic research in mycology will help decide the direction of applied antifungal research and which of the pathways above will be taken, for there is no doubt that there are vast gaps in our knowledge of fungal biology and biochemistry. Compared to bacteriology, it is as though mycology has sprung from the stone age to the space age, completely by-passing the middle ages, baroque and all that comes between. The molecular biology and biotechnology of fungi are better understood than many aspects of their basic biochemistry.

6.1   Improving established drugs

Azoles

Studies of the mode of action of existing drugs are an obvious source of information that can lead to the discovery of new, better variations. Not only does finding out exactly how a drug works help to design better drugs, but it also allows the problems of resistance and toxicity to be approached on a more rational basis. Furthermore, it often allows new substances to be better evaluated at an early stage, thus aiding decisions on when to embark upon costly and time-consuming development. Nowhere is such research being carried out more intensively than in the area of the azole derivatives, but despite all that has been done there is still much that is not known about the way the azoles work, and many aspects of their action are still under discussion.

Any number of reviews have summarized what is known or postulated [7, 10, 68, 305]. That the primary attack of these inhibitors is on the cytochrome P450-dependent 14α-sterol demethylase is without doubt, and the mechanism of this interaction has been, and still is being, studied in detail [306–309]. Sophisticated structure – function analysis and computer graphics are used in the design of new substances in this structural class [310]. The enzyme has been purified from *Candida albicans* and the amino acid sequence is known [311, 312]. However, recent reports that ketoconazole and itraconazole additionally inhibit the 4α-demethylation of sterols in *Histoplasma capsulatum* show that even at the molecular level knowledge is not complete. This result could explain the high efficacy of azoles against dimorphic fungi, as the inhibition of two enzymes in one biosynthetic pathway is obviously particularly effective.

How this enzyme inhibition actually leads to inhibition of fungal growth has been much discussed, but despite many theories and much good work is still not really clear. What is certain is that many factors are involved, and it has long been accepted that there is considerable variation between individual azoles [313]. The traditional explanation is that the alteration of the composition of the fungal membrane not only affects its permeability and other physical properties, but also disturbs the function of many membrane bound enzymes. Thus chitin synthesis appears to be deregulated, fatty acid synthesis and respiration are affected, and accumulation of toxic peroxides has been observed. However, the most recent publications on the subject show that uncertainty still abounds. Vanden Bossche, probably the leading expert in matters concerning the mode of action of azoles, has always been of the opinion that accumulation of lanosterol or other unusual sterols under the influence of sterol biosynthesis inhibitors, rather than depletion of ergosterol, is the decisive factor in the action of azoles. However, recent work on morpholines from Karst's group leads to the opposite conclusion [314]. The case for the destructive effect of unusual sterols in the membrane seems to be stronger for the allylamines, which accumulate the straight chain molecule squalene, obviously very different structurally to the post-cyclization sterols.

The basis of the selectivity of the class has also recently been called into question [355] with the suggestion that an inherent difference in sensitivity of the target enzyme is not the deciding factor, but that a protective effect of other P450 enzymes in mammalian cells plays the major role. Unfortunately, the evidence is far from convincing, and a rather unusual silicon-containing azole was used in the study from which a general conclusion was drawn, but the hypothesis is interesting and deserves further investigation.

The molecular basis of resistance to azoles has also been investigated by several different approaches. For instance, various strains of *S. cerevisiae* have been used to study the effect of cytochrome P-450 levels on azole sensitivity [316], and the same group have provided evidence that a defective C5–6 desaturation step can allow the fungal cells to remain viable despite inhibition of their C-14 demethylation [317]. Other studies with cytochrome P-450 deficient mutants of *C. albicans* have confirmed that strains that can grow without the C-14 demethylase are resistant to azole drugs, and have also pointed to a possible role for hyphal formation in the determination of azole sensitivity [318]. A mutant of *S. cerevisiae* that has a defective demethylase due to a point mutation is a further example of this mechanism of azole resistance. By contrast, a *Candida glabrata* strain resistant to fluconazole proved to have an elevated level of ergosterol in the membrane, and a higher P-450 activity leading to a higher rate of ergosterol synthesis [vanden Bossche in ref. 7].

Although beyond the scope of this review, mode of action studies on azoles have had a further interesting spin-off. A study of the molecular basis of the side effects of azoles has opened up new possibilities for the treatment of hormonal disorders [319], and ketoconazole has in fact been used in the treatment of hirsutism as well as having been shown to potentiate interleukin 1 α mediated antitumor effects [320].

Amphotericin B

The mechanism of action of Amp B has naturally been the subject of a great deal of interest during the three decades since it became available. This interest has, if anything, increased during recent years, perhaps because of the realization that Amp B is not after all about to be replaced as the most effective antimycotic available for systemic mycosis. Much of the work has understandably been directed towards reducing the toxicity, but a greater understanding of how polyene antibiotics work could help the development of new drugs of this class.

The mode of action of Amp B is subject to periodic review [7, 69] but it is clear that it is far from well understood at the molecular level. The effects on the membrane bound proteins of the fungal cell seem similar to those induced by ergosterol biosynthesis inhibitors, a general imbalance being introduced [321]. The traditional hypothesis that the differential complex forming ability of Amp B with ergosterol and cholesterol has been supported by studies of calcium ion influx and carboxyfluorescein release using phospholipid vesicles [322, 323], and also by molecular mechanics studies [324], but other work in similar systems has been interpreted as arguing against the sterol-dependent pore hypothesis of Amp B activity [325]. However, evidence is mounting that fine details of the structure of both polyenes and sterols are responsible for their selective toxicity [326, 327]. The actual mechanics of Amp B toxicity is nevertheless still at the hypothesis stage [328–330], and if a clearer picture could be obtained it might lead to advances in the design and use of this class of drug.

That there is interaction between Amp B and drugs used in the treatment of cancer has been known for many years, but this has mostly been looked at from the point of view of Amp B enhancing the effect of these drugs. This has been used in clinical situations, and is at least to some extent related to the permeabilizing effects of Amp B [for example 331–333]. More recently however, the situation has been examined from the antifungal point of view [334–337]. The interactions are complex, and although progress has been made in understanding and predicting these interactions, the extent of their usefulness in the clinic is far from clear.

Another facet of Amp B that is coming to the attention of medical mycologists is its potential as an immune stimulant. This again has been reported and investigated for over 15 years, but direct investigation of the antifungal consequences have been relatively rare [338–344]. Interest in this area is continuing, and it is interesting that it is being suggested that the antifungal efficacy of not only Amp B and its derivatives, but also of triazoles, may to a certain extent depend on their effect on the host immune system [N. Henry-Toulné in ref. 6, J. Bolard in ref. 7].

An interesting story to appear in the literature recently concerns the reduction of Amp B toxicity by vascular decongestants. Attempts to elucidate the mechanism of Amp B nephrotoxicity led to the observation that pentoxifylline can help to reduce these side effects, at least in part due to its properties as a vascular decongestant [345]. Further studies in a murine model of candidosis showed that treatment of infected mice with Amp B together with another such compound, the methylxanthine analog HWA-138, resulted in a remarkably increased clearance of *Candida* from the kidneys [346]. The next installment is eagerly awaited.

So although many clinicians, and presumably a good many patients, would like to be shot of Amp B as soon as possible, the number of new ideas that are coming out of research on this old drug suggest that it still has a lot to offer.

6.2   New inhibitors of old targets

Apart from the cell membrane as a physical entity which is directly attacked by polyene-type antibiotics, the only "old target" for antifungal drugs is the ergosterol biosynthesis pathway. Those working in the field within the pharmaceutical industry are often asked "Why do you keep on plugging away at sterol biosynthesis? Why don't you do something new?" The answer is that quite apart from the lack of basic biochemical knowledge and the high risk factors involved in entering a whole new target area, sterol biosynthesis inhibitors (SBIs) really do still look the best bet for making progress. Although research into other possibilities goes on, up until now nothing has come of attempts to attack new targets. With all their drawbacks, the azoles are very good antimycotics, and the allylamines and morpholines must be judged outstanding against susceptible fungi. Substances attacking other biochemical pathways always seem to have a narrower spectrum and greater toxicity problems, and the success of current SBIs is such that increasing attention is being paid to the sterol biosynthesis targets that have not yet yielded marketable antimycotics.

While the early enzymes of the pathway are of more interest to those working on the control of cholesterol synthesis in mammalian cells, the post-squalene steps have remained predominantly the sphere of the antifungal researcher. Squalene epoxidase inhibitors seem not to be generally active against the pathogens causing deep mycoses, but both allylamine and thiocarbamate derivatives occasionally give hope that this is not a universal phenomenon [347, 348]. A recent report of a squalene epoxide inhibitor that is specific for mammalian cells, in direct contrast to all those previously known, suggests that this enzyme holds more possibilities than have as yet been explored [349].

The next enzyme in the pathway, the 2,3-oxidosqualene-lanosterol cyclase, has been the subject of study for many years without getting beyond the "appears to be a promising target stage" [350–354]. However, recent efforts at F. Hoffmann-La Roche seem to be leading in the right direction. Although no substances with in vivo activity have as yet been reported, for the first time inhibitors of this enzyme with genuine broad in vitro activity have been synthesized [355, 356]. The cloning and characterization of the gene for this enzyme, which has not yielded much information about itself to date, by a group at the Squibb Institute promised to help efforts in this direction, but no further work seems to be in progress [357].

At a recent colloquium dedicated solely to post-squalene inhibitors of sterol biosynthesis, Benveniste summarized the considerable amount of both theoretical and practical work that he and others have carried out on mechanism-based inhibitors of practically all steps of the pathway [358], a useful summary of work in this field. The Δ_{14}-reductase and the Δ_8-Δ_7-isomerase, mentioned at the same meeting, are simultaneously inhibited by several classes of compound, including the morpholine class of antifungals [A. Polak in ref. 2, 359], but these two enzymes could each be a target in its own right. The Δ_{24}-sterol methyltransferase has also long been considered a possible target, and still seems to be under consideration [360, 361].

Perhaps it is only because it has been so much better characterized than other aspects of fungal biochemistry, but the sterol biosynthesis pathway is still considered a major hope for the design of new antimycotis, despite the calls for novel modes of action.

6.3   New targets

There are naturally a good many possible targets that may be considered when the search for, or design of, new antifungal drugs is under discussion. Nonetheless, the greater similarity of the eucaryotic fungal cell to the host cell, together with the incomplete understanding of fungal biochemistry and metabolism, serves to reduce their number relative to those available in the bacterial cell. So what remains? Where should we look for targets for the innovative antimycotics of the next generation? In order to follow a rational approach one should ideally look at metabolic processes where the enzymes are well characterized. Where there are differences in structure, sequence, kinetic parameters, etc, there is hope for specificity. Another general criterion for possible target enzymes is their location.

Proteins with their active site on the outside of the cell membrane are obviously more easily reached than those which require a drug to penetrate the membrane. However, the cell wall is a very unpredictable barrier, allowing the penetration of a molecule as large as Amp B while proving impermeable to much smaller molecules.

The cell wall is in theory an excellent target for antifungal drugs as it is essential for the fungus and has no mammalian counterpart. The three main components of the cell wall are chitin, glucan and mannoprotein, and the inhibition of their synthesis has received a fair amount of attention over the years. Apart from polymoxin D, which has been developed as an agricultural fungicide in Japan, and the Nikkomycins no inhibitor of chitin synthesis has appeared a likely candidate. Much effort was expended on the enzyme chitin synthetase until it was found not in fact to be essential for chitin synthesis and septum formation [361]. It is now known that a second chitin synthase exists [362, 363], and that it is an essential enzyme [365], but this illustrates well the dangers inherent in the rational approach to drug design when the biochemical background is insufficient. It is likely that a protease is involved in the regulation of chitin synthesis activity, but studies in this direction have not yet progressed to the stage of its inhibition. Other enzymes in the chitin synthesis pathway could also be targeted, and glucosamine-6-phosphate synthetase has already been mentioned, but the earlier the intervention in any biosynthesis the greater are the chances that selectivity will become a problem. The complementary enzyme, chitinase, which is thought to play a role in morphogenesis by controlled lysis of the cell wall, has also been termed an ideal target. The antibiotic allosamidin has been found to inhibit the activity of chitinase derived from *Candida albicans,* but its failure to effect the growth of whole fungal cells in vitro suggests either that it does not penetrate to the location of the enzyme, or that the target is not after all as ideal as it appears [366].

The synthesis of mannoproteins is perhaps rather too similar in mammalian and fungal cells to assume that selectivity of inhibition is possible until it has been demonstrated, but the disruption of the synthesis of mannan itself has always looked more promising. Here is a system of many steps, some of the enzymes involved are well characterized, and it could be seen in the same light as peptidoglycan synthesis in bacteria. Glucan synthesis has received a lot of attention. There is a great deal of literature on various groups of inhibitors such as the echinocandins, aculeacins and papulacandins, and the echinocandin B derivative cilofungin almost made it onto the market. But the similarity in the mode of action of all the known inhibitors, and their narrow spectrum, makes one begin to wonder if this pathway will lead anywhere.

Attacks on the fungal cell membrane have obviously been very successful, but up to now have concentrated on ergosterol synthesis or direct attack. However, there is no reason why lipid or phospholipid synthesis should not also be a relevant target. It is just that nobody seems to have tried it as yet.

There are a very limited number of targets that exist in fungi but not at all in man, and the next best idea would seem to be to seek a target that is non-conserved in the evolutionary sense. The maximum change in structure but the minimum change of function gives the best chance of selective inhibition. This consideration advises against enzymes involved in DNA, RNA or protein synthesis as antifungal targets, although there are individual cases where there are indications that specificity could be achieved, such as DNA polymerase, topoisomerase II and elongation factor 3. Penetration to the site of these targets also appears to be a problem, and very little in the way of a rational approach in the search for inhibitors of such enzymes has appeared in the literature.

The synthesis in fungi of the essential amino acids of man should be a target with a high specificity. The substance RI-331 has been mentioned above, and there seems to be increasing activity in this area. The in vivo relevance of the antagonism by amino acids that has been observed in vitro is not fully clear, and this may or may not be a practical problem. Most activity in this area has been found in amino acid analogs discovered by microbiological screening, and this will probably continue to be the case in the immediate future. Although the metabolic pathways are reasonably well known, the enzymes involved have not yet been well characterized at the molecular level.

Polyamine biosynthesis also offers the possibility of specific inhibition of essential enzymes in fungi. (α)-difluorodimethyl ornithine inhibits the action of ornithine decarboxylase, probably the best studied system of polyamine biosynthesis. Several other substances have been described [367, 368], but a sufficient level of in vivo activity has not yet been achieved in fungi, although the activity against protozoa is most satisfactory.

Folate antagonists are well known as therapeutic agents, and the enzyme dihydrofolate reductase (DHFR) has long been a target for antibacterial and antineoplastic drugs [369]. Despite some effort [370], no DHFR inhibitor has yet been found that is sufficiently active and specific to be of clinical use, but the search is being intensified. The enzyme from *C. albicans* has been characterized [371], and that from *S. cerevisiae* even more intensively studied and sequenced [372, 373]. Investigation of thymidilate synthase is also in progress [374], and this may also prove a valid target for antifungals. Although fungi seem to be more resistant than bacteria to the folate antagonists that are as yet available, the fact that they lack a salvage pathway for thymine and thymidine should render this class of antimetabolite particularly effective if suitable inhibitors could be found [375].

And so one could continue. Microtubular formation, carbohydrate metabolism, electron transport – all these and many more have been considered as antifungal targets at one time or another, and remain as potential approaches to the problem of killing fungi.

Possibly the most expanding area of medical science at the present is immunology, where our knowledge of the defences against infection which Nature has provided is growing rapidly. Turning this knowledge into practical therapeutic possibilities has proved more difficult. Knowledge of the immunology of fungal infections is also growing, but has by no means reached maturity. The title of a lecture given to the 1990 Annual Meeting of the British Society for Mycopathology by J. Domer, a leading worker in this field, perhaps summarizes the present state of affairs: "The host-parasite relationship in candidiasis: many theories, few proofs." The somewhat empirical use of immune modulators has begun, as described above, but basic knowledge is still being sought. Both the interactions of fungi with the immune system and the immunological properties of present antifungal drugs are being investigated along with the search for new substances for immunotherapy [376–378], and one can only hope that the early promise of this line of attack against fungal infection will be fulfilled.

An aspect of mycoses that is receiving considerable attention at the moment is pathogenicity. What factors are responsible for the differing pathogenicity of fungi, the differences even among strains of the same species? Can we influence these factors, and is this a real possibility for preventing fungal infection? Just as the state of the host has become accepted as of decisive importance in the occurrence and outcome of mycoses, it is now recognized that a fungus does not cause disease just by being there. Which of its properties contribute to its virulence and pathogenicity is not known in any detail, but a good

deal of information is emerging and the outline of a picture is forming. As with so many aspects of medical mycology, most is known
about *Candida albicans,* although studies of *Cryptococcus neoformans*
have increased with its emergence as a frequent pathogen in AIDS.
The factors which are of greatest importance for the pathogenicity of
Candida albicans, at least if judged in terms of published work, are adherence, morphology, and phospholipase and protease production
[379–382]. The matter of adherence is still controversial, and despite
much study one has the impression that the mechanisms by which it
influences pathogenicity are in no way clear. Morphology is clearly of
significance, but understanding of the way in which it actually influences the virulence of fungi is still in its infancy. Even the assumption
that hyphal formation is linked to the pathogenicity of *C. albicans* has
not stood up to closer examination. The work of D. Soll on morphology switching suggests that this property of *Candida* could be of importance, but again details have not yet become clear. Proteinase
excretion has been found to correlate with pathogenicity in vaginal
and deep candidosis, and considerable work is in progress to elucidate the molecular mechanisms involved. The same also applies to
phospholipase production, the inhibition of which has been shown to
reduce the virulence of *C. albicans.*

The importance of *Cryptococcus neoformans* infections in AIDS has
stimulated research into the factors that make it the most pathogenic
of yeasts. Although the growth rate and the production of some enzymes play a role, the capsule seems crucial for virulence which depends not only on its existence but also on its composition [7]. The
pigment melanin is also a factor in *Cryptococcus* as well as in the dematiaceous fungi, where it has been shown to play an important role
in the virulence and course of infection [380]. As with so much in this
area, the details are poorly understood and studies at the molecular
level are only now beginning to yield results.

Clearly, much more knowledge is required before attenuation of
pathogenicity becomes a method of prophylaxis or treatment of fungal diseases, but a start has been made. One of the most interesting
aspects of such research is the suggestion that modification of pathogenicity by present antifungal drugs could play a more important role
in their efficacy than has been hitherto realized [380].

So there seems, in fact, to be a sufficient choice of targets for the development of new antifungal drugs. But the fact is that no antifungal

drug has yet been discovered as the result of a rational approach. All have been found by "serendipity" or screening, and it is small wonder that many still have more faith in screening procedures for the identification of new lead structures. The factors involved in deciding whether a particular chemical structure will be an active, specific antifungal that penetrates to its target in fungi but is not toxic to man are extremely involved. The idea that at least some of the "design problems" can be left to nature is thus attractive, and much effort is being put into microbiological screening programs. Naturally, these can also be rationalized, and the target area narrowed by suitable selection of procedures, but one still needs luck. The targets attacked by compounds identified by screening procedures are, not surprisingly, the same as those identified by researchers wishing to embark on rational drug design, but there is a running discussion concerning the real chances of success, the optimists pointing to the new substances constantly being found, the pessimists reminding them how often the same substances turn up, and both quoting statistical calculations as to the exhaustibility or inexhaustibility of Nature's store of antifungals.

But in the midst of such considerations of rational approaches to drug design one can be brought up short by simplicity itself. Recent studies have confirmed the usefulness of hyperthermic treatment of chromomycosis and sporotrichosis, both in conjunction with chemotherapy and alone [M. Hiruma and J. A. Conte-Diaz in ref. 7]. It is a sobering thought that while so much effort is being put into expanding our arsenal of drugs, simply warming the infected area has proved so effective.

7   *Pneumocystis carinii*

It is difficult to write anything in the field of mycology nowadays without at least a paragraph on *Pneumocystis carinii*. The problem is where to put it! The controversy about whether this organism should be classified as a fungus or not is likely to be with us for a considerable time, and is regularly reviewed [383, 384]. Perhaps it says something about the arrogance of mankind that it is regarded as so vital that an organism be strictly classified within the order he himself has imposed on Nature. A most relevant result in favor of a fungal status is the ribosomal RNA sequence homology determined by Stringer et al., but the fact that this organism has separate thymidylate synthase and DHFR activities rather than the bifunctional enzyme found in protozoa is also telling [385–387]. The characterization of these enzymes will aid the search for new drugs as folate synthesis appears one of the most promising targets [388, 389]. At present, treatment is difficult and often associated with considerable side effects, and prophylaxis plays an important role. This is most often effected with pentamidine inhalation or trimethoprim-sulphamethoxazole combination. This latter has also been associated with toxicity problems, but reports at the 1990 ICAAC in Atlanta suggested that doses sufficiently low to avoid toxicity still provide the required protection. It has also been reported [8, 390] that antifungals such as cilofungin that inhibit the synthesis of cell wall components are active against *P. carinii,* which is interesting in view of the fact that imidazole antifungals are ineffective [391]. Fungus or not, *P. carinii* remains a very troublesome pathogen.

8   Conclusion – Are we winning?

We have tried to put together relevant information on the present state of antifungal chemotherapy, particularly of deep mycoses [summarized in Table 2], and on recent and expected advances in the field. We have also expressed our thoughts on how further progress could be made. We hope that this is sufficient for the reader to answer for himself the question of the title, and to stimulate discussion on the subject. There are sufficient avenues to be explored to give hope that some of them will lead to new, more effective antimycotics, be it through "rational" drug design or via leads obtained from screening programs. It is going to be a long hard battle either way.

A question of some relevance is "who is going to do the fighting?". The increase in the significance of mycoses as an indication area has made it more interesting to the pharmaceutical industry, where a reasonable hope of profitability is necessary to justify research effort, at least in most cases. But the antimycotic cake is never going to be large enough for extensive basic research programs to be carried out or financed by industry, and a great deal of basic research is necessary to fill the gaps in the knowledge of fungal biochemistry upon which applied research must be based. For this reason genuinely novel approaches to discover new antifungal drugs are likely to be seen less

Table 2
Indications of antifungal agents on the market[a]

	First choice of therapy	Alternative or unclear
Amph B	all fungal infections unknown fever	–
Amph B + 5-FC	candidosis cryptococcosis in AIDS and non AIDS unknown fever	–
Miconazole	Pseudallescheria boydii	–
	vaginal candidosis mucocutaneous candidosis infections due to true pathogenic fungi	prophylaxis
Itraconazole	maintenance therapy of cryptococcosis in AIDS aspergilloma sporotrichosis histoplasmosis chromomycosis (sometimes combined with 5-FC)	aspergillosis maintenance for aspergillosis
Fluconazole	vaginal candidosis oropharyngeal candidosis maintenance therapy cryptococcosis in AIDS	unknown fever

[a] The authors' interpretation of the current literature.

often than will probably be the case in the antibacterial field.

A most encouraging sign, however, is the growth of interest in medical mycology. Even if it takes time to bear fruit, more pharmaceutical firms and academic and medical laboratories are contributing to the progress in the field.

A final quote from M. Rinaldi, speaking about new and emerging mycoses to a packed auditorium at the 1990 ICACC: *"Even five years ago you could have held this whole meeting in the men's room, and now nobody can even get in here. This is terrific for mycology."*

Such an increasing interest in the problem of antifungal chemotherapy must surely lead to an acceleration of the rate of progress in the field.

Since the completion of the manuscript, another two hopes for the future have fallen by the wayside. Schering has suspended development of genaconazole because of carcinogenicity in long-term toxicology studies. This is a great blow for hopes of improvement in the therapy of systemic mycoses. Most recently, Bristol-Myers Squibb is reported to have discontinued development of pramicidin A, and Janssen has also dropped Saperconazole. At the moment, the cupboard is bare.

References

Literature taken into account to October 1990

1   P. D. Hoeprich: Progress in Drug Research *33*, 317 (1989).
2   J. F. Ryley (ed.): Chemotherapy of Fungal Diseases, Springer-Verlag (1990).
3   T. J. Walsh, P. A. Pizzo: Diagnosis and Therapy of Systemic Fungal Infections, Holmberg K. & Meyer R. D. (eds.), Raven Press New York (1989), p. 47.
4   H. A. Gallis, R. H. Drew, W. W. Pickard: Rev. Infect. Dis. *12* (Suppl. 2), 308 (1990).
5   A. M. Sugar, J. J. Stern, B. Dupont: Rev. Infect. Dis. *12* (Suppl. 3), 338 (1990).
6   Abstracts of the International Congress of Bacteriology and Mycology (IUMS) Osaka, Japan, 16–22 September, 1990.
7   Abstracts of the First International Conference on Antifungal Chemotherapy, Oiso, Japan, 24–26 September, 1990.
8   Abstracts of the 1990 Interscience Conference on Antimicrobial Agents and Chemotherapy (ICAAC) Atlanta, USA, 22–24 October, 1990.
9   H. J. Scholer and A. Polak: Antimicrobial Drug Resistance, Chapter 14 "Resistance to Systemic Antifungal Agents". Academic Press Inc., New York (1984) p. 393.
10 A. Polak: Handbook of Experimental Pharmacology, Vol. *96*, Chemotherapy of Fungal Diseases, Chapter 6, Springer-Verlag Berlin, Heidelberg 1990, p. 153.
11 W. M. Artis, B. M. Odle and H. E. Jones: Arch. Dermatol. *117*, 16 (1981).
12 D. Handtschke and H. Götz: Z. Hautkr. *56*, 1326 (1981).
13 N. Ryder: Antimicrob. Agents Chemother. *27*, 252 (1985).
14 J. R. Lever, P. J. Dykes, R. Thomas and A. Y. Finlay: J. Dermatol. Treatm. *1* (Suppl. 2), 23 (1990).
15 J. C. Jensen: J. Dermatol. Treatm. *1* (Suppl. 2), 15 (1990).
16 M. J. D. Goodfield, N. R. Rowell, R. A. Forster, E. G. V. Evans and A. Raven: Brit. J. Dermatol. *121*, 753 (1989).
17 H. Mieth: Proceedings of the First International Conference on Antifungal Chemotherapy (ICAFC), Oiso, Japan, 24–26 September, 1990 (in press).
18 A. Polak: Sabouraudia *21*, 205 (1983).
19 A. Polak: Infection *17* (4), 203 (1989).
20 W. Melchinger, A. Polak, J. Müller: Mykosen (in press).
21 A. Polak: Bull. Soc. Fr. Mycol. Méd. *3*, 175 (1974).
22 E. Rohde, M. Zaug, D. Hartmann: Recent Trends in the Discovery, Development and Evaluation of Antifungal Agents. R. A. Fromtling (ed.), J. R. Prous Science Publishers, S. A. (1987), p. 575.
23 A. Polak, M. Zaug: Handbook of Experimental Pharmacology, Vol. *96*, Chemotherapy of Fungal Diseases, Chapter 21, Springer-Verlag Berlin, Heidelberg (1990), p. 506.
24 J. S. Wilkinson: Lancet *2*, 448 (1849).
25 C. J. Carroll, R. Hurley, V. C. Stanley: J. Obstet. Gynaecol. Por. Common. W. *80*, 258 (1973).
26 K. V. Ratnam, C. T. Lee, T. W. Wong: Ann. Acad. Med. Singapore, *16* (2), 306 (1987).
27 S. S. Witkin, J. Jeremias, W. J. Ledger: J. Med. Vet. Mycol. *27*, 57 (1989).
28 S. S. Witkin, J. Jeremias, W. J. Ledger: J. Allergy Clin. Immunol. *81*, 412 (1988).
29 D. A. Levy, J. M. Bohbot, F. Catalan, G. Normier, A. M. Pinel, D. Dussourd, L. Hinterland: Vaccine *7*, 337 (1989).

30 D. Rigg, M. M. Miller, W. J. Metzger: Am. J. Obstet. Gynecol. *162*, 332 (1990).

31 S. S. Witkin, J. Hirsch, W. J. Ledger: Am. J. Obstet. Gynecol. *155*, 790 (1986).

32 D. J. Trumbore, J. D. Sobel: Obstetr. Gynecol. *67*, 810 (1986).

33 F. C. Odds: Candida and Candidosis, Leicester University Press, Leicester (1979).

34 J. D. Sobel: New Engl. J. Med. *315*, 1455 (1986).

35 J. D. Sobel, C. Schmitt, C. Meriwether: Obstet. Gynecol. *73*, 330 (1989).

36 T. E. Bushell, E. G. Evans, J. D. Meaden, J. D. Milne, D. W. Warnock: Genitourin. Med. *64*, 335 (1988).

37 M. J. Balsdon, J. M. Tobin: Genitourin. Med. *64*, 124 (1988).

38 J. M. Lailla-Vicens: Med. Clin. (Barc) *94*, 337 (1990).

39 A. Schaffner: Mycoses *32*, 499 (1989).

40 J. N. Aucott, J. Fayen, H. Grossnicklas, A. Morrissey, M. M. Lederman, R. A. Salata: Rev. Infect. Dis. *12*, 406 (1990).

41 A. Naficy, H. Murray: J. Infect. Dis. *161*, 1041 (1990).

42 N. A. Rotowa, H. J. Shadomy, S. Shadomy: Mycoses *33*, 203 (1990).

43 O. Male: Curr. Probl. Dermatol. *18*, 241 (1989).

44 M. R. Ujhelyi, R. H. Raasch, C. M. van der Horst, W. D. Mattern: Rev. Infect. Dis. *12*, 621 (1990).

45 E. J. Anaissie, G. P. Bodey, M. G. Rinaldi: Eur. J. Clin. Microbiol. Infect. Dis. *8*, 323 (1989).

46 T. J. Walsh, G. P. Melcher, M. G. Rinaldi, J. Lecciones, D. A. McGough, P. Kelly, J. Lee, D. Callender, M. Rubin, P. A. Pizzo: J. Clin. Microbiol. *28*, 1616 (1990).

47 R. J. Blinkhorn, D. Adelstein, P. J. Spagnuolo: J. Clin. Microbiol. *27*, 236 (1989).

48 K. Spitzer, T. Painter, W. Kobayashi, G. Medoff: J. Infect. Dis. *162*, 258 (1990).

49 W. L. Whelan, D. R. Kirsch, K. J. Kwon-Chung, S. M. Wahl, P. D. Smith: J. Infect. Dis. *162*, 513 (1990).

50 R. Kappe: Mycoses *32*, 24 (1987).

51 R. Hafner, G. Schaer: Schweiz. Med. Wochenschr. *118*, 42 (1988).

52 R. Rüchel: Mycoses *32*, 627 (1989).

53 G. Quindós, J. Pontón, R. Cisterna, D. W. R. Mackenzie: Eur. J. Clin. Microbiol. Infect. Dis. *9*, 178 (1990).

54 G. P. Bodey, S. Vartivarian: Europ. J. Clin. Microb. Infect. Dis. *8*, 413 (1989).

55 K. A. Haynes, J. P. Latge, T. R. Rogers: J. Clin. Microbiol. *28*, 2040 (1990).

55a J. van Cutsem, L. Meulemans, F. van Gerven, D. Stynen: Mycoses *33*, 61 (1990).

56 B. Wong, K. L. Brauer, J. R. Clemens, S. Beggs: Infect. Immun. *58*, 283 (1990).

57 C. E. Musial, F. R. Cockerill III, G. D. Roberts: Clin. Microb. Rev. *1*, 349 (1988).

58 P. M. Spencer, G. G. Jackson: J. Antimicrob. Chemother. *23* (Suppl. A), 107 (1989).

59 G. P. Bodey, E. J. Anaissie: Eur. J. Clin. Microbiol. Infect. Dis. *8*, 855 (1989).

60 M. Thaler, B. Pastakia, T. H. Shawker, T. O'Leary, P. A. Pizzo: Ann. Int. Med. *108*, 88 (1988).

61 J. Bross, G. H. Talbot, G. Maislin, S. Hurwitz, B. L. Strom: Am J. Med. *87*, 614 (1989).

62 J. M. Wiley, N. Smith, B. G. Leventhal, M. L. Graham, L. C. Strauss, C. A. Hurwitz, J. Modlin, D. Mellits, R. Baumgardner, B. J. Corden, C. I. Civin: J. Clin. Oncol. *8*, 280 (1990).

63 Reviews of Infectious Diseases, Vol. *11* (Suppl. 7), November–December, 1989.

64 Y. Fukazawa, K. Kagaya: Microbiol. Sciences *5*, 124 (1988).

65 Y. Nozawa, Y. Kitajiama, T. Sekiya and Y. Ito: Biochim. Biophys. Acta *367*, 32 (1974).

66 G. Medoff and G. A. Kobayashi: Antifungal Chemotherapy, Wiley, New York (1980), p. 3.

67 J. Kotler-Brajtburg, H. D. Price, G. Medoff, D. Schlessinger and G. S. Kobayashi: Antimicrob. Agents Chemother. *5*, 377 (1974).

68 D. Kerridge: Adv. Microb. Physiol. *27*, 1 (1986).

69 J. Brajtburg, W. G. Powderly, G. S. Kobayashi and G. Medoff: Antimicrob. Agents Chemother. *34*, 183 (1990).

70 H. J. Scholer, F. Gloor und L. Dettli: Hefepilze als Krankheitserreger bei Mensch und Tier, Springer-Verlag Berlin (1973), p. 78.

71 E. Drouhet: Med. Treatm. *7*, 539 (1970).

72 D. Pappagianis, M. S. Collins, R. Hector and J. Remington: Antimicrob. Agents Chemother. *16*, 123 (1979).

73 R. Guinet, J. Chanas, A. Gouillier, G. Bonnefoy and P. Ambroise-Thomas: J. Clin. Microbiol. *18*, 443 (1983).

74 D. J. Drutz and R. I. Lehrer: Am. J. Med. Sci. *276*, 77 (1978).

75 W. G. Merz and G. R. Sandford: J. Clin. Microbiol. *9*, 677 (1979).

76 J. D. Dick, W. G. Merz and R. Saral: Antimicrob. Agents Chemother. *18*, 158 (1980).

77 W. G. Powderly, G. S. Kobayashi, G. P. Herzig and G. Medoff: Am. J. Med. *84*, 826 (1988).

78 M. K. Sachs, R. G. Paluzzi, J. H. Moore Jr., H. S. Fraimow, D. Ost: Lancet *335*, 1475 (1990).

79 K. Jakab, E. Kelemen, G. Prinz, I. Török: Lancet *335*, 473 (1990).

80 M. S. Maddux, S. L. Barriere: Drug Intell. Clin. Pharm. *14*, 177 (1980).

81 J. D. Cleary, D. Weisdorf, C. V. Fletcher: Drug Intell. Clin. Pharm. *22*, 769 (1988).

82 L. Loomer, J. Cruz, B. Powell, R. Capizzi, J. Peacock: Proc. Am. Soc. Clin. Oncol. *7*, 285 (1988).

83 W. A. Bowler, H. E. Hill, P. I. Weiss, L. A. Hoffmeister, A. R. Blackey, E. C. Oldfield III. In: Abstracts of the 1990 Interscience Conference on Antimicrobial Agents and Chemotherapy (ICAAC) Atlanta, USA, 22–24 October, 1990.

84 Y. Yoshiyama, S. Nakano, T. Kobayashi, F. Tomonaga. Abstracts of the First International Conference on Antifungal Chemotherapy, Oiso, Japan, 24–26 September, 1990.

85 M. Arning, R. E. Scharf: Klin. Wochenschr. *67*, 1020 (1989).

86 A. Ohnishi, T. Ohnishi, W. Stevenhead, R. D. Robinson, A. Glick, D. M. O'Day, R. Sabra, E. K. Jackson, R. A. Branch: Antimicrob. Agents Chemother. *33*, 1222 (1989).

87 R. S. Stein, K. Albridge, R. K. Lenox, W. Ray, J. M. Flexner: South Med. J. *81*, 1095 (1988).

88 P. D. Hoeprich: J. Infect. *19*, 173 (1990).

89 G. Kokren, A. Lau, J. Klein, C. Golas, M. B. Campenau, S. Soldin: J. Pediatr. *113*, 559 (1988).

90 M. A. Fisher, G. H. Talbot, G. Maislin, B. P. McKeon, K. P. Tynan, B. L. Strom: Am. J. Med. *87*, 546 (1989).

91 J. K. S. Chia, E. J. McManus: Antimicrob. Agents Chemother. *34*, 906 (1990).

92 J. Chia: Clin. Res. *37*, 425 A (1989).

93 H. J. Schmitt, D. Armstrong: Current Therapy in Infectious Diseases, 3rd Ed. E. H. Kass and R. Platt (eds.), B. C. Decker, Philadelphia (1990), p. 12.

94   J. M. Benson, M. C. Nahata: Clin. Pharm. *7*, 424 (1988).
95   A. Polak, H. J. Scholer: Rev. Inst. Pasteur *13*, 233 (1980).
96   E. Drouhet, L. Mercier-Soucy, S. Montplaisir: Ann. Microbiol. *126* B, 25 (1975).
97   R. L. Stiller, J. E. Bennett, H. J. Scholer, M. Wall, A. Polak, D. A. Stevens: Antimicrob. Agents Chemother. *22*, 482 (1982).
98   M. O. Fasoli, D. Kerridge, J. F. Ryley: J. Med. Vet. Mycol. *28*, 27 (1990).
99   W. L. Whelan, P. T. Magee: J. Bacteriol. *145*, 896 (1981).
100 A. Polak: Chemotherapy *28*, 461 (1982).
101 A. Polak: Chemotherapy *33*, 381 (1987).
102 A. Polak: Mycoses *33*, 353 (1990).
103 R. B. Diasio, D. E. Lakings, J. E. Bennett: Antimicrob. Agents Chemother. *14*, 903 (1978).
104 M. C. Malet-Martino, R. Martino, M. de Forni, J. P. Armand: Proc. Am. Ass. Cancer Res. *31*, Abstr. 1249 (1990).
105 B. E. Harris, B. W. Manning, T. W. Federle, R. B. Diasio: Antimicrob. Agents Chemother. *29*, 44 (1986).
106 C. A. Kauffmann, P. T. Frame: Antimicrob. Agents Chemother. *11*, 244 (1977).
107 A. M. Stamm, R. B. Diasio, W. E. Dismukes, S. Shadomy, G. A. Cloud, C. A. Bowles, G. H. Karam, A. Espinel-Ingroff: Am. J. Med. *83*, 236 (1987).
108 W. E. Dismukes, G. Cloud, H. A. Gallis, T. M. Kerkering et al.: New Engl. J. Med. *317*, 334 (1987).
109 M. Kissling, P. Keller, M. Fernex: Mycoses *31*, 107 (1988).
110 Aspergillus and Aspergillosis. H. Vanden Bossche, D. W. R. Mackenzie, G. Cauwenbergh (eds.), Plenum Press New York, London (1988).
111 K. J. Smith, D. W. Warnock, C. T. Kennedy, E. M. Johnson, V. Hopwood, J. Van-Cutsem, H. Vanden Bossche: J. Med. Vet. Mycol. *24*, 133 (1986).
112 S. Thorsen, L. R. Mathiesen: Scand. J. Infect. Dis. *22*, 375 (1990).
113 B. D. Albertson, K. L. Frederick, N. C. Maronian, P. Feuillan, S. Schorer, J. F. Dunn, D. L. Loriaux: Res. Comm. Chem. Pathol. Pharmacol. *61*, 17 (1988).
114 B. D. Albertson, N. C. Maronian, K. L. Frederick, M. DiMattina, P. Feuillan, J. F. Dunn, D. L. Loriaux: Res. Comm. Chem. Pathol. Pharmacol. *61*, 27 (1988).
115 A. M. Sugar, S. Alsip, J. N. Galgiani, J. R. Graybill, W. E. Dismukes, G. A. Cloud, P. C. Craven, D. A. Stevens: Antimicrob. Agents Chemother. *31*, 1874 (1987).
116 N. Sonino: New Engl. J. Med. *317*, 812 (1987).
117 A. P. Farwell, J. T. Devlin, J. A. Stewart: Am. J. Med. *84*, 1063 (1988).
118 H. A. Gallis, R. H. Drew, W. W. Pickard: Rev. Infect. Dis. *12*, 308 (1990).
119 F. Meunier, J. Klastersky: Eur. J. Cancer Clin. Oncol. *24*, 539 (1988).
120 R. A. Larsen: J. Infect. Dis. *162*, 727 (1990).
121 P. A. Burch, J. E. Karp, W. G. Merz: J. Clin. Oncol. *5*, 1985 (1987).
122 National Institute of Allergy and Infectious Diseases Mycoses Study Group: Ann. Int. Med. *103*, 861 (1985).
123 D. W. Denning, D. A. Stevens: BMJ *299*, 407 (1989).
124 Reviews of Infectious Diseases. Vol. *12*, Supplement 3 (1990).
125 S. M. Grant, S. P. Clissold: Drugs *37*, 310 (1989).
126 S. M. Grant, S. P. Clissold: Drugs *39*, 877 (1990).
127 E. M. Bailey, D. J. Krakovsky, M. J. Rybak: Pharmacother. *10*, 146 (1990).
128 G. Cauwenbergh, P. De Doncker: Recent Trends in the Discovery, Development and Evaluation of Antifungal Agents. J. R. Prous, Barcelona (1987), p. 273.
129 R. Negroni: Antifungal Drugs. V. St. Georgiev (ed.), Ann. NYC Acad. Sci. *544* (1988), p. 497.

130 A. Restrepo, A. Gonzalez, I. Gomez, M. Arango, C. de Bedout: Antifungal Drugs. V. St. Georgiev (ed.), Ann. NYC Acad. Sci. *544* (1988), p. 504.

131 D. Borelli: Ref. Infect. Dis. *9* (Suppl. 1), 557 (1987).

132 M. A. Viviani, A. M. Tortorano, R. Woenstenberghs, R. Cauwenbergh: Mykosen *30,* 233 (1988).

133 D. W. Denning, R. M. Tucker, L. H. Hanson, D. A. Stevens: Am. J. Med. *86,* 791 (1989).

134 A. Schaffner: Therapeutische Umschau *47,* 664 (1990).

135 A. Viviani: J. Am. Acad. Dermatol. (1990) (in press).

136 D. W. Denning, R. M. Tucker, L. H. Hanson, J. R. Hamilton, D. A. Stevens: Arch. Intern. Med. *149,* 2301 (1989).

137 I. de Gans, J. K. M. Eeftinck Schattenkerk, R. J. van Ketel: Br. Med. J. *296* (6618), 339 (1988).

138 G. Dupont, W. Drouhet: Ann. Intern. Med. *106,* 778 (1987).

139 J. J. Stern, B. J. Hartman, P. Sharkey, V. Rowland, D. Squires, H. W. Murray, J. R. Graybill: Am. J. Med. *85,* 447 (1988).

140 P. A. Robinson, A. K. Knirsch, J. A. Joseph: Rev. Infect. Dis. *12* (Suppl. 3), S349 (1990).

141 R. A. Larson, M. A. E. Leal, L. S. Chan: Ann. Int. Med. *113,* 183 (1990).

142 P. L. Gaut, W. T. W. Ching, R. D. Meyer: Clin. Res. *38,* 152A (1990).

143 A. M. Sugar, C. Saunders: Am. J. Med. *85,* 481 (1988).

144 F. Meunier, M. Aoun, M. Gerard: Ref. Infect. Dis. *12* (Suppl. 3), S364 (1990).

145 R. J. Hay: Rev. Infect. Dis. *12* (Suppl. 3), S334 (1990).

146 C. L. S. Leen, E. M. Dunbar, M. E. Ellis, B. K. Mandal: J. Infect. *21,* 55 (1990).

147 R. M. Tucker, J. N. Galgiani, D. W. Denning, L. H. Hanson, J. R. Graybill, K. Sharkey, M. R. Eckman, C. Salemi, R. Libke, R. A. Klein, D. A. Stevens: Ref. Infect. Dis. *12* (Suppl. 3), S380 (1990).

148 M. Cruciani, G. di Perri, E. Concia, D. Bassetti, A. Bonora, E. Mecca, G. Panozzo, L. Tomazzoli: J. Antimicrob. Chemother. *25,* 718 (1990).

149 D. W. Warnock, J. Burke, N. J. Cope, E. M. Johnson, N. A. von Fraunhofer, E. W. Williams: Lancet *II,* No. 8623, 1310 (1988).

150 K. J. Smith, D. W. Warnock, C. T. C. Kennedy, E. M. Johnson, V. Hopwood, J. Van Cutsem, H. Vanden Bossche: J. Med. Vet. Mycol. *24,* 133 (1986).

151 Ch. A. Hitchcock, K. J. Barrett-Bee, N. J. Russel: J. Med. Vet. Mycol. *25,* 329 (1987).

152 J. D. Lazar, K. D. Wilner: Rev. Inf. Dis. *12* (Suppl. 3), S327 (1990).

153 K. L. M. Lavrijsen, J. M. G. van Houdt, D. M. J. van Dyck, W. E. G. Meuldermans, J. J. P. Heykants: Antimicrob. Agents Chemother. *34,* 402 (1990).

154 N. Doble, R. Shaw, C. Rowland-Hill, M. Lush, D. W. Warnock, E. E. Keal: J. Antimicrob. Chemother. *21,* 633 (1988).

155 P. Collignon, B. Hurley, D. Mitchell: Lancet *I,* No. 8649, 1262 (1989).

156 M. R. Kramer, S. E. Marshall, D. W. Denning, A. M. Keogh, R. M. Tucker, J. N. Galgiani: Ann. Intern. Med. *113,* 327 (1990).

157 R. A. Blum, J. H. Wilton, D. M. Hilligoss, M. J. Gardner, E. B. Chin., J. J. Schentag, N. Y. Buffalo: Clin. Pharmacol. Ther. *47,* 182 (1990).

158 I. La Delfa, Q. M. Zhu, T. F. Blaschke: Clin. Res. *36,* 365A (1988).

159 N. Collette, P. van der Auwera, A. Pascual Lopez, C. Heymans, F. Meunier: Antimicrob. Agents Chemother. *33,* 362 (1989).

160 J. Brajtburg, W. G. Powderly, G. S. Kobayashi, G. Medoff: Antimicrob. Agents Chemother. *34,* 381 (1990).

161 C. W. M. Grant, K. S. Hamilton, K. D. Hamilton, K. R. Barber: Biochim. Biophys. Acta *984,* 11 (1989).

162 S. Jullien, A. Contrepois, J. E. Sligh, Y. Domart, P. Yeni, J. Brajtburg, G. Medoff, J. Bolard: Antimicrob. Agents Chemother. *33,* 345 (1989).

163 S. Jullien, J. Brajtburg: Biochim. Biophys. Acta M *1021,* 39 (1990).

164 J. Brajtburg, S. Elberg, G. S. Kobayashi, G. Medoff: J. Infect. Dis. *153,* 623 (1986).

165 R. T. Mehta, G. Lopez-Berestein: G. Lopez-Berestein, I. J. Fidler (eds.) Liposomes in Therapy of Infectious Diseases and Cancer. Alan R. Liss Inc., New York (1989), p. 263.

166 R. Kirsh, R. Goldstein, J. Tarioff, D. Parris, J. Hook, N. Hanna: J. Infect. Dis. *158,* 1065 (1988).

167 C. Tasset, F. Goethals, V. Preat, M. Roland: Int. J. Pharm. *58,* 41 (1990).

168 A. S. Janoff, L. T. Boni, M. C. Popescu, S. R. Minchey, P. R. Cullis, T. D. Madden, T. Taraschi, S. M. Gruner, E. Shyamsunder, M. W. Tate, R. Mendelsohn, D. Bonner: B. Proc. Natl. Acad. Sci. USA *85,* 6122 (1988).

169 I. Gruda, E. Gauthier, S. Elberg, J. Brajtburg, G. Medoff: Biochem. Biophys. Res. Commun. *154,* 954 (1988).

170 T. F. Patterson, P. Miniter, J. Dijkstra, F. C. Szoka Jr., J. L. Ryan, V. T. Andriole: J. Infect. Dis. *159,* 717 (1989).

171 J. A. Gondal, R. P. Swartz, A. Rahman: Antimicrob. Agents Chemother. *33,* 1544 (1989).

172 K. M. Wasan, K. Vadiei, G. Lopez-Berestein, D. R. Luke: J. Infect. Dis. *161,* 562 (1990).

173 I. Ahmad, A. K. Sarkar, B. K. Bachhawat: Ind. J. Biochem. Biophys. *26,* 351 (1989).

174 R. L. Taylor, D. M. Williams, P. C. Craven, J. R. Graybill, D. J. Drutz, W. E. Magee: Am. Rev. Respir. Dis. *145,* 748 (1982).

175 J. R. Graybill, P. C. Craven, R. L. Taylor, D. M. Williams, W. E. Magee: B. J. Infect. Dis. *145,* 748 (1982).

176 G. Lopez-Berestein, R. Mehta, R. L. Hopfer, K. Mills, L. Kasi, K. Mehta, V. Fainstein, M. Luna, E. M. Hersh, R. Juliano: B. J. Infect. Dis. *147,* 939 (1983).

177 G. Lopez-Berestein: G. Lopez-Berestein, I. J. Fidler (eds.) Liposomes in Therapy of Infectious Diseases and Cancer. Alan R. Liss, New York (1989), p. 317.

178 V. J. Wiebe, M. W. DeGregorio: Rev. Infect. Dis. *10,* 1097 (1988).

179 G. Lopez-Berestein, V. Fainstein, R. Hopfer, K. Mehta, M. P. Sullivan, M. Keating, M. G. Rosenblum, R. Mehta, M. Luna, E. M. Hersh, J. Reuben, R. L. Juliano, G. P. Bodey: J. Infect. Dis. *151,* 704 (1985).

179a L. Pisarik, V. Joly, S. Jullien, C. Carbon, P. Yeni: J. Infect. Dis. *161,* 1041 (1990).

180 D. R. Hospenthal, A. L. Rogers, G. L. Mills: Mycopathol. *101,* 37 (1988).

181 D. R. Hospenthal, A. L. Rogers, E. S. Beneke: Antimicrob. Agents Chemother. *33,* 16 (1989).

182 G. Lopez-Berestein, V. Fainstein, R. Hopfer, K. Mehta, M. P. Sullivan, M. Keating, M. G. Rosenblum, R. Mehta, M. Luna, E. M. Hersh, J. Reuben, R. L. Juliano, G. P. Bodey: J. Infect. Dis. *151,* 704 (1985).

183 G. Lopez-Berestein, G. P. Bodey, L. S. Frankel, K. Mehta: J. Clin. Oncol. *5,* 310 (1987).

184 G. Lopez-Berestein. Antifungal Drugs. Ann. NYC Acad. Sci. *544* (1988), p. 590.

185 F. Meunier, J. P. Sculier, A. Coune, C. Brassinne, C. Heyman, C. Laduron, N. Collette, C. Hollaert, D. Bron, J. Klastersky. Antifungal Drugs. Ann. NYC Acad. Sci. *544* (1988), p. 598.

186 F. Meunier: Ref. Infec. Dis. *11* (Suppl.) S1605 (1989).

187 F. Meunier, J. P. Sculier, A. Coune, C. Brassinne, C. Haymans, C. Laduron et al.: Ann. NYC Acad. Sci. *544,* 598 (1988).

188 G. Lopez-Berestein, G. P. Bodey, V. Fainstein, M. Keating, L. S. Frankel, B. Zeluff, L. Gentry, K. Mehta: Arch. Intern. Med. *149*, 2533 (1989).

189 A. Polak: J. Chemother. *24*, 221 (1990).

190 A. Polak: Mykoses *31* (Suppl. 2), 45 (1988).

191 M. Thaler, J. Bacher, T. O'Leary: J. Infect. Dis. *158*, 80 (1988).

192 C. E. Hughes, R. L. Peterson, W. H. Beggs, D. N. Gerding: J. Antimicrob. Chemother. *18*, 45 (1986).

193 T. J. Walsh, S. Aoki, F. Mechinaud, G. Foulds, M. Rubin, P. A. Pizzo: Microbiol. *406*, F88 (1988).

193a R. Allendoerfer, A. J. Marquis, M. Rinaldi, J. R. Graybill: Antimicrob. Agents Chemother. *35*, 726 (1991).

194 J. E. Bennett, W. E. Dismukes, R. J. Duma, G. Medoff, M. A. Sande, H. Gallis, J. Leonhard, B. T. Fields, M. Bradshaw, H. Haywood, Y. A. McGee, Th. R. Cate, C. G. Cobbs, J. F. Warner, D. W. Alling: New Engl. J. Med. *301*, 127 (1979).

195 H. Heidemann, W. Krich, J. Gerkens, R. Branch: Verh. Ges. Inn. Med. *89*, 921 (1983).

196 H. Heidemann, E. Jacqz, E. Ohnhaus, W. Ray, R. Branch: Recent Advances in Chemotherapy. Antimicr. Section 3 (Proc. 14th Int. Congr. Chemother. Kyoto) (1985), p. 2628.

197 R. D. Mayer, K. Holmberg: H. Holmberg, R. D. Meyer (eds.) Diagnosis and Therapy of Systemic Fungal Infections (1989), p. 79.

198 D. N. Chernoff, M. A. Sande: Paper presented at the Conférence Internationale sur le SIDA, Paris (1986) Abstr. 543.

199 F. Staib, G. Roegler, L. Pruefer-Kraemer, M. Seibold, D. Eichenlaub, H. D. Pohle: Dtsch. Med. Wochenschr. *111*, 1061 (1986).

200 R. A. Larsen, S. Bozzette, J. A. McCutchan, J. Chiu, M. A. Leal, D. D. Richmann and the California Collaborative Treatment Group. Ann. Int. Med. *111*, 125 (1989).

201 S. L. Chuck, M. A. Sande: New Engl. J. Med. *321*, 794 (1989).

202 V. Tozzi, E. Bordi, S. Galgani, G. C. Leoni, P. Narciso, P. Sette, G. Visco: Am. J. Med. *87*, 353 (1989).

203 G. Just-Nübling, C. Laubenberger, E. B. Helm, S. Falk, W. Stille: Forschg. Praxis *9*, 6 (1990).

204 D. Armstrong. Holmberg, R. D. Meyer (ed.) Diagnosis and Therapy of Systemic Fungal Infections (1989), p. 149.

205 M. v. Eiff, M. Essink, N. Roos, W. Hiddemann, Th. Buechner, J. van de Loo: Zeitschr. Antimicrob. Antineoplast. Chemother. Suppl. 1, 1 (1989).

206 E. Haron, R. Feld, P. Tuffnell, B. Patterson, R. Hasselback, A. Matlow: Am. J. Med. *83*, 17 (1987).

207 I. K. P. Cheng, G. X. Fang, T. M. Chan, P. C. K. Chan, M. K. Chan: Quart. J. Med. New Series *71*, 407 (1989).

208 A. Slingeneyer, B. Laroche, F. Stec, B. Canaud, J. J. Beraud, C. Mion: Perit. Dial. Bull. *4* (Suppl.), S. 60 (1984).

209 T. Walsh, P. A. Pizzo: Holmberg, R. D. Meyer (eds.) Diagnosis and Therapy of Systemic Fungal Infections (1989), p. 47.

209a B. Dupont: J. Am. Acad. Dermatol. *23*, 607 (1990).

210 G. P. Bodey, S. Vartivarian: Eur. J. Clin. Microbiol. Inf. Dis. *8*, 413 (1989).

211 D. N. Atukorala, G. M. Pothupitiya: Ceylon Med. J. *30*, 193 (1985).

212 G. Moulin, Th. Cognat, E. Ferrier, H. Alligier: J. Dermatol. de Paris *14*, 54 (1989).

212a R. B. Ashman, J. M. Papadimitriou, A. K. Ott, J. R. Warmington: Immunol. Cell. Biol. *68*, 1 (1990).

213 J. W. Van't Wout, J. W. M. Van der Meer, M. Barza, Ch. A. Dinarello: Eur. J. Immunol. *18*, 1143 (1988).

214   R. A. Pecyk, E. B. Fraser-Smith, T. R. Matthews: Infect. Immun. *57*, 3257 (1989).

215   G. S. Deepe Jr., C. L. Taylor, J. E. Harris, W. E. Bullock: Infect. Immun. *53*, 6 (1986).

216   I. Bleiberg, Y. Kletter, I. Riklis, I. Fabian: Exp. Hematol. *17*, 895 (1989).

217   B. A. Wu-Hsieh, D. H. Howard: Infect. Immun. *55*, 1014 (1987).

218   J. Y. Djeu, D. K. Blanchard, D. Halkias, H. Friedman: J. Immunol. *137*, 2980 (1986).

219   E. Brummer, D. A. Stevens: Clin. Exp. Immunol. *70*, 520 (1987).

220   I. E. A. Flesch, G. Schwamberger, S. H. E. Kaufmann: J. Immunol. *142*, 3219 (1989).

221   H. W. Murray, G. L. Spitalny, C. F. Nathan: J. Immunol. *134*, 1619 (1985).

222   L. Beaman: Infec. Immun. *55*, 2951 (1987).

223   Ch. J. Morrison, E. Brummer, D. A. Stevens: Infect. Immun. *57*, 2953 (1989).

224   R. K. Maheshwari, R. N. Tandon, A.-R. Feuilette, G. Mahouy, G. Badilett, R. M. Friedman: J. Interferon Res. *8*, 35 (1988).

225   D. Arenberg, E. Navarro, E. Roilides, V. Thomas, J. Peter, J. W. Lee, P. S. Francis, P. A. Pizzo, T. J. Walsh: Ann. Meeting of the American Society for Microbiology *1990*, Abstract F-90 (1990), p. 423.

226   M. Matsumoto, S. Matsubara, T. Matsuno, M. Tamura, K. Hattori, H. Nomura, M. Ono, T. Yokota: Infect. Immun. *55*, 2715 (1987).

227   S. Matsubara, M. Matsumoto, T. Matsuno, M. Tamura, K. Hattori, H. Nomura, M. Ono: Exp. Hematol. *15*, 558 (1987).

228   H. Yasuda, Y. Ajiki, T. Shimozato, M. Kasahara, H. Kawada, M. Iwata, K. Shimizu: Infect. Immun. *58*, 2502 (1990).

229   R. W. Frenck, G. Sarman, T. E. Harper, E. S. Buescher: J. Infect. Dis. *162*, 109 (1990).

230   G. M. Silver, R. L. Gamelli, M. O'Reilly: Surgery *106*, 452 (1989).

231   M. S. Cairo, D. Mauss, S. Kommareddy, K. Norris, C. van de Ven, H. Modanlou: Ped. Res. *27*, 612 (1990).

232   E. Anaissie, E. Wong, G. P. Bodey, S. Obrien, J. Gutterman, S. Vadhan: Abstracts of the ICAAC 1989, Houston, Texas. Abstract 73.

233   P. Martino, G. Meloni, A. Cassone: Ann. Int. Med. *112*, 966 (1990).

234   B. D. Cheson: Drugs News Perspect. *3*, 154 (1990).

235   J. E. Groopman: Seminars in Oncol. *17* (Suppl. 1), 31 (1990).

236   D. Metcalf: Cancer *65*, 2185 (1990).

237   G. S. Kobayashi, S. J. Travis, M. G. Rinaldi, G. Medoff: Antimicrob. Agents Chemother. *34*, 524 (1990).

238   J. Defaveri, S. H. Sun, J. R. Graybill: Antimicrob. Agents Chemother. *34*, 663 (1990).

239   K. V. Clemons, L. H. Hanson, A. M. Perlman, D. A. Stevens: Antimicrob. Agents Chemother. *34*, 928 (1990).

240   B. I. Restrepo, J. Ahrens, J. R. Graybill: Antimicrob. Agents Chemother. *33*, 1242 (1989).

241   J. R. Perfect, K. A. Wright, M. M. Hobbs, D. T. Durack: Antimicrob. Agents Chemother. *33*, 1735 (1989).

242   T. J. Walsh, C. Lester-McCully, M. G. Rinaldi, J. E. Wallace, F. M. Balis, J. W. Lee, P. A. Pizzo, D. G. Poplack: Antimicrob. Agents Chemother. *34*, 1281 (1990).

243   A. M. Sugar, M. Picard, L. Noble: Antimicrob. Agents Chemother. *34*, 896 (1990).

244   T. J. Walsh, J. W. Lee, J. Lecciones, P. Kelly, J. Peter, V. Thomas, J. Bacher, P. A. Pizzo: Antimicrob Agents Chemother. *34*, 1560 (1990).

245   T. Tanio, N. Ohashi, T. Saji, M. Fukusawa: Abstracts of the First International Conference on Antifungal Chemotherapy, Oiso, Japan, 24–26 September, 1990.

246 J. van Cutsem, F. van Gerven, P. A. J. Janssen: Drugs of the Future *14* (12), 1187 (1989).

247 J. van Cutsem, F. van Gerven, P. A. J. Janssen: Antimicrob. Agents Chemother. *33* (12) (1989).

248 R. S. Gordee, D. J. Zeckner, L. C. Howard, W. E. Alborn, M. Debona: Ann. N. Y. Acad. Sci. *544*, 294 (1988).

249 M. Pfaller, J. Riley, T. Koerner: Eur. J. Clin. Microbiol. Infect. Dis. *8*, 1067 (1989).

250 C. S. Taft, A. N. Stark, C. P. Selitrenikoff: Antimicrob. Agents Chemother. *32*, 1901 (1988).

251 K. R. Smith, K. M. Lank, C. G. Cobbs, G. A. Cloud, W. E. Dismukes: Antimicrob. Agents Chemother. *34*, 1619 (1990).

252 C. J. Morrison, D. A. Stevens: Antimicrob. Agents Chemother. *34*, 746 (1990).

253 A. Padula, H. F. Chambers: Antimicrob. Agents Chemother. *33*, 1822 (1989).

254 J. R. Perfect, M. M. Hobbs, K. A. Wright, D. T. Durack: Antimicrob. Agents Chemother. *33*, 1811 (1989).

255 A. N. Bulo, S. F. Bradley, C. A. Kauffmann: Mycoses *32*, 151 (1988).

256 M. Plempel, K. H. Büchel: Rev. Iber. Micolog. *6* (Suppl.) (1988), Abstracts 0–7.

257 M. Plempel, D. Berg, K. H. Büchel, W. Ritter, D. Berg, M. Plempel (eds.), Sterol Biosynthesis Inhibitors. Pharmaceutical and Agrochemical Aspects. Ellis Horwood, Chichester (1988), p. 349.

258 A. W. Fothergill, D. A. McGough, M. G. Rinaldi: 1989 Interscience Conference on Antimicrobial Agents and Chemotherapy (ICAAC), Houston, Texas, USA 1989.

259 D. Pappagianis, B. L. Zimmer, G. Theodoropoulos, M. Plempel, R. F. Hector: Antimicrob. Agents Chemother. *34*, 1132 (1990).

260 R. F. Hector, E. Yee: Antimicrob. Agents Chemother. *34*, 448 (1990).

261 J. F. Ryley, S. McGregor, R. G. Wilson: Ann. N. Y. Acad. Sci. *544*, 310 (1988).

262 M. Konishi, M. Nishio, K. Saitoh, T. Miyaki: J. Antibiot. *42*, 1749 (1989).

263 T. Oki, M. Hirano, K. Tomatsu, K. Numata: J. Antibiot. *42*, 1756 (1989).

264 M. Levy, U. Zehavi, M. Naim, I. Polacheck: J. Agric. Food Chem. *34*, 960 (1986).

265 I. Polacheck, U. Zehavi, M. Naim, M. Levy, R. Evron: Antimicrob. Agents Chemother. *30*, 290 (1986).

266 I. Polacheck, U. Zehavi, M. Naim, M. Levy, R. Evron: Zentralbl. Bakteriol. Mikrobiol. Hyg. Ser. A *261*, 481 (1986).

267 R. Evron, I. Polacheck, M. Guizie, M. Levy, U. Zehavi: Antimicrob. Agents Chemother. *32*, 1586 (1988).

268 R. Evron, M. Guizie, U. Zehavi, I. Polacheck: Antimicrob. Agents Chemother. *34*, 1600 (1990).

269 T. Oki, M. Konishi, K. Tomatsu, K. Tomita, K. Saitoh, M. Tsunakawa, M. Nishio, T. Miyaki, H. Kawaguchi: J. Antibiot. *XLI*, 1701 (1988).

270 T. Oki, O. Tenmyo, M. Hirano, K. Tomatsu, H. Kamei: J. Antibiot. *XLIII*, 763 (1990).

271 Y. Sawada, M. Nishio, H. Yamamoto, M. Hatori, T. Miyaki, M. Konishi, T. Oki: J. Antibiot. *XLIII*, 771 (1990).

272 T. Takeuchi, T. Hara, H. Naganawa, M. Okada, M. Hamada, H. Umezawa, S. Gomi, M. Sezaki, S. Kondo: J. Antibiot. *XLI*, 807 (1988).

272a Y. Sawada, K. Numata, T. Murakami, H. Tanimichi, S. Yamamoto, T. Oki: J. Antibiot. *XLIII*, 715 (1990).

273 R. F. Hector, B. L. Zimmer, D. Pappagianis: Antimicrob. Agents Chemother. *34*, 587 (1990).

274   S. Hedges: New Scientist, November 1989, p. 31.
275   C. P. Schaffner: Recent Trends in the Discovery, Development and Evaluation of Antifungal Agents. R. A. Fromtling (ed.) J. R. Prous Science Publ. (1987), p. 595.
276   C. P. Schaffner, E. Borowski: Antibiot. Chemother. *11*, 724 (1961).
277   H. Lechevalier, E. Borowski, J. O. Lampen, C. P. Schaffner: Antibiot. Chemother. *11*, 640 (1961).
278   G. Ragni, W. Szybalski, E. Borowski, C. P. Schaffner: Antibiot. Chemother. *11*, 797 (1961).
279   W. Mechlinski, C. P. Schaffner: J. Antibiot. *25*, 256 (1972).
280   C. P. Schaffner, O. J. Plescia, D. Pontani, D. Sun, A. Thornton, R. C. Pandey, P. S. Sarin: Biochem. Pharmacol. *35*, 4110 (1986).
281   D. P. Bonner, R. P. Tewari, M. Solotorovsky, W. Mechlinski, C. P. Schaffner: Antimicrob. Agents Chemother. *7*, 724 (1975).
282   R. M. Lawrence, P. D. Hoeprich: J. Infect. Dis. *133*, 168 (1976).
283   H. H. Gadebusch, F. Panski, C. Klepner, R. Schwind: J. Infect. Dis. *134*, 423 (1976).
284   G. R. Keim, Jr., P. L. Sibley, Y. H. Yoon, J. S. Kulesza, I. H. Zaidi, M. M. Miller, J. W. Poutsiaka: Antimicrob. Agents Chemother. *10*, 687 (1976).
285   P. D. Hoeprich: Scand. J. Infect. Dis. Suppl. *16*, 74 (1978).
286   P. D. Hoeprich, M. M. Kawachi, K. K. Lee, C. P. Schaffner: Curr. Chemother. Infect. Dis. Proc. 11th Int. Congr. Chemotherapy and 19th Int. Conf. Antimicrob. Agents Chemother. Am. Soc. Microbiol. Washington, 972 (1980).
287   P. C. Schaffner: Macrolide Antibiotics, Chemistry, Biology and Practice. S. Omura (ed.), Academic Press New York (1984), p. 457.
288   S. P. Racis, O. J. Plescia, H. M. Geller, C. P. Schaffner: Antimicrob. Agents Chemother. *34*, 1360 (1990).
289   P. D. Hoeprich, N. M. Flynn, M. M. Kawachi, K. K. Lee, R. M. Lawrence: Clin. Res. *36*, 621A (1988).
290   L. Falkowski, J. Golik, P. Kolodziejczyk, J. Pawlak, J. Zielinski, T. Ziminski, E. Borowski: J. Antibiot. *28*, 244 (1975).
291   L. Falkowsi, A. Jarzebski, B. Stefanska, E. Bylec, E. Borowski: J. Antibiot. *33*, 103 (1980).
292   A. Czerwinski, T. Zieniawa, E. Borowski: J. Antibiot. *XLIII*, 680 (1990).
293   J. Grzybowska, E. Borowski: J. Antibiot. *XLIII*, 907 (1990).
294   S. Milewski, H. Chmara, E. Borowski: Arch. Microbiol. *135*, 130 (1983).
295   S. Milewski, H. Chmara, E. Borowski: Arch. Microbiol. *145*, 234 (1986).
296   R. Andruszkiewicz, H. Chmara, S. Milewski, E. Borowski: Int. J. Peptide Protein Res. *27*, 449 (1986).
297   S. Milewski, H. Chmara, R. Andruszkiewicz, E. Borowski: Drugs Exptl. Clin. Res. *XIV*, 461 (1988).
298   R. Andruszkiewicz, S. Milewski, T. Zieniawa, E. Borowski: J. Med. Chem. *33*, 132 (1990).
299   S. Milewski, H. Chmara, E. Borowski: Drugs Exptl. Clin. Res. *XII*, 577 (1986).
300   C. Rapp, G. Jung, W. Katzer, W. Loeffler: Angew. Chem. Int. Ed. Engl. *27*, 1733 (1988).
301   M. Focke, A. Feld, H. K. Lichtenthaler: FEBS *261*, 106 (1990).
302   S. Yoshida, S. Kasuga, N. Hayashi, T. Ushiroguchi, H. Matsuura, S. Nakagawa: Appl. Environ. Microbiol. *53*, 615 (1987).
303   G. San-Blas, F. San-Blas, F. Gil, L. Marino, R. Apitz-Castro: Antimicrob. Agents Chemother. *33*, 1641 (1989).
304   L. E. Davis, J.-K. Shen, Y. Cai: Antimicrob. Agents Chemother. *34*, 651 (1990).

305 P. A. J. Janssen: in: Frontiers in Microbiology, E. de Clenq (ed.), Martinus Nijhoff Publ. (1987), pp. 29.
306 C. A. Hitchcock, S. B. Brown, E. G. V. Evans, D. J. Adams: Biochem. J. *260,* 549 (1989).
307 C. A. Hitchcock, K. Dickinson, S. B. Brown, E. G. V. Evans, D. J. Adams: Biochem. J. *266,* 475 (1990).
308 R. T. Fischer, S. H. Stam, P. R. Johnson, S. S. Ko, R. L. Magolda, J. L. Gaylor, J. M. Trzaskos: J. Lipid Res. *30,* 1621 (1989).
309 G. D. Wright, T. Parent, J. F. Honek: Biochim. Biophys. Acta *1040,* 95 (1990).
310 Y. Aoyama, Y. Yoshida, Y. Sonoda, Y. Sato: Biochim. Biophys. Acta *1006,* 209 (1989).
311 C. A. Hitchcock, K. Dickinson, S. B. Brown, E. G. V. Evans, D. J. Adams: Biochem. J. *263,* 573 (1989).
312 M. H. Lai, D. R. Kirsch: Nucl. Acid Res. *17,* 804 (1989).
313 I. J. Sud, D. S. Feingold: Antimicrob. Agents Chemother. *20,* 71 (1981).
314 C. Marcireau, M. Guilloton, F. Karst: Antimicrob. Agents Chemother. *34,* 989 (1990).
315 J. M. Trzaskos, M. J. Henry: Antimicrob. Agents Chemother. *33,* 1228 (1989).
316 S. Kenna, H. F. J. Bligh, P. F. Watson, S. L. Kelly: J. Med. Vet. Mycol. *27,* 397 (1989).
317 P. F. Watson, M. E. Rose, S. W. Ellis, H. England, S. L. Kelly: Biochem. Biophys. Res. Comm. *164,* 1170 (1989).
318 N. D. Lees, M. C. Broughton, D. Sanglard, M. Bard: Antimicrob. Agents Chemother. *34,* 831 (1990).
319 H. Vanden Bossche, G. Willemsens, D. Bellens, I. Roels, P. A. J. Janssen: Biochem. Soc. Trans. *18,* 10 (1990).
320 P. G. Braunschweiger, N. Kumar, I. Constantinidis, J. P. Wehrle, J. D. Glickson, C. S. Johnson, P. Furmanski: Cancer Res. *50,* 4709 (1990).
321 M. Mpona-Minga, J. Coulon, R. Bonaly: Res. Microbiol. *140,* 95 (1989).
322 H. Ramos, A. Attias de Murciano, B. E. Cohen, J. Bolard: Biochim. Biophys. Acta *982,* 303 (1989).
323 J. Milhaud, M.-A. Hartmann, J. Bolard: Biochimie *71,* 49 (1989).
324 M. Baginski, A. Tempczyk, E. Borowski: Eur. Biophys. J. *17,* 159 (1989).
325 S. C. Hartsel, W. R. Perkins, G. J. McGarvey, D. S. Cafiso: Biochem. *27,* 2656 (1988).
326 C. M. Gary-Bobo: Biochim. *17,* 37 (1989).
327 M. Hervé, J. C. Debouzy, E. Borowski, B. Cybulska, C. M. Gary-Bobo: Biochim. Biophys. Acta *980,* 261 (1989).
328 F. Z. Gil, G. Malnic: Eur. J. Physiol. *413,* 280 (1989).
329 A. Binet, J. Bolard: Biochem. J. *253,* 435 (1988).
330 R. E. Schell, N. V. Tran, J. S. Bramhall: Biochem. Biophys. Res. Comm. *159,* 1165 (1989).
331 F. Valeriote, G. Medoff, J. Dieckman: Cancer Res. *39,* 2041 (1979).
332 C. A. Presant, C. Klahr, R. Santala: Ann. Int. Med. *86,* 47 (1977).
333 N. Henry, J. Bolard: Biochim. Biophys. Acta *854,* 84 (1986).
334 D. W. Warnock, E. M. Johnson, J. Burke, R. Pracharktam: J. Antimicrob. Chemother. *23,* 837 (1989).
335 M. A. Ghannoum, K. H. Abu-Elteen, M. S. Motawy, M. A. Abu-Hatab, A. S. Ibrahim, R. S. Criddle: Chemother. *36,* 308 (1990).
336 M. A. Ghannoum, M. S. Motawy, M. A. Abu-Hatab, K. H. Abu Elteen, R. S. Criddle: Antimicrob. Agents Chemother. *33,* 726 (1989).
337 M. A. Ghannoum, M. S. Motawy, M. A. Abu-Hatab, A. S. Ibrahim, R. S. Criddle: Antimicrob. Agents Chemother. *33,* 717 (1989).

338 H.-S. Lin, G. Medoff, G. S. Kobayashi: Antimicrob. Agents Chemother. *11*, 154 (1977).

339 S. F. Shirley, J. R. Little: J. Immunol. *123*, 2878 (1979).

340 S. F. Shirley, J. R. Little: J. Immunol. *123*, 2883 (1979).

341 S. H. Stein, J. R. Little, K. D. Little: Cell. Immunol. *105*, 99 (1987).

342 N. Henry-Toulmé, M. Seman, J. Bolard: Biochim. Biophys. Acta *982*, 245 (1989).

343 F. Bistoni, A. Vecchiarelli, R. Mazzolla, P. Puccetti, P. Marconi, E. Garaci: Antimicrob. Agents Chemother. *27*, 625 (1985).

344 J. Brajtburg, S. Elberg, G. S. Kobayashi, G. Medoff: J. Antimicrob. Chemother. *24*, 333 (1989).

345 K. M. Wasan, K. Vadiel, G. Lopez-Berestein, R. R. Verani, D. R. Luke: Antimicrob. Agents Chemother. *34*, 241 (1990).

346 D. R. Luke, K. M. Wasan, T. J. McQueen, G. Lopez-Berestein: J. Inf. Dis. *162*, 211 (1990).

347 K. Iwata, T. Yamashita, H. Uehara: Antimicrob. Agents Chemother. *33*, 2118 (1989).

348 T. Morita, K. Iwata, Y. Nozawa: J. Med. Vet. Mycol. *27*, 17 (1989).

349 M. Horie, Y. Tsuchiya, M. Hayashi, Y. Iida, Y. Iwasawa, Y. Nagata, Y. Saswasaki, H. Fukuzumi, K. Kitani, T. Kamei: J. Biol. Chem. *265*, 18075 (1990).

350 L. Cattel, M. Ceruti, G. Balliano, F. Viola, G. Grosa, F. Schuber: Steroids *53*, 363 (1989).

351 L. Cattel, M. Ceruti, F. Viola, L. Delprino, G. Balliano, A. Duriatti, P. Bouvier-Navé: Lipids *21*, 31 (1986).

352 M. Ceruti, G. Balliano, F. Viola, L. Cattel, N. Gerst, F. Schuber: Eur. J. Med. Chem. *22*, 199 (1987).

353 A. Duriatti, P. Bouvier-Navé, P. Benveniste, F. Schuber, L. Delprino, G. Balliano, L. Cattel: Biochem. Pharmacol. *34*, 2765 (1985).

354 E. I. Mercer, P. K. Morris, B. C. Baldwin: Comp. Biochem. Physiol. *80B*, 341 (1985).

355 S. Jolidon, A. Polak, P. Guerry, P. Hartman: Biochem. Soc. Transact. *18*, 47 (1990).

356 S. Jolidon, A. Polak, P. Guerry, P. Hartman: Pesticide Sci. 1990 (in press).

357 R. Kelly, S. M. Miller, M. H. Lai, D. R. Kirsch: Gene *87*, 177 (1990).

358 A. Rahier, M. Taton, P. Benveniste: Biochem. Soc. Transact. *18*, 48 (1990).

359 M. Taton, P. Benveniste, A. Rahier: Eur. J. Biochem. *185*, 605 (1989).

360 A. S. Narula: J. Am. Chem. Soc. *103*, 2408 (1981).

361 M. A. Ator, S. J. Schmidt, J. L. Adams, R. E. Dolle: Biochem. *28*, 9633 (1989).

362 C. E. Bulawa, M. L. Slater, E. Cabib, J. Au-Young, A. Sburlati, W. L. Adair, P. W. Robbins: Cell *46*, 213 (1986).

363 A. Sburlati, E. Cabib: J. Biol. Chem. *261*, 15147 (1986).

364 P. Orlean: J. Biol. Chem. *262*, 5732 (1987).

365 S. J. Silverman, A. Sburlati, M. L. Slater, E. Cabib: Proc. Natl. Acad. Sci. *85*, 4735 (1988).

366 K. Dickinson, V. Keer, C. A. Hitchcock, D. J. Adams: J. Gen. Microbiol. *135*, 1417 (1989).

367 M. A. Pfaller, J. Riley, T. Gerarden: Mycopathol. *112*, 27 (1990).

368 S. A. Foster, D. R. Walters: J. Gen. Microbiol. *136*, 233 (1990).

369 B. I. Schweitzer, A. P. Dicker, J. R. Bertino: FASEB J. *4*, 2441 (1990).

370 W. T. Colwell, J. I. Degraw, K. J. Ryan, J. A. Lawson, A. Cheng: in: H. C. Curtius et al. (ed.) Chemistry and Biology of Pteridines, Pteridines and Folic Acid Derivatives. 9th Int. Symp. 1989 Zürich, Walter de Gruyter Berlin (1990), pp. 1052.

371 D. P. Baccanari, R. L. Tansik, S. S. Joyner, M. E. Fling, P. L. Smith, J. H. Freisheim: J. Biol. Chem. *264*, 1100 (1989).

372 M. E. Fling, J. Kopf, C. A. Richards: Gene *63*, 165 (1988).

373 B. J. Barclay, T. Huang, M. G. Nagel, V. L. Misener, J. C. Game, G. M. Wahl: Gene *63*, 175 (1988).

374 S. C. Singer, C. A. Richards, R. Ferone, D. Benedict, P. Ray: J. Bacteriol. *171*, 1372 (1989).

375 B. J. Barclay, B. A. Kunz, J. C. Little, R. H. Haynes: Can. J. Biochem. *60*, 172 (1982).

376 Immunology of Fungal Disease. E. Kurstak (ed.), Marcel Dekker Inc., New York, 1989.

377 J. R. Perfect, D. L. Granger, D. T. Durack: J. Inf. Dis. *156*, 316 (1987).

378 E. Roilides, T. J. Walsh, M. Rubin, D. Venzon, P. A. Pizzo: Antimicrob. Agents Chemother. *34*, 196 (1990).

379 M. Borg, R. Rüchel: J. Med. Vet. Mycol. *28*, 3 (1990).

380 R. Rüchel, B. Ritter, M. Schaffrinski: Zbl. Bakt. *273*, 391 (1990).

381 A. Polak: Mycoses *33*, 215 (1989).

382 K. J. Kwong-Chung, I. Polacheck, T. J. Popkin: J. Bacteriol. *150*, 1414 (1982).

383 H. Masur, H. C. Lane, J. A. Kovacs, C. J. Allegra, J. C. Edman: Ann. Int. Med. *111*, 813 (1989).

384 W. T. Hughes: Eur. J. Epidemiol. *5*, 265 (1989).

385 S. L. Stringer, J. R. Stringer, M. A. Blase, P. D. Walzer, M. T. Cushion: Exp. Parasitol. *68*, 450 (1989).

386 U. Edman, J. C. Edman, B. Lundgren, D. V. Santi: Proc. Natl. Acad. Sci. *86*, 6503 (1989).

387 J. C. Edman, U. Edman, M. Cao, B. Lundgren, J. A. Kovacs, D. V. Santi: Proc. Natl. Acad. Sci. *86*, 8625 (1989).

388 J. A. Kovacs, C. J. Allegra, J. Beaver, D. Boarman, M. Lewis, J. E. Parrillo, B. Chabner, H. Masur: J. Inf. Dis. *160*, 312 (1989).

389 S. Merali, Y. Zhang, D. Sloan, S. Meshnick: Antimicrob. Agents Chemother. *34*, 1075 (1990).

390 D. M. Schmatz, M. A. Romancheck, L. A. Pittarelli, R. E. Schwartz, R. A. Fromtling, K. H. Nollstadt, F. L. Vanmiddlesworth, K. E. Wilson, M. J. Turner: Proc. Natl. Acad. Sci. *87*, 5950 (1990).

391 M. S. Bartlett, S. F. Queener, J. W. Smith: Int. Congr. Inf. Dis. Montreal, July 1990. Abstr. 138.

The hopanoids, bacterial triterpenoids, and the biosynthesis of isoprenic units in prokaryotes

By Michel Rohmer, Philippe Bisseret and Bertrand Sutter

Ecole Nationale Supérieure de Chimie de Mulhouse,
3 rue Alfred Werner, 68093 Mulhouse Cédex, France

1   Introduction

For a long time prokaryotes were thought to be unable to synthesize polycyclic triterpenes. However, biomarkers possessing the triterpenic hopane (**1**) skeleton were found in the organic matter of all sediments and petroleums, independently of their age, nature and origin [1]. They are the most abundant natural products of defined structure on earth, their carbon representing more than all the carbon accumulated in the biosphere [2]. Hopanoids are present in a few scattered taxa of higher plants as well as in several cryptogames. However this rather rare occurrence in living higher organisms and the C_{30} skeleton of these eukaryotic hopanoids could not account for the ubiquity of the geohopanoids possessing extended side-chains with up to five additional carbon atoms. The wide distribution of these geolipids as well as the early identification of simple C_{30} hopanoids in a few prokaryotes led to the following hypothesis: these molecular fossils may originate from still unknown lipids of ubiquitous microorganisms, *i.e.* most probably from prokaryotes [3, 4]. The rather fortuitous discovery of the C_{35} bacteriohopanetetrols in *Acetobacter aceti* ssp. *xylinum* in 1973 [5] was the first report of a new series of long undisclosed and completely overlooked prokaryotic membrane components and conforted the hypothesis of the prokaryotic origin of the geohopanoids.

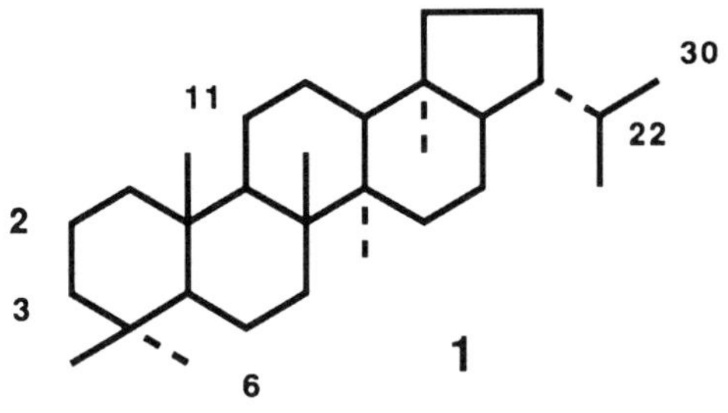

Figure 1
Hopane (**1**)

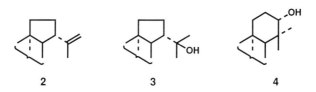

Figure 2
Diploptene (**2**), diplopterol (**3**) and tetrahymanol (**4**).

2   Structures of bacterial hopanoids
2.1   Hopanoids with the basic C_{30} triterpenic skeleton

The most easily detected hopanoids are a C_{30} olefin, diploptene (**2**), and a C_{30} tertiary alcohol, diplopterol (**3**) [3, 6]. They were the first hopanoids identified in the late 60's and are present, at least as minor compounds, in nearly all hopanoid synthesizing bacteria [7]. In the phototrophic bacterium *Rhodopseudomonas palustris,* diplopterol is accompanied by its isomer, the quasi-hopanoid tetrahymanol (**4**). This is up to now the only record of a triterpene of the gammacerane series from a prokaryote. Tetrahymanol has been reported from very few eukaryotes: ciliates of the genus *Tetrahymena,* a fern and an anaerobic fungus. However, the wide distribution of molecular fossils of the gammacerane series in marine and hypersaline sediments suggests a much broader distribution [8].

2.2   The C_{35} bacteriohopane skeleton

The most abundant prokaryotic hopanoids possess the C_{35} bacteriohopane skeleton, named by the groups of Colvin and Biemann who detected these triterpenoids for the first time in the acetic acid bacterium *Acetobacter aceti* ssp. *xylinum* [5]. In these compounds, the C_{30} triterpenic hopane skeleton is linked via its C-30 carbon atom to a polyhydroxylated C_5 *n*-alkyl chain. Bacteriohopanepolyols can differ one from each other by several structural features.
– The stereochemistry at C-22 is usually unique and identical in all bacteriohopane derivatives (*i.e.* 22 *R* for tetrol (**5a**) and 22 *S* for aminopentol (**11**) corresponding to the same absolute configuration) [9–11]. However, the 22*S*-tetrol (**5b**) of opposite configuration can occasionally be found, for instance in all *Acetobacter* species [9].
– The configurations of the chiral centers of the side-chain have been determined for the tetrol (**5a**) and aminotriol (**9**) from several bacteria and are usually always identical [12–15]. On the other hand again in the *Acetobacter* species, the two stereoisomers at C-34 (**5a** and **6**) are present (B. Peiseler and M. Rohmer, unpublished results).
– Double-bonds can be found in the pentacyclic moiety, either at C-6, or at C-11, or even in both positions [16, 17].
– An extra methyl group can be present either at C-2β or at C-3β [17–22].

– Additional hydroxy groups can be found in the side-chain at C-30 or/and at C-31 (*e.g.* as in **7, 8, 10** or **11**) [16, 20].
– Finally the primary hydroxy group at C-35 can be replaced by an amino group (*e.g.* as in **9, 10** and **11**) [11, 23, 24], but polyols, and up to now, aminopolyols have never been found in a same bacterium.

2.3 Composite bacteriohopane derivatives: glycosides, ethers, peptides, nucleosides

In many hopanoid synthesizing bacteria, free polyols or aminopolyols are not the major hopanoids. They are linked to polar moieties which are representative of all major classes of natural products, *i.e.* carbohydrates, amino acids or nucleosides. On the one hand, bacteriohopanetetrol can be linked via a glycosidic bond to a glucosamine (**12**) or

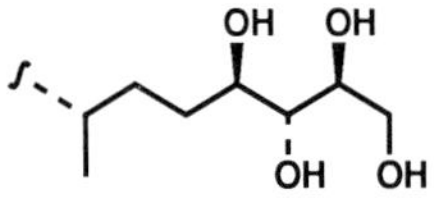

5a 22R
5b 22S

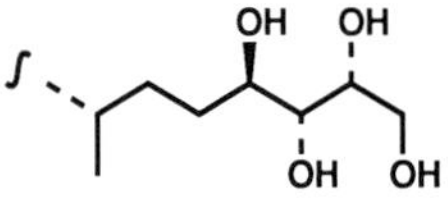

6

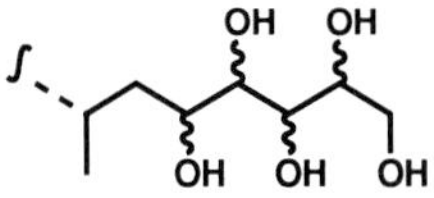

7

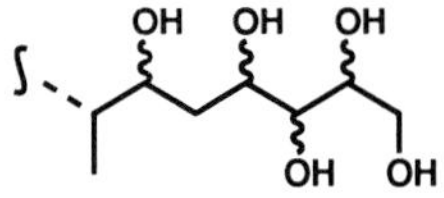

8

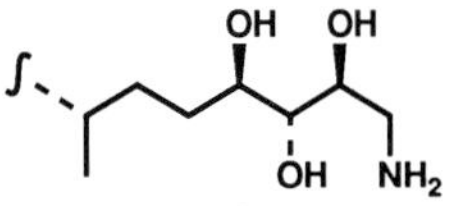

9

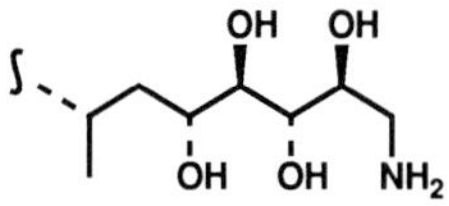

10

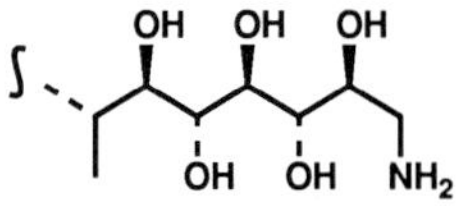

11

Figure 3
Side-chains of bacteriohopanepolyols and aminobacteriohopanepolyols.

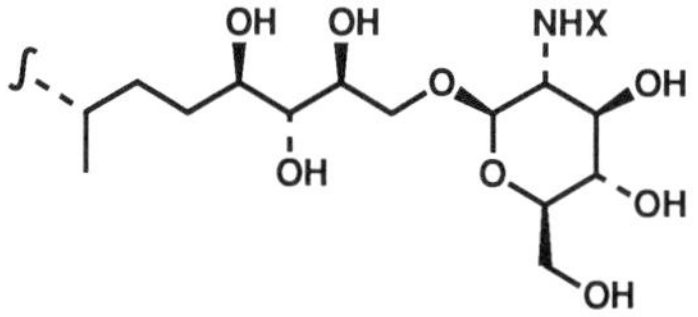

Figure 4
Composite bacteriohopane derivatives.

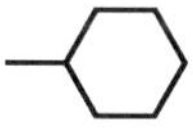

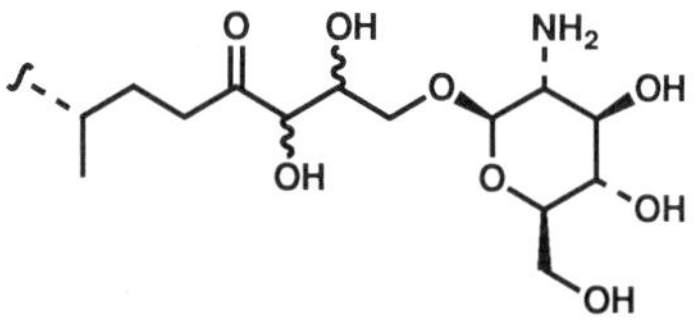

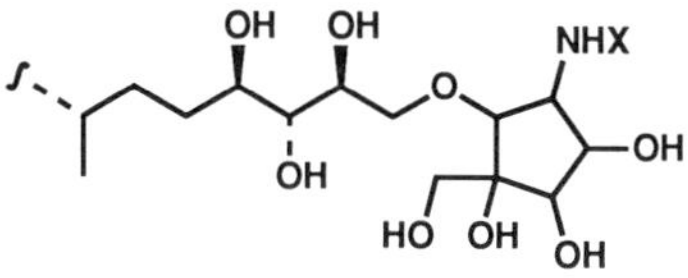

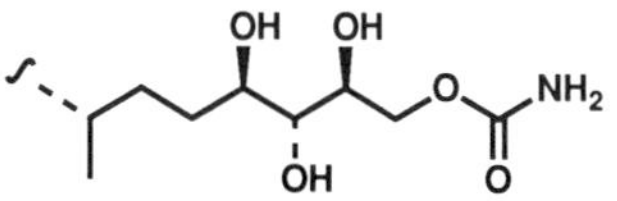

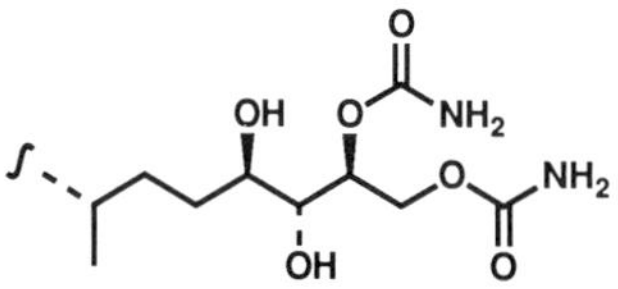

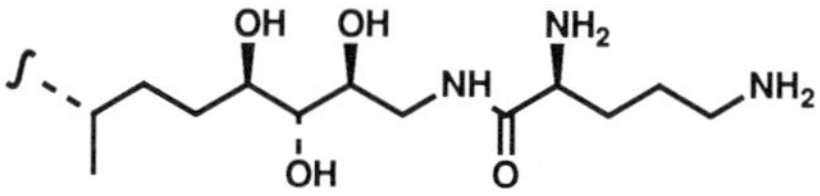

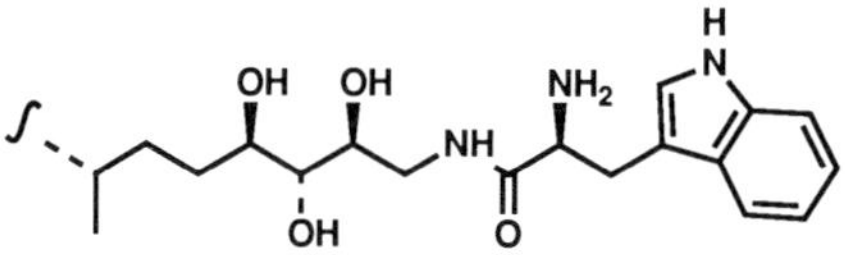

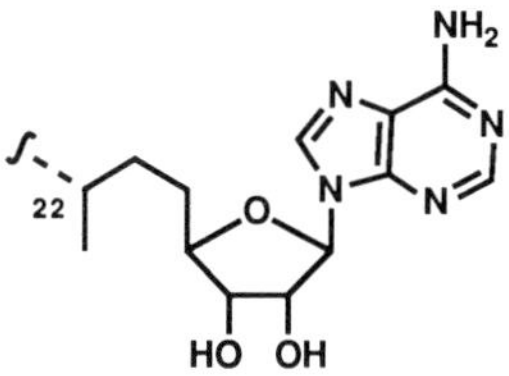

an *N*-acylglucosamine (**14**) [25–27], or via an ether bond to a novel type of carbapseudopentose like cyclitols (**15** and **16**) [12, 26, 27]. Carbamoyl groups can be found either at C-35, or at C-35 and C-34 (**17** and **18**) [12]. On the other hand, aminobacteriohopanetriol can be linked via a peptidic bond to ornithine or tryptophane (**19** and **20**) [24]. The most striking features are however the structures of adenosylhopanes (**20**) and (**21**) [12, 28]. These nucleoside analogues are the first compounds possessing a C-C bond between a triterpene and a carbohydrate derivative.

The significance of this structural diversity is not yet understood and will be discussed in section 5 and in the conclusion.

3   The distribution of hopanoids in prokaryotes

Owing to the numerous structurally different bacteriohopane side-chains, there is no simple and rapid method permitting the direct identification of all complex hopanoids, as those can be isolated from a crude bacterial extract only after acetylation and most often tedious chromatographic procedures [24, 26, 29]. In order to determine the total hopanoid content of a bacterium, one has to get rid of these side-chains. This can be efficiently done by periodic acid cleavage of the polyols, followed by $NaBH_4$ reduction, resulting in primary alcohols (Fig. 5) which can be readily isolated and quantitated by gas chromatography and high performance liquid chromatography [7, 9, 30]. This method is probably the best one for a reliable detection of these triterpenoids in bacteria. For periodic acid oxidation, however, the presence of two vicinal hydroxy groups is required. Adenosylhopanes for instance can not be detected by this method, and this restriction must be kept in mind.

Hopanoids are widespread amongst prokaryotes. However, no clear cut rules from their presently known distribution could be defined [7,

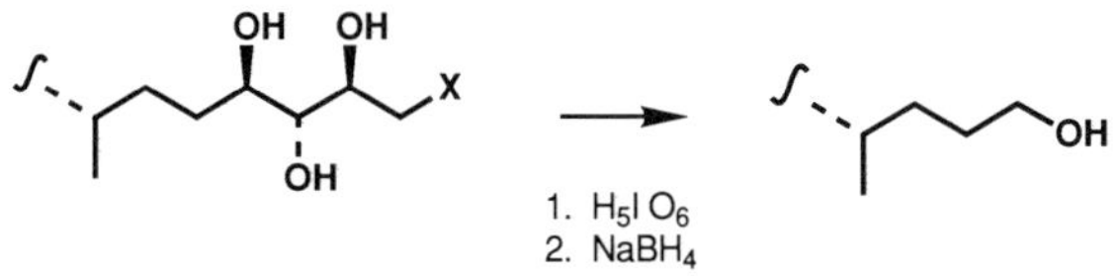

Figure 5
Cleavage of bacteriohopanepolyol side-chains.

31]. Hopanoids have been thus found in nearly all analyzed cyanobacteria, in many Rhodospirillaceae (but not in all of them), in obligate methylotrophs, in gram-negative (*e.g. Acetobacter* spp., *Zymomonas mobilis,* some *Pseudomonas* spp., *Azotobacter*...) or gram-positive (*e.g.* some thermotolerant *Bacillus,* some *Streptomyces*...) chemoheterotrophs. Many taxa are devoid of any detectable hopanoids: they have for instance never been found in Archaebacteria or in strict anaerobes (but very few strains have been analyzed).

They are apparently more common in bacteria living free in environments where they are exposed to rather harsh physiological conditions (variations of temperature, osmotic pressure and/or pH, presence of ethanol or acetic acid as for *Zymomonas* and *Acetobacter*). They have never been found in the many analyzed enterobacteria or in pathogenic bacteria, reflecting possibly their physically and chemically rather stable life conditions. As hopanoids act as membrane stabilizers (see further, Section 5), it is reasonable to assume that the former hopanoid producers possessing compounds capable of modulating the permeability and the fluidity of their membrane systems developed or maintained this metabolic pathway in response to environmental pressure. The presently known distribution of biohopanoids is furthermore in full accordance with the ubiquity and abundance of their molecular fossils in sediments.

The hopanoid concentration in prokaryotic cells (ca. 0.5–3 mg/g, dry weight) is of the same order of magnitude as those reported for sterols in eukaryotes [7]. Despite numerous reports in the literature concerning the presence of sterols in prokaryotes, it seems that these microorganisms are unable to synthesize these terpenoids *de novo* [31]. Indeed in most cases the reported concentrations were so low that no structural role could be devoted to these compounds. We analyzed several strains reported to contain sterols, and our conclusion was rather pessimistic: the greater the precautions against contaminants, the lower the amount of detected sterols of the same order of magnitude as those from blank experiments performed without bacterial cells [32]. For two bacteria only *(Methylococcus capsulatus* and *Nannocystis exedens)* large amounts of uncommon sterols have been detected and the *de novo* biosynthesis clearly documented [33–35].

4   Biosynthesis

4.1   Isoprenic unit biosynthesis in prokaryotes: an overlooked problem?

Incorporation of (1-^{13}C)- or (2-^{13}C)acetate into the hopanoids of several bacteria *(Methylobacterium organophilum, Rhodopseudomonas palustris* and *Rhodopseudomonas acidophila)* [36] or of specifically ^{13}C labeled glucose (either at C-1, C-2, C-3, C-5 or C-6) into those of *Zymomonas mobilis* [37, 38] shed some light on an unexpected problem. The following conclusions could be drawn from these labeling experiments.

– Exogenous acetate was not directly incorporated into the terpenoid biosynthetic pathway as expected from similar experiments performed on eukaryotic cells, although it was "normally" incorporated into poly-β-hydroxybutyrate and carbohydrates. Similar results were obtained in the case of feeding experiments with *Zymomonas mobilis* with specifically ^{13}C labeled glucose. Glucose was incorporated, as expected, into amino acids, fatty acids or carbohydrates, but the hopanoid labeling pattern could not be explained by the incorporation of acetate units derived from known glucose catabolic pathways. In all cases no ^{13}C scrambling could be observed.

– Assuming that the same isoprenic biosynthetic pathway is operating in eukaryotes as well as in prokaryotes, and that HMGCoA, the precursor of mevalonate, is formed by the condensation of three acetylcoenzyme A units, the former C_2 unit donors have to come from two different pools in the case of the bacteria utilized for the acetate labelling experiments and even from three in the case of *Zymomonas mobilis*. Such a compartmentation of acetate pools, which can not be fully excluded at this stage, seems however very unlikely in prokaryotic cells without organelles.

– This might point to a possible new, still unknown biosynthetic pathway for prokaryotic isoprenoids. This question has been mostly completely overlooked. Indeed, experiments concerning the biosynthesis of prokaryotic isoprenoids (carotenoids, acyclic polyprenols and isoprenic quinones) involved nearly always incorporation of radioactive precursors, usually without localization of the labeled positions in the metabolites. In two cases however (incorporation of [^{14}C]acetate into ubiquinone from *Escherichia coli* [39] or of [^{13}C]-acetate into the phytanyl chains from *Halobacterium cutirubrum* phospholipids [40]), the labeling patterns of these isoprenoids did not correspond with those expected from a direct acetate incorporation into the "classical" biosynthetic pathway.

4.2   The origin of the bacteriohopanepolyol side-chain

The presence of an extra C_5 *n*-alkyl polyhydroxylated side-chain linked to the triterpenic hopane skeleton is a unique feature found only in the bacteriohopane derivatives. According to the side-chain labeling patterns observed after feeding experiments with ^{13}C-labeled acetate [36] or glucose [37, 38], the precursor of this side-chain is a D-pentose derivative arising from the non-oxidative pentose phosphate pathway and linked via its C-5 carbon to the hopane skeleton. According to the stereochemistries of tetrol (**5a**) and aminotriol (**9**) this precursor might be a D-ribose derivative [12–15]. For tetrol (**6**) with a different configuration at C-34, it might be a D-arabinose derivative. In spite of numerous attempts, no data concerning the mechanism of the enzymatic reaction permitting this linkage or the structure of the precursor for the triterpene and carbohydrate moieties could be collected. Adenosylhopanes (**21**) and (**22**) might represent possible precursors as after loss of the base, reduction or reductive amination they could afford tetrols (**5a** and **5b**) as well as aminotriol (**9**).

4.3   Squalene cyclase: the formation of the pentacyclic skeleton

Squalene cyclase is the only enzyme which has been studied in the hopanoid biosynthetic pathway. Whereas all eukaryotic 3-hydroxytriterpenes are derived from the cyclization of squalene oxide, the bacterial hopane framework of diploptene (**2**) and diplopterol (**3**) (which are 3-desoxytriterpenes) derives from a direct enzyme-catalyzed, proton-initiated cyclization of squalene itself. This enzymatic activity has been been characterized in several bacteria [41–44], and the enzyme itself has been purified and isolated from the thermoacidophilic *Bacillus acidocaldarius* [45–47], permitting the determination of the amino acid sequence [48].

Compared to eukaryotic squalene oxide cyclases which cyclize solely the (3*S*) enantiomer of squalene oxide (**24**) into 3β-hydroxytriterpenes (**26**) leaving the other enantiomer and squalene unattacked [49],

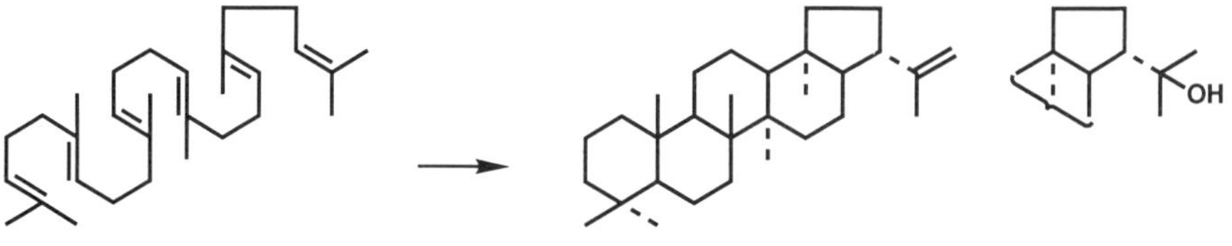

23   **2**   **3**

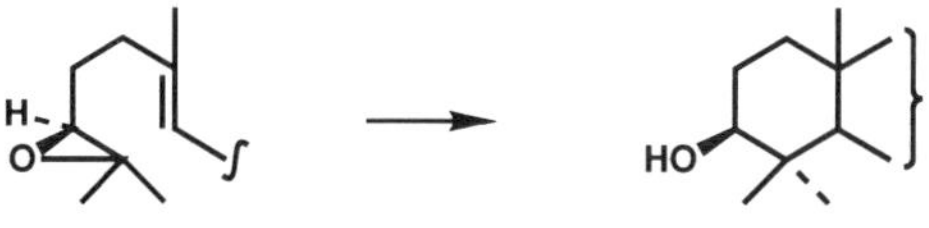

24   **26**

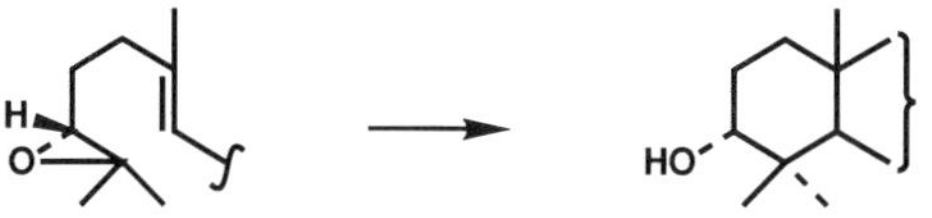

25   **27**

Figure 6
Cyclization of squalene (**23**), (3S)-squalene oxide (**26**) and (3R)-squalene oxide (**27**)
by bacterial cyclases.

the prokaryotic cyclases show little specificity toward the substrate.
They cyclize squalene, their normal substrate, as well as both enantiomers of squalene oxide which are normally absent in bacterial
cells: the (3S)-enantiomer (**24**) gives thus 3β-hydroxyhopanoids (**26**)
(as expected from the knowledge of eukaryotic cyclases), whereas the
unnatural (3R) enantiomer (**25**) gives the 3α-hydroxyhopanoids (**27**)
[40–42]. Concerning the formation of ring A, the former reaction

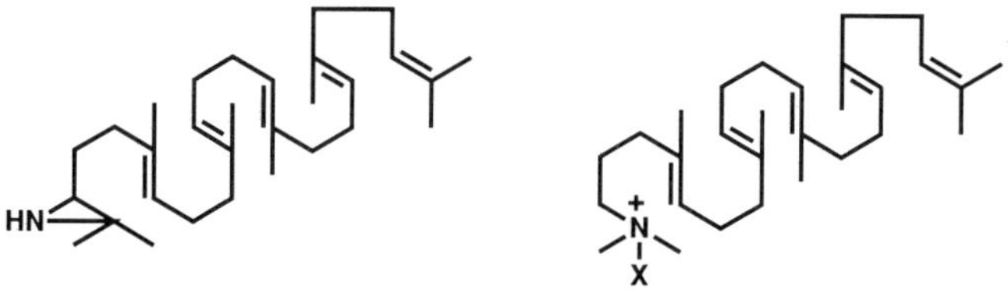

X = H
X = CH₃
X = O⁻

Figure 7
Inhibitors of squalene and squalene
oxide cyclases.

corresponds to a pre-chair conformation of the substrate, and the latter to a pre-boat conformation [50].

Like for eukaryotic squalene cyclases, squalene analogues mimicking putative high energy intermediates of the enzymatic cyclization are also potent inhibitors of bacterial cyclases ($I_{50} < 1$ μM). These compounds inhibit also selectively the growth of hopanoid-producing bacteria at low concentrations (ca. 1 μM) and do not affect the growth of hopanoidless bacteria at the highest tested concentration, *i.e.* 200 mM [44]. This observation suggests that hopanoids are essential metabolites for the bacteria producing them.

5   Hopanoids as membrane stabilizers
5.1   Effect on biological membrane models

Bacteriohopane derivatives, like cholesterol, are amphiphilic molecules, with a planar, rigid, hydrophobic, polycyclic ring system and a length similar to those of the acyl chains of fatty acid and permitting thus their insertion in phospholipid bilayers. Do these structural similarities reflect similar biological roles as membrane stabilizers [51]? Indeed, the hopanoids of the gram-negative bacterium *Zymomonas mobilis* have been tentatively localized in the cytoplasmic as well as in the outer membrane [52]. The effects of bacteriohopane derivatives have been tested on several biological membrane models by the groups of Poralla and Ourisson. When bacteriohopanetetrol (**5a**) or its glycoside (**14**) were incorporated into monolayers of phosphatidylcholine containing either linear, branched or ω-cyclohexyl fatty acyl chains, lipid condensation and quenching of the phase transition occurred [53–56]. By differential scanning calorimetry, it could be shown that a 40 % molar concentration of bacteriohopanetetrol completely abolishes the phase transition in multilamellar dispersions of phosphatidylcholine [55]. Black lipid membranes are a model of phospholipid bilayers permitting the evaluation of membrane permeability. 2β-Methyldiplopterol and tetrol *N*-acylglycoside lowered both the permeability of this membrane toward lipophilic ions or lipophilic neutral peptides [57]. Finally, hopanoids (diplopterol, natural bacteriohopanetetrol mixture from *Acetobacter* or tetrol *N*-acylglycoside) induced a reduced permeability toward glycerol in liposomes [57] or toward water into unilamellar vesicles [58].

All these experiments suggest that hopanoids have a sterol-like function in prokaryotic membranes; the effects on membrane models observed with hopanoids are in all cases qualitatively similar to those obtained with sterols, although usually somewhat smaller.

5.2   Effect in living cells

The first equivalence between sterols and hopanoids was deduced from studies on the ciliate *Tetrahymena pyriformis*. Indeed, when grown in the absence of sterols, it synthesizes a quasi-hopanoid tetrahymanol and incorporates this triterpene mainly into its cytoplasmic membrane. When grown in the presence of sufficient amounts of sterols, tetrahymanol biosynthesis is fully inhibited, and sterols are incorporated into the membranes, usually after slight modifications [59]. This was the first evidence for identical roles of two different triterpenoid series. Furthermore, this protozoon does not grow in the presence of triparanol, an hypocholesterolemic drug also inhibiting the cyclization of squalene into tetrahymanol. Sterols, hopanoids as well as several other polyterpenoids restored growth and permitted survival of the cells in the presence of the drug, showing again the equivalence of both series [60]. Similar experiments have been performed with *Mycoplasma mycoides,* a parasitic wall-less prokaryote requiring cholesterol for its growth. In the absence of the sterol, a hopanoid, diplopterol, supported the growth suggesting again that diplopterol can fulfill a sterol-like function in *Mycoplasma* membranes [61].

Further evidence was obtained with other bacterial cells. The higher the temperature of cultures of the thermoacidophilic *Bacillus acidocaldarius,* the higher the hopanoid content of the cells [62]. *Zymomonas mobilis* is an ethanol-producing bacterium. It can tolerate an up to 14 % high concentration of this solvent, which is much higher than any bacterium can tolerate; in this case too, the higher the ethanol concentration, the higher the hopanoid content of the cell membranes [63]. It seems thus that hopanoids have a membrane-stabilizing effect, counterbalancing in these two last examples a probable temperature or solvent-induced destabilization of the membranes.

6   **Conclusion. Other possible roles for hopanoids. A view to new antibacterial agents?**

The sole structural role of hopanoids as membrane stabilizers does not probably account for the structural variety of the polyfunctionalized side-chains from all known bacteriohopane derivatives. This diversity might reflect other possible physiological roles which could not be examined primarily because of the rather small amounts of free native hopanoids available up to now.

Some of the most striking features to be discovered through hopanoid biochemistry are the unexpected anomalies found in the biosynthesis of prokaryotic hopanoids. They might point out differences between eukaryotes and prokaryotes either at the level of the regulation of isoprenoid biosynthesis, or at the level of the biosynthetic pathway itself. If these observations are of general scope and concern all prokaryotes and all prokaryotic isoprenoids (including the nearly ubiquitous undecaprenol implied in cell wall biosynthesis or the isoprenic quinones of the cellular oxido-reduction systems), isoprenoid biosynthesis could represent a new target for specific antibacterial drugs.

Acknowledgments

Work on hopanoids was supported by the *Centre National de la Recherche Scientifique (Unité de Recherche Associée 135)* and by the *Ministère de l'Education Nationale* (Réseau Européen de Laboratoires).

References

1   G. Ourisson, P. Albrecht and M. Rohmer: Pure Appl. Chem. *51*, 709 (1979) and references cited therein.
2   G. Ourisson, P. Albrecht and M. Rohmer: Sci. Am. *251*, 44 (1984).
3   C. W. Bird, J. M. Lynch, S. J. Pirt and W. W. Reid: Tetrahedron Lett. 3190 (1971).
4   A. Ensminger, P. Albrecht, G. Ourisson, B. J. Kimble, J. R. Maxwell and G. Eglinton: Tetrahedron Lett. 3861 (1972).
5   H. J. Förster, K. Biemann, W. G. Haigh, N. H. Tattrie and J. R. Colvin: Biochem. J. *135*, 133 (1973).
6   M. de Rosa, A. Gambacorta, L. Minale and J. Bu'Lock: J. Chem. Soc. Chem. Commun. 619 (1979).
7   M. Rohmer, P. Bouvier-Navé and G. Ourisson: J. Gen. Microbiol. *130*, 1137 (1984).

8   G. Kleemann, K. Poralla, G. Englert, H. Kjosen, S. Liaaen-Jensen, S. Neunlist and M. Rohmer: J. Gen. Microbiol. *136,* 2251 (1990), and references cited therein.

9   M. Rohmer and G. Ourisson: Tetrahedron Lett. 3633 (1976).

10   M. Zundel and M. Rohmer: FEMS Microbiol. Lett. *28,* 61 (1985).

11   S. Neunlist and M. Rohmer: Biochem. J. *231,* 635 (1985).

12   S. Neunlist, P. Bisseret and M. Rohmer: Eur. J. Biochem. *171,* 245 (1988).

13   P. Bisseret and M. Rohmer: J. Org. Chem. *54,* 2958 (1989).

14   S. Neunlist and M. Rohmer: J. Chem. Soc. Chem. Commun. 830 (1988).

15   P. Zhou, N. Berova, K. Nakanishi and M. Rohmer: J. Chem. Soc. Chem. Commun. 256 (1991).

16   M. Rohmer and G. Ourisson: Tetrahedron Lett. 3637 (1976).

17   M. Rohmer and G. Ourisson: J. Chem. Res. (*S*) 356, (*M*) 3037 (1986).

18   M. Rohmer and G. Ourisson: Tetrahedron Lett. 3641 (1976).

19   M. Zundel and M. Rohmer: Eur. J. Biochem. *150,* 23 (1985).

20   P. Bisseret, M. Zundel and M. Rohmer: Eur. J. Biochem. *150,* 29 (1985).

21   A. Babadjamian, R. Faure, M. Laget, G. Duménil and P. Padieu: J. Chem. Soc. Chem. Commun. 1657 (1987).

22   M. Zundel and M. Rohmer: Eur. J. Biochem. *150,* 35 (1985).

23   S. Neunlist and M. Rohmer: Biochem. J. *131,* 1363 (1985).

24   S. Neunlist, O. Holst and M. Rohmer: Eur. J. Biochem. *147,* 561 (1985).

25   T. A. Langworthy, W. R. Mayberry and P. F. Smith: Biochem. biophys. Acta *431,* 550 (1976).

26   J.-M. Renoux and M. Rohmer: Eur. J. Biochem. *151,* 405 (1985).

27   G. Flesch and M. Rohmer: Biochem. J. *262,* 673 (1989).

28   S. Neunlist and M. Rohmer: Biochem. J. *228,* 769 (1985).

29   H. Schulenberg-Schell, B. Neuss and H. Sahm: Analyt. Biochem. *181,* 120 (1989).

30   K. D. Barrow and J. O. Chuck: Analyt. Biochem. *184,* 395 (1990).

31   G. Ourisson, K. Poralla and M. Rohmer: Ann. Rev. Microbiol. *41,* 301 (1987), and references cited therein.

32   P. Bouvier: Ph. D. Thesis. Université Louis Pasteur, Strasbourg, France (1978).

33   C. W. Bird, J. M. Lynch, S. J. Pirt, W. W. Reid and C. J. W. Brooks: Nature, *230,* 473 (1971).

34   P. Bouvier, M. Rohmer and G. Ourisson: Biochem. J. *159,* 267 (1976).

35   N. Kohl, A. Gloe and H. Reichenbach: J. Gen. Microbiol. *129,* 1629 (1983).

36   G. Flesch and M. Rohmer, Eur. J. Biochem. *175,* 405 (1988).

37   M. Rohmer, B. Sutter and H. Sahm: J. Chem. Soc. Chem. Commun. 1471 (1989).

38   B. Sutter: Ph. D. Thesis, Université de Haute Alsace, Mulhouse, France (1991).

39   S. Pandian, S. Saendjan and T. S. Raman: Biochem. J. *196,* 675 (1981).

40   I. Ekiel, G. D. Sprott and I. P. Smith: J. Bacteriol. *166,* 559 (1986).

41   C. Anding, M. Rohmer and G. Ourisson: J. Am. Chem. Soc. *90,* 3563 (1976).

42   M. Rohmer, C. Anding and G. Ourisson: Eur. J. Biochem. *112,* 541 (1980).

43   M. Rohmer, P. Bouvier and G. Ourisson: Eur. J. Biochem. *112,* 557 (1980).

44   G. Flesch and M. Rohmer: Arch. Microbiol. *147,* 100 (1987).

45   S. Neumann and H. Simon: Biol. Chem. Hoppe-Seyler: *367,* 723 (1986).

46   B. Seckler and K. Poralla: Biochim. Biophys. Acta *881,* 356 (1986).

47   D. Ochs, C. H. Tappe, P. Gärtner, R. Kellner and K. Poralla: Eur. J. Biochem. *194,* 75 (1990).

48   D. Ochs: Ph. D. Thesis, Universität Tübingen, Tübingen, FRG (1990).

49 D. H. R. Barton, T. R. Jarman, K. C. Watson, D. A. Widdowson, R. B. Boar and K. Damp: J. Chem. Soc. Perkin I, 1134 (1975).
50 P. Bouvier, Y. Berger, M. Rohmer and G. Ourisson: Eur. J. Biochem. *112*, 549 (1980).
51 M. Rohmer, P. Bouvier and G. Ourisson: Proc. Natl. Acad. Sci. USA *76*, 847 (1979).
52 Y. Tahara, H. Yuhara and Y. Yamada: Agric. Biol. Chem. *52*, 607 (1988).
53 E. Kannenberg and K. Poralla: Naturwissenschaften *67*, 458 (1980).
54 K. Poralla, E. Kannenberg and A. Blume: FEBS Lett. *113*, 107 (1980).
55 E. Kannenberg, A. Blume, R. N. McElhaney and K. Poralla: Biochim. Biophys. Acta *733*, 111 (1983).
56 E. Kannenberg, A. Blume, K. Geckeler and K. Poralla: Biochim. Biophys. Acta *817*, 170 (1985).
57 R. Benz, D. Hallmann, K. Poralla and H. Eibl: Chem. Phys. Lipids *34*, 7 (1983).
58 P. Bisseret, G. Wolff, A.-M. Albrecht, T. Tanaka, Y. Nakatani and G. Ourisson: Biochim. Biophys. Res. Commun. *110*, 320 (1983).
59 R. L. Conner, J. R. Laudrey, C. H. Burns and F. B. Mallory: J. Protozool. *15*, 600 (1968).
60 D. Raederstorff and M. Rohmer: Biochim. Biophys. Acta *960*, 190 (1988).
61 E. Kannenberg and K. Poralla: Arch. Microbiol. *133*, 100 (1982).
62 K. Poralla, T. Härtner and E. Kannenberg: FEMS Microbiol. Lett. *23*, 253 (1984).
63 A. Schmidt, S. Bringer-Meyer and H. Sahm: Appl. Microbiol. Biotechnol. *25*, 32 (1986).

Isosterism and bioisosterism in drug design

By Alfred Burger

University of Virginia, Department of Chemistry,
Charlottesville, Virgina 22901, USA

1   Methods of drug discovery
1.1   The discovery of "lead" compounds

In every scientific undertaking that is to break new ground, one has to have a goal, a working hypothesis, or a leading idea or fact. This will encourage research and help in the pursuit of a worth-while objective, be it the enrichment of knowledge or the elaboration of a practical purpose. A medicinal scientist who hopes to find a new biologically active drug will have to be guided by such considerations.

When Nature presented itself to primitive human societies as a mysterious and clouded vision, people had no choice but to try its offerings, one after another, to discover some material that would help them to alleviate pain, heal diseases, and delay inevitable death, meanwhile maintaining an individual in tolerable health. Components of rocks, soils and minerals were tried by self-appointed medicine men and healers, and plants and animal tissues were applied or consumed as potential therapeutic materials. This random and wasteful process of trial and error was conducted both for the treatment of reasonably well-defined illnesses or, in the last two centuries, in biological model experiments with a bearing on the pathological condition that was to be halted, alleviated, or cured.

As more and more natural materials from the animal and plant kingdoms were screened and tested, and the successes and failures of these trials were recorded in ancient philosophical treatises, a therapeutic folklore developed as a tentative, selective guide for future medicinal experimentation. Some plant families could be recommended as sources of medicines for certain diseases, and other members of these families could then be expected to provide similar therapeutic powers. It was not a reliable method because ancient diagnoses of diseases could not often be trusted. At least there was a possibility of taking totally aimless randomness out of searches for natural drugs. Interestingly, the pharmacognosists of our day still screen plants and crude plant extracts and soil samples randomly if the biological test method is informative, quick, and inexpensive. Exotic botanical materials can now be transported rapidly from previously inaccessible regions. They can be purified by new isolation techniques and their structure elucidated quickly. They offer the never-ending hope that they may cure hitherto untreatable diseases, and provide novel sources of unexpected "lead" structures.

With the ascendency of synthetic organic chemicals, screening processes turned to available samples of such compounds. If a compound shows promise in a given test, structurally related substances will be chosen as test candidates. They will often also be screened for side effects or other activities that might enhance their therapeutic potential. Once in a while, an unexpected biological effect may turn up during such trials and call attention to a possible activity quite different from the original screening purpose. At this point the biological discovery assumes some aspects of drug design. A classical case of such a study was the discovery of significant antihypertensive activities of certain heterocyclic sulfonamides and sulfonylureas that had been conceived and tested as antibacterials. The design portion involved molecular modifications such as the displacement of the *p*-amino group, which is essential for bacteriostasis, by alkyl or halogen and incorporation of the sulfamyl groups into hetero rings. These measures suppress antibacterial activity and allow the new activity to come to the fore.

Other examples of useful side effects include the observation that propranolol, which was designed to block β-adrenergic impulses and to counteract angina, can be used to lower blood pressure. Phenobarbital was conceived as a hypnotic but became important in controlling epilepsy. Imipramine, originally planned to be a neuroleptic, was found to be an antidepressant in clinical trials. The local anesthetic, lidocaine, can stabilize cardiac arrhythmias. In some of these cases no molecular modification was needed to emphasize the new useful activity. In other instances, extensive molecular modification was required to convert a former side effect to a desirable therapeutic activity.

An important biochemically-based search for "lead" compounds arises from a study of metabolites. Thousands of metabolites of animals are known and some of them have been recognized as protecting the body against disease aberrations. By contrast, metabolites of invasive or infectious organisms are causative agents of the invasive or infectious diseases. They may be counteracted by metabolite analogs produced by molecular modification.

1.2   Molecular modification

The second stage of drug development involves the fine-tuning of a "lead" structure by molecular modification. Analogs resulting from molecular modification must still be screened for biological behavior, and in most cases must be modified further to maximize the desired biological activity and specificity. The time of random structural variations in molecular modification ("molecular roulette") prevalent throughout the first three decades of the twentieth century is past. Molecular modification now always involves drug design as far as the state of the art permits. This article centers on one widely used approach to drug design with ramifications to other contributions in our understanding of rationality in medicinal chemistry. This does not rule out serendipity and empirical trials guided by "experience".

1.3   What is biological activity?

One of the most important goals of chemistry is the elucidation of the relationships of chemical structure and various physical properties, such as solubility, electrical conductance, plasticity, optical properties, etc. The relationships between chemical structure and color and dyestuff properties have been studied extensively; colored compounds as well as dyestuffs must contain a chromophore, commonly an unsaturated system of conjugated double bonds. Biological activity has been correlated with the presence of pharmacophores, i.e. sections of a molecule containing atoms and linkages responsible for the activity. Great caution is necessary not to generalize too much about such pharmacophores, because biological activity is much too diffuse a term. It may depend upon the presence of ionizable groups of atoms, or on unsaturated or potentially unsaturated functions, and on the shape and chirality of a molecule. Indeed, since biologically active substances must interact with active sites of flexible macromolecules such as enzymes, bioreceptors and nucleic acids, the shape of biosubstrates and drugs is of greatest importance. If it is complementary to a section of an active site, it offers functional atoms or groups of the approaching molecule a close fit at macromolecular sites, and thereby an opportunity to ligate to the macromolecule and rapidly interact with it.

In most cases, biological activity is much more complex than the biochemical reaction between an enzyme, receptor or polynucleotide with a usually relatively small-sized substrate or drug molecule. In order to produce a biological effect (motion, sound, pain, etc.) a cascade of interdependent reactions must take place which amplifies the energy liberated by each participating system until an overt action can be registered. The "biological activity" of a substrate therefore depends on some reaction that contributes a small increment to such biochemical cascades, at best setting in motion a sequence of biochemical events [1].

It is therefore necessary to understand what is meant by "biological activity" in each case. Studies of structure-activity relationships (SAR) are meaningful only if the same biological, and preferably biochemical phenomenon or reaction is affected by two compounds to be compared. Most drugs are inhibitors of enzyme systems or substrate antagonists. All too often the ability of a test substance to "lower blood pressure", to "affect diuresis", to "increase the pain threshold", and to produce similar pharmacological phenomena serves as a basis for comparison with another structurally similar chemical without referring to the very mechanism of the observed overall results. It is even worse to compare structurally unrelated compounds using qualitative pharmacological observations because such substances have a good chance of producing these test data by different biochemical mechanisms. That means, they may react at different active sites of the same or different receptors, or they may interfere with different enzymes in cascade systems which manifest themselves in the same biological end-occurrence.

The ideal comparison of the biochemical activity of two compounds should therefore be based on the effect of the compounds on the same mechanisms in enzymatic, receptor-ligating and other reactions with the biomacromolecules of the same organism. This goal is difficult to attain in therapeutic areas in which the causative biochemical agents have not yet become known. In tests involving invasive or infectious conditions, one will search for differences between isozymes of the host and those of the disease-causing cells. For some infectious and invasive pathogens, isozymes of dihydrofolate reductase have been purified and candidate drugs could be screened for cytostatic activity against the isozyme of the pathogen. For some viruses, their unique retropolymerases have become the target of drug tests. Bioisosteres of metabolites of such pathogens have become effective drugs for the inhibition of life processes of the damaging cells.

The requirement of searching for a drug that will act exactly like a known prototype is often relaxed for practical reasons. Especially in the pharmaceutical industry where the vast majority of therapeutic agents is developed, one tries almost always to design compounds with enhanced potency, selectivity, and fewer side effects. In other words, one digresses voluntarily from a strictly scientific search for mechanistically matching drugs to a search for compounds with improved *in vitro* and *in vivo* properties. Needless to say such investigations dilute comparative knowledge and complicate the ultimate aims of biochemically based drug design.

Working with macromolecular biochemical and with cellular and tissue-oriented systems, one encounters complexities which stretch our contemporary understanding of biological phenomena to the limit. If such knowledge is to be heightened, one has to reduce these complexities radically. This does not often appeal to experimental biologists in the industry who confront tantalizing complex questions in their chosen sciences and hope to dent these uncertainties at perhaps one point in their lifetime. Physical chemists realize that even in such simple systems as diatomic molecules, let alone the much more complicated and biologically unavoidable molecules of water, $(H_2O)_n$, enough problems of intra- and interatomic forces have remained unsolved to provide fundamental research topics for a long time to come. If biological mechanisms in drug design are to be elucidated on the molecular or ionic levels, one had better revert first to very simple chemical structures in which molecules have been reduced to a bare minimum and the complexities of larger or very large molecules have been stripped off as far as possible.

1.4   Isosterism

An early attempt to compare chemical and physical properties of diatomic molecules such as N_2 and CO was made by Moir [2, 3]. His reasonings about "isomerism" of these two gases are no longer compatible with present-day views; nevertheless, his ideas were expanded by Hinsberg [4] who applied them to partial structures of organic compounds. He defined groups which can be exchanged for each other in aromatic ring systems without considerable change of the physical properties of the resulting compounds as ring equivalents, citing benzene, thiophene and pyridine as examples. A -CH=CH- group in benzene is replaced by divalent sulfur, -S-, in thiophene, or its -CH= by trivalent nitrogen, -N=, in pyridine. Indeed, benzene boils at 81.1° (760 mm), thiophene at 84.4° (760 mm), but pyridine digresses from these similar data, boiling at 115–116° (760 mm). In those early days, it was actually difficult to fractionate benzene and thiophene from coal tar benzene. Hinsberg suggested that sulfur must resemble -C = C- in its external shape. The bothersome hydrogen atoms were disregarded as unimportant compared to the much larger aromatic carbon atoms. Hückel [5] then advanced other examples of ring equivalents, comparing the imino group, -NH-, to oxygen, -O-, in organic compounds such as pyrrole and furan. He also equated methyl, CH_3, with fluorine, and methylene, $= CH_2$, with nitrogen as seen in diazomethane, CH_2N_2, which was compared to ethylene, $CH_2 = CH_2$.

The physicist Grimm [6–8] called groups such as OH and NH_2 "pseudoatoms". He assumed that a proton (H^+O-; H^+NH-) penetrated the electron shell of the larger atom and was "submerged" in it and did not have much effect on the interatomic ligating power of the heavier atom (O, N). This submergence of hydrogen – the smallest atom – appeared to be allowed [9] for small atoms. It could be interpreted as a combination with the orbitals of the outer valence electrons. The inner orbitals must not be affected. Of course, hydrogen bridging was not yet understood.

Compounds that contained pseudoatoms were predictably similar physically although quite different in their chemical reactivity, provided that their molecular size and overall charge distribution were similar and not affected by dipole moments. In an effort to imitate the periodic table of the elements and apply analogous ideas to molecules, Grimm arranged a number of elements in a Table which lists progressive increases in proton attachments, and which he called the "hydride displacement law". The last word must be regarded as excessive, because it is an illustration rather than a law of physics. As one descends diagonally from the left to the right in Table 1 representing this idea, one H is added after another, and the elements and groups in the vertical columns become "pseudoatoms". For the chemist searching for lines of comparison between functional groups, columns 2, 3, and 4 are particularly instructive.

Table I
Grimm's "hydride displacement law"

C	N	O	F	Ne
	CH	NH	OH	FH
		CH_2	NH_2	OH_2
			CH_3	NH_3

Among simple compounds which contain pseudoatoms would be such pseudohalogen molecules as hydrogen peroxide (HOOH), hydrazine (H_2NNH_2), and ethane (CH_3CH_3). The actual location, motion, and resonance of electrons in orbitals was not considered in this early picture.

In 1919, the American Nobelist, Irving Langmuir, published two papers [10] that were designed to develop the then emerging octet rule for electron shell stability. The second of these articles was entitled "Isomorphism, Isosterism and Covalences". The concept of electron orbitals had not yet taken hold, but it was known that the elements in the vertical groups of the periodic table owed their similarities to the identity of their outer electron shells. In molecules with similar physical properties, an analogous arrangement could be expected. Langmuir coined the term isosteres ($\iota\sigma\acute{o}\varsigma$ = like, $\sigma\tau\epsilon\rho\epsilon\acute{o}\varsigma$ = shape) for such pairs of molecules and offered 21 examples for this concept. He quoted some inorganic isosteres, among them the negative ions, ClO_4^-, SO_4^{2-}, and PO_4^{3-}. Such groups are not isoelectric, they do not have the same electric charge. Some others are isoelectric, however, and they are the ones that are most similar to one another. Among them, three pairs were listed: CO and N_2; N_2O and CO_2; and azide, N_3^-, and isocyanate (NCO^-) ions. Diazomethane was now compared to a proposed molecule, ketene ($CH_2=C=O$) which had not yet been discovered, and not to ethylene [5]. The prediction of the similarity of diazomethane and ketene was confirmed 18 years later [11].

The definition of isosterism underwent a number of changes as the picture of electron orbitals emerged. It became necessary to include other properties that were to be compared, especially those that could be measured more easily at different stages of instrumental evolution. To begin with, they included similarities in boiling points, densities of liquids, melting points, molecular weights, and critical pressures (C_p), temperatures (C_t), and volumes (C_v). The more such physical properties could be measured and compared, the more accurate did such comparisons become. For example, C_p/C_v values for diphenylmethane and diphenyl ether ($=CH_2$ versus $O=$) had approximately the same collision areas [12–14], i.e. the same shape and spatial volume. Additional observations concerned similar mobilities of isosteric ions [15, 16], densities of complex ions [17], ionic radii [18], and parachors [19].

If one of the main characteristics of isosteres is equality of molecular volumes and great similarity of shape, two such compounds should be isomorphic, that is, similar in crystal habits and probably their ability to form mixed crystals. A study of the behavior of about 200 pairs of compounds demonstrated that only one-fourth of these formed mixed crystals over the whole range of percentage composition, and only an additional 17 % over part of this range. In other words, isomorphism does not necessarily imply mixed crystal formation [20–23]. It seems that mixed crystal formation may require also similarity of polarization, and this property is not always found in isosteres. Therefore, requiring mixed crystal formation is unrealistic to qualify for isosterism. Hans Erlenmeyer of the University of Basel [22, 24] suggested an extension of the concept of pseudoatoms, principally of pseudohalogens, to include groups mentioned by Birckenbach [15, 16, 25–27] such as -CN, -OCN, -N(CN)$_2$, -C(CN)$_3$, -SCN, and -SeCN. A number of other possibilities such as the comparison of C_6H_5COCl, $C_6H_5N_2{}^+Cl^-$, and C_6H_5MgCl, did not capture the attention of organic chemists either for synthetic purposes or other applications.

Erlenmeyer whose career included some time in the pharmaceutical industry before he returned to academic pursuits was quite naturally interested in the biological properties of organic compounds and the relationships of the structure of these substances to their biological activities. This interest was compounded by the research then flourishing all around him, especially in Switzerland and Germany, on the chemistry of vitamins, hormones and various drugs. The biological manifestations of almost all organic compounds were gross descriptions of activities in various pharmacological test systems at that time and were not yet based on biochemical reactions affected by the test substances. Trying to apply rigorous criteria to his explanations of biological observations, Erlenmeyer turned to a test system known for its specificity. The immunologist Karl Landsteiner [28] had shown that artificial antigens, formed by coupling aromatic diazonium ions to proteins, could be injected into animals and there provoked formation of specific antibodies as seen in combination and/or precipitation of the azoprotein. The immune reaction is highly specific, depending on the structure of the hapten portion, i. e. the aromatic azo moiety. Even minor changes in this portion of the antigen molecule prevent reaction with a given antibody. In Erlenmeyer's experiments [21, 29], the aromatic portion was represented by p-C_6H_5-O-C_6H_4-, p-C_6H_5-NH-C_6H_4-, and p-C_6H_5-CH_2-C_6H_4-, the groups linking the aromatic nuclei corresponding to the third vertical column of Grimm's Table of pseudoatoms. All three azoproteins containing these coupling components showed similar antigenic properties. This demonstrated the application of isosteric replacements in a demanding biochemical situation. Similarly, the azoprotein haptens derived from p-benzamidophenyldiazonium *(1)* and p-(2-thienyl) carboxamidophenyldiazonium *(2)* ions were serologically indistinguishable and so were

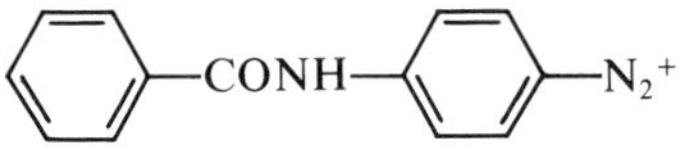

1 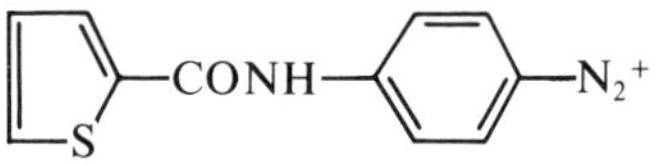   2

the azoproteins containing aryl groups with p-sulfonic *(3)* and p-selenoic acid *(4)* substituents [29, 30]. When the strongly polar substituents

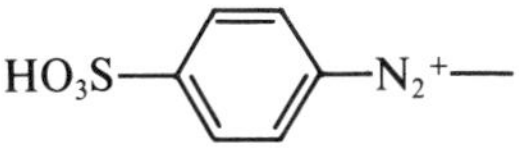

3 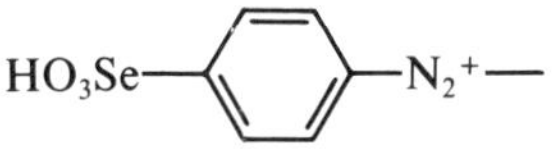   4

were replaced by less polar groups such as p-$HO_2SC_6H_4N_2$, the resulting azoproteins did not overlap with the antibody of the p-sulfonic acid derivative. Similarly, the azoproteins synthesized from p-aminobenzenephosphonic and -arsonic acid had the same antigen activity [30–32] but the corresponding stibionic acid analog behaved differently, perhaps because stibionic acids exist only in a polymeric form.

When it became apparent that comparisons of one or two physical properties might not be adequate to classify compounds as isosteres in the classical sense proposed by Grimm [6–8] and by Erlenmeyer [33], other additional properties were contemplated even though some of them were harder to measure. In all these studies, too many exceptions were noted to use the comparison as a firm basis of classification. For example, only a few functional derivatives of benzene and thiophene, respectively, have similar boiling points [34, 35]. The ionization potentials and the decomposition voltage of compounds containing pseudohalogens (F, OH, NH_2, CH_3) do not show steady trends

[36]. When the conductivity of compounds containing pseudohalogens was measured, differences arose because of an unequal degree of hydration [16]. The acid dissociation constants of isosteric heterocyclic acids, which depend on the dipole moments of the compounds, cannot be compared readily either [37]. Such dissociation constants increase with an increase of electron-attracting (electronegative) groups present, as observed for aryl and heteroaryl-substituted sulfanilamides, p-$H_2NC_6H_4SO_2NH$-R, where R represents such substituents [38]. Some regularities have been encountered when wavelength absorptions were compared but only to some extent such as the occurrence of maxima and minima in otherwise non-overlapping curves [39]. The optical activity of the thiophene isostere of cocaine is similar to that of the natural alkaloid [40].

All the difficulties in arriving at binding directives that make two compounds isosteric show that molecules cannot be compared as strictly as elementary particles. Every nuance of analogy of shells of outer electrons with the accompanying accumulation of regions of high and low electron density can be fitted into the views proposed by Langmuir and elaborated by Grimm, Erlenmeyer and others. Similarity of overall molecular shape and stereochemistry must be observed as a prime prerequisite. The most important practical application of the concept of isosterism, diluted by the uncertainties just presented, has been in drug design. Even though regretfully it does not provide an accurate guide, it has led to the design of compounds which should have, and often do have, affinity to a given biochemical reaction system. Such compounds either activate such biochemical reactions, i.e. they are agonists of recognized substrates, or else deactivate the same biochemical system by reacting with it at rates faster than the substrate or by interdicting access of the substrate to catalytic sites by bulky steric blockade of the reactive biochemical. In that case they are antagonists. A steady transition from agonists to antagonists remains a weakness in designing a biologically active molecule on the basis of isosterism.

Agonists have a high intrinsic activity; competitive antagonists have low or no intrinsic activity whereas non-competitive antagonists lack structural features that are needed for a close fit at the receptor. They therefore attach themselves to non-binding sites of the receptor protein or polynucleotide. Agonist molecules are usually smaller than competitive antagonists which cover areas larger than the active site.

1.4.1   Bioisosterism

To deal with all these divergent possibilities and difficulties in interpretation, Harris L. Friedman [41] coined the term bioisosterism for the relationship of compounds "which fit the broadest definition of isosteres and have the same type of biological activity". In other words, bioisosterism should account for structure-activity relationships (SAR) of biologically active chemicals. The purpose of SAR studies is the elucidation of the reasons for equivalence or nonequivalence of biologically active compounds.

Friedman's definition is less restrictive than Erlenmeyer's postulate that isosteres are atoms, ions or molecules in which the peripheral layers of electrons can be considered to be identical. This becomes untenable if "identical" is enforced in the light of modern electron theory, and makes it less predictive and explanatory in medicinal drug design. The "broadest definition of isosteres" as suggested by Friedman provides such wide interpretation of SAR that it becomes scientifically too vague, but in another sense it is of great help: it permits the medicinal chemist to roam towards structures that are somewhat similar to a prototype.

Hansch [42] tried to extricate this vagueness of language by defining bioisosteres as "compounds causing identical biochemical or pharmacological response in a standard test system. The system might be an enzyme, membrane, mouse or man". This would probably hold if the test uses an enzyme as a target, but for biological activity measured in isolated tissues, not to speak of whole animals including man, too many variables could interfere. Absorption, metabolism [43], attack at different stages of a multireactional cascade of events, and especially different mechanisms of action which may present an overall identical therapeutic effect would have to be factored into the definition.

We would like to suggest an expanded statement which takes into account biochemical views of biological activity. "Bioisosteres are compounds or groups that possess near-equal molecular shapes and volumes, approximately the same distribution of electrons, and which exhibit similar physical properties such as hydrophobicity. Bioisosteric compounds affect the same biochemically associated systems as agonists or antagonists and thereby produce biological properties that are related to each other."

A subdivision of bioisosteres is now also in use. The cases that satisfy the conditions set forth by Langmuir, Grimm, and Erlenmeyer are called classical bioisosteres if biochemical or pharmacological interactions are concerned. Nonclassical bioisosterism [44–46] refers to a more widely applicable set of compounds which cause qualitatively similar agonistic or antagonistic biochemical or pharmacological responses at the molecular level. Hansch recommended for such compounds the term partial bioisosteres but "nonclassical bioisosteres" is used more often.

Bioisosteres are also found abundantly in nature. Many alkaloid-bearing plants contain series of chemically related alkaloids whose individual structures and biological activities overlap or differ only marginally. In animals, the many closely related adrenergic, steroid, thyroid, oxytocic, and other hormonal families can be classified as bioisosteres. Inter-species bioisosteres have also been observed, for example, the insulins isolated from the pancreases of different animals.

1.4.2   Physical properties

With the improvements in many branches of instrumentation, it has become possible to measure physical properties of chemicals which could barely have been attempted a few decades ago. This holds for many analytical methods and particularly for spectroscopic determinations (UV, IR, NMR, mass spectra, Raman spectra, X-ray diffraction spectra) and computational devices, often coupled with spectroscopic methods. The resulting savings in time and effort have made most of these measurements available for routine laboratory work. In another area, chromatographic distribution and separation procedures can be used rapidly by technicians to determine partition coefficients of chemicals between different solvent systems. Largely through the work of Hansch and his school, the lipophilicity, hydrophobicity and hydrophilicity of biologically active substances have been documented extensively [47–50]. The partition coefficients of thousands of substances have been determined conveniently in a 1-octanol – water system [51–53] and have probably become the most widely quoted physical property of biological test substances. They are criteria of the transport of a test compound through body liquids and cell membranes to their receptors, an important aspect of drug action. The value of hydrophobicity in explaining the action of a drug at its receptor is less certain.

Interactions of substrates or drugs at biomacromolecules could be electrostatic, steric (blockade or repulsion), and hydrophobic and dispersive. Since partition coefficients are so easily determined, they can indicate what other compounds with similar numerical values one should choose in planning molecular modifications. Sometimes, agreement between partition coefficients has been calculated only after a series of molecular analogs had been prepared and tested intuitively. In any event, if two compounds exhibit the same degree of hydrophobicity, isosterism could be involved.

Despite all this work, the calculation of *log P* still involves many empirical data and variables. For aromatic compounds, should one use π values from benzene and σ values for regression equations? If benzene and pyridine isosteres are to be compared, the hydrogen-bonding nitrogen of pyridine will have to be incorporated in the equation. Moreover, the *log P* values will differ in their σ values for each of the isomeric positions of the pyridine ring, and thus lead to a large number of variables.

1.4.3   QSAR methods

Quantitative structure-activity relationships (QSAR) try to transform the chemical structure of a compound into quantitative numerical values that describe properties relevant to a given biological activity. Hansch [42] felt that organic formulas are "a terrible hindrance to progress in relating structure to activity" because "there is no dynamic message for those who are interested in rate processes". As pointed out above, the detailed organic reaction scheme of a drug with its receptor – be that the active site of an enzyme, an antibody [54, 55], or a high-molecular weight polynucleotide receptor region – makes good use of organic formulas and conveys to an experienced organic biochemist a set of properties, reaction possibilities, and steric effects that would require extensive correlation of physical data to summarize the same information.

An example of the advantage of emphasizing rate processes over comparisons of structures has been described by Hansch [42]. Two pairs of compounds, *5* and *6*, and *7* and *8*, respectively, increase the membrane potential of the mollusc basal ganglion by 20 mV [56]. In spite of irreconcilable differences in structure, identical concentrations (log 1/C; C is the molar concentration causing the 20 mV increase in membrane

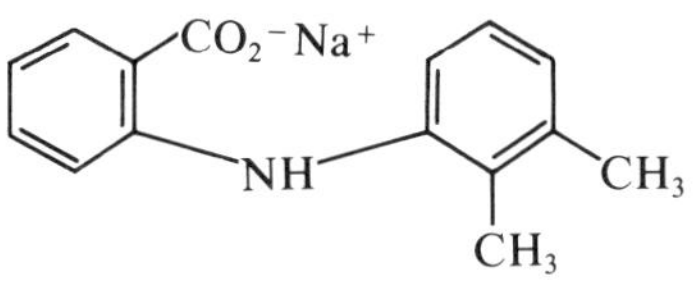

5

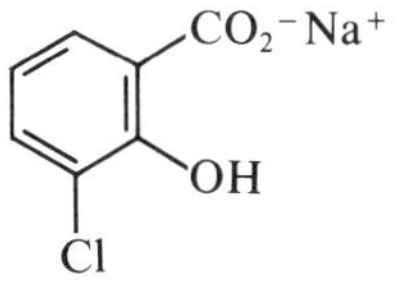

log 1/C	3.48
log P	0.28

6

3.48
0.23

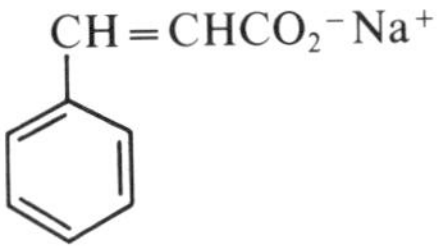

7

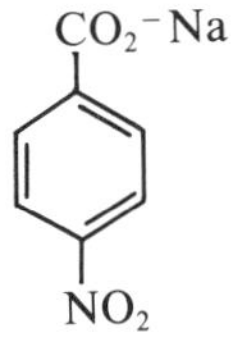

log 1/C	1.48
log P	−2.23

8

1.48
−2.21

potential) for pair *5–6*, and the pair *7–8* produce identical biological responses in the test system, that is, they are isosteric on the basis of Hansch's definition.

The SAR is shown in equation (1):

$$\log 1/C = 0.839\,(\pm 0.07)\,\log \text{P-ion} + 3.308\,(\pm 0.10)\quad \begin{array}{ccc} n & r & s \\ 30 & 0.979 & 0.177 \end{array}\quad (1)$$

where P-ion is the 1-octanol/water partition coefficient of the sodium salts *5* to *8*, n is the number of measured data points, r is the correlation coefficient, and s is the standard deviation. Figures in parentheses are the 95 % confidence intervals; the slope of near 1 may be expected for membrane perturbation [49]. But although the pairs have the same log P, to be sure, this was discovered by screening various test compounds, and not by prediction based on these calculations [56]. This does not mean that once the predictive value of a partition coefficient has been confirmed that this measurement should not be used in every other case to support and explain biological evaluation. Another illustration of the Hansch equation is a variation of a simple substituent, such as a group on an aromatic ring. This substituent will have several parameters, leading to equation (2) where *C* again is the concentration of the compound

$$\log (1/C) = X(\pi) + Y(\sigma) + Z(E_s) \qquad (2)$$

needed for a given biological effect; π is Hansch's partition coefficient from which the lipophilic character can be determined; σ is Hammett's value for the electronic property of the substituent; and E_s is Taft's steric parameter which indicates the size of the substituent.

If Y and Z are zero for a given structural series, then the potency would be a function of π only, and the old and new substituent on the ring would be truly bioisosteric. If these substituents are structurally unimportant, even a significant numerical size of X, Y, and Z will not affect selective activity too much. If the values for σ, E_s, hydrogen bonding, pK_a and other measurable parameters are taken into account, then structural groups with analogous π values could be called isolipophilic [42].

Tables of σ, π, and E_s values have been published by Topliss [57] and Hansch and his associates [58, 59].

The interpretation of quantitative numerical data to express biological activity will be colored by the principal inclination of the investigating scientists. Physical and physical-organic chemists will approach the problem by studying physical measurements of the chemicals involved and arranging them in summarizing equations. Organic and especially medicinal chemists who think in terms of reaction mechanisms, likely transformations, and also the biological potential of their compounds will try to make generalizations that reflect their main expertise. This may explain the approach taken by James W. Wilson, a medicinal organic chemist, in collaboration with S. M. Free, a biostatistician. The Free-Wilson method [60] has the advantage that one does not need physicochemical measurements of the compounds, but of course one can therefore not make predictions based on such properties. The procedure assumes that introducing a given substituent at a particular position of the molecule always produces a quantitatively similar effect on the biological potency of the rest of the molecule [61]. In equation (3), i is the number of the position of substitution, j is the number of the substituent

$$\log (1/C) = x + \overset{m,\,n}{\Sigma} a_{ij} G_{ij} \tag{3}$$

at that position, m is the total number of substituted positions, and n is the number of substituents. The value a_{ij} represents the presence (1.0) or absence (0.0) of the substituent ij. The values G_{ij} are group contributions; they are obtained by multiple regression analysis. Examples may be found in a monograph by Yvonne Martin [62] and a review by Kubinyi [63].

The proposal that there is a skeletal center of a molecule (a pharmaco-phore) equipped with substituents and that these substituents make additive quantitative contributions to the biological activity has been in the minds of medicinal chemists for a long time. Indeed, it can be read into the 1868 statement by Crum Brown and Frazer [64] that the physiological activity of a compound is a function of its chemical structure. Later, Meyer [65], Overton [66] and others suggested that partition coefficients, solubility data, the vapor pressure and other physical properties had an effect on toxicity, narcotic, microbicidal and hemolytic activities. They thought first of general anesthetics such as ether and chloroform whose action must be based on their partition coefficients between blood (i.e. water) and nervous tissue lipids. Even the element xenon is a safe and potent clinical anesthetic, and since it is chemically inert these actions must be related to its par-tition coefficient.

Bruice et al. [67] correlated the thyromimetic activity of 47 analogs *(9)* of thyroxine with their sustituent constants *f* of R, R′, X and Y which

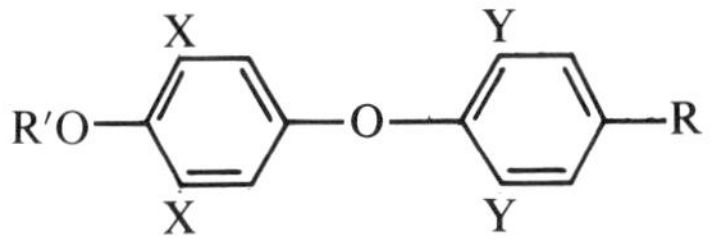

9

were derived from Hammett σ constants. The correlation was ex-pressed by equation (4). Other examples can be found in reference [63].

$$\text{log of \% of thyromimetic activity} = k.\Sigma f + c \qquad (4)$$

A simplification of the Free-Wilson equation was proposed by Fujita and Ban [68]. Many investigators now combine their modified Free-Wilson method with the extrathermodynamic approach by Hansch to arrive at mathematical formulations of QSAR. These ideas and other developments leading up to present-day usage have been summarized by Tute [69].

No attempt will be made here to describe all aspects of QSAR, its suc-cesses and failures. The goal of QSAR studies is to delineate more pre-cisely the reasons for the equivalence or nonequivalence of biological activity than is possible by intuitive experience. This can decrease the average number of analogs one may have to test by 2.5–3-fold during the inevitable process of molecular fine-tuning. Since the concept of bioisosterism relies so heavily on SAR, quantitation of SAR inevitably must sharpen up our view of bioisosteres.

Additional understanding of bioisosterism can be gained by the emerging application of X-ray diffractometry to the identification of hydrophobic regions of a drug molecule, especially in the process of binding to a macromolecular site. This can involve the measurement of likely hydrogen bonds and the adaptation of a sterically flexible molecule to a sterically compatible macromolecule. If one remembers the postulate that similar shape is a precondition of isosterism, any change in the shapes of molecules participating in mutual recognition, attraction and ligating can modify our concept of bioisosterism. Uncertainty about molecular conformation impairs the predictability of potency of a drug but could be removed by X-ray diffraction studies. It is not surprising that the most successful mapping of drug-receptor interactions, and hence a better understanding of the biological activity of a drug, has been achieved in series of relatively rigid drug molecules [70–72]. NMR spectroscopy can complement X-ray diffraction to reveal conformational changes of substrate and receptor protein during ligating processes in solution.

1.4.4   Stereochemical differences

The effect of steric differences is seen most clearly in stereoisomers. They may differ quantitatively in biological activity, occasionally also qualitatively. This includes rigid geometric and also chiral RS-isomers. Since in such pairs even antagonism has been observed occasionally, recommendations have been adopted that at least future drugs that can exist as optical isomers will have to be resolved and administered to the patient in a single steric conformation.

Non-chiral flexible compounds such as acetylcholine can assume a preferred and essential conformation during complexation with muscarinic receptors. In the case of L(−)threo-chloramphenicol (10) NMR coupling constants indicate that the hydrogen atoms of the alcoholic hydroxyls are in the gauche position. Apparently, there is hydrogen bonding between these groups. This conformation corresponds to that of uridine 5'-phosphate (11) in size, orientation of the hydroxyl groups, and distribution of negative charges.

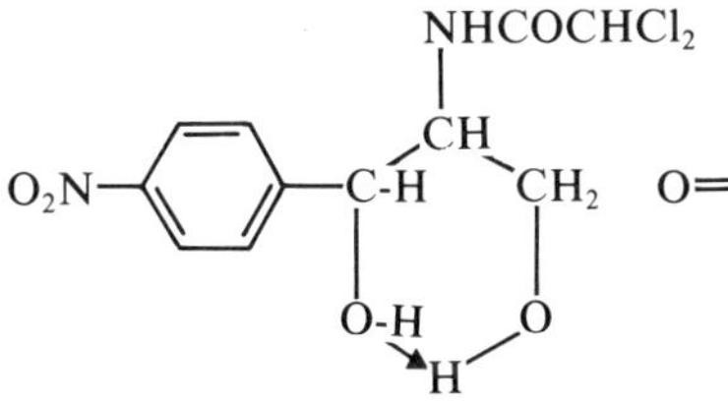

10 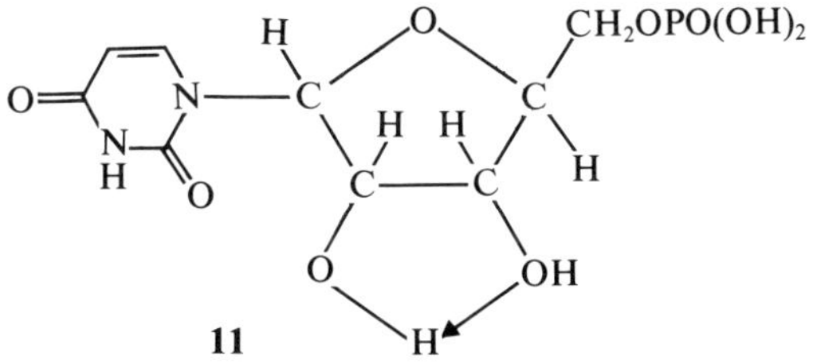   **11**

In bioisosteres, compounds with the same absolute configuration or with steric relationships are compared most meaningfully. The importance of a uniform test method for compounds of divergent structure and steric arrangements is illustrated in *12–16* [73]. All these substances, clonidine *(12)*, lofexidine *(13)*, guanabenz *(14)*, lidamidine *(15)*, and rolgamidine *(16)*, are potent antidiarrheal drugs when administered subcutaneously. Both inhibition of the propulsive activity of the gut, and of hypersecretion play a role in their action, the latter being mediated by an adrenergic α_2-agonist mechanism. There is a formal chemical relationship between *12*, *13*, and *14*, and also between *15* and *16*. The best separation of the two antidiarrheal mechanisms was achieved in *17*, a bioisostere of *14* with an α_2-agonist activity, by introducing a phenolic hydroxyl group.

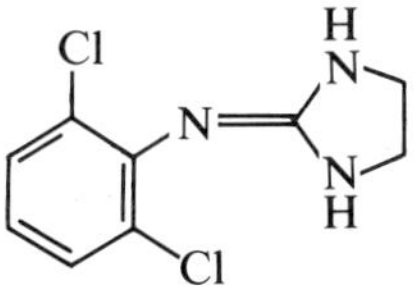

12 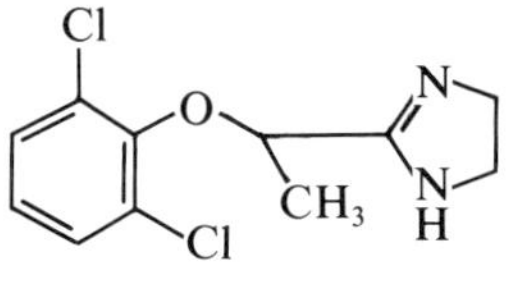   **13** 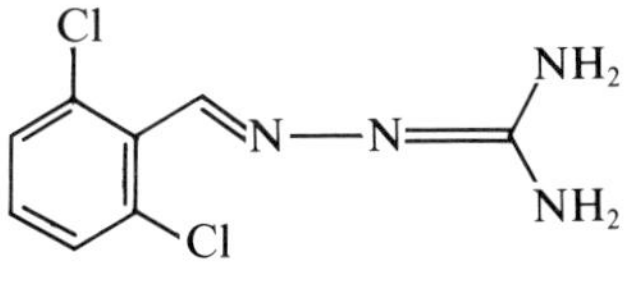   **14**

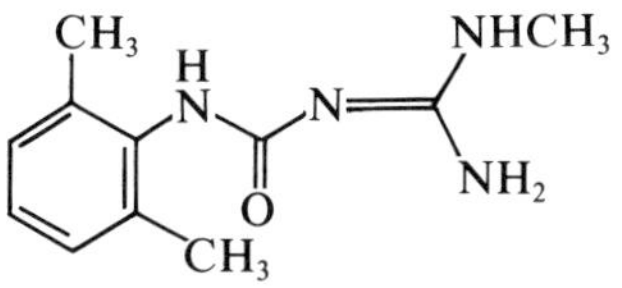

15 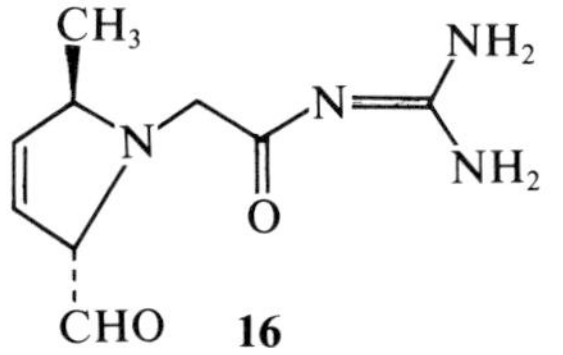   **16** 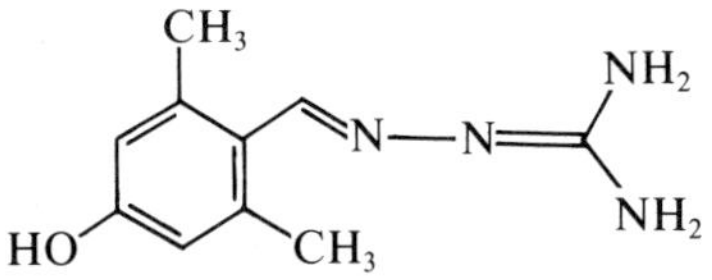   **17**

1.5   Examples of classical bioisosteres

Many examples of bioisosterism from the early chemical and pharmacological literature suffer from a lack of measurements of the biological activity of the reported compounds. Terms such as "similarity of activity", or "both compounds possess a given activity" would no longer be adequate for meaningful comparisons. Methods for quantitative biological evaluations developed slowly over the years, and biochemical comparisons lagged behind even further. One must commend the pharmaceutical industry for creating so many useful drugs during those days.

Classical bioisosterism is seen in aminopyrine and its analog *18* in which -$CH_2CH(CH_3)_2$ replaces -$CH_2N(CH_3)_2$ to give great similarity of antipyretic action and toxicity. The isopropyl derivative *18* was potent enough to be tested clinically for a short while [30, 31, 33, 74, 75].

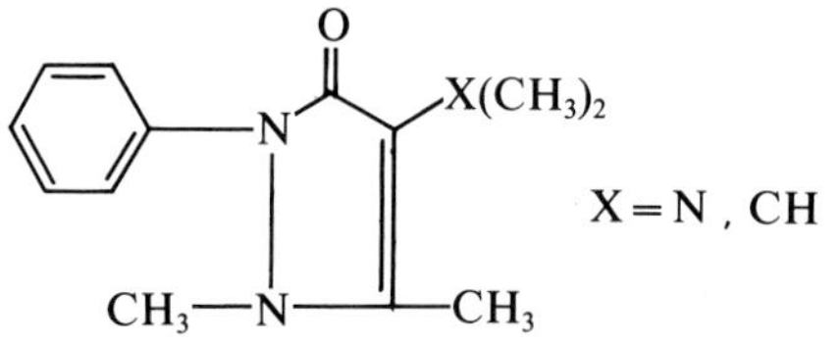

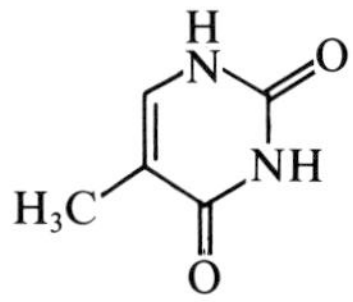

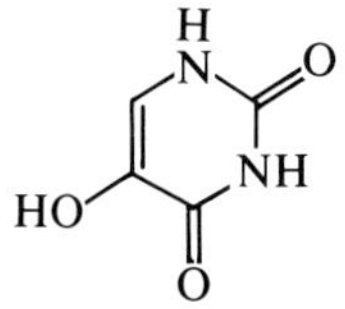

Replacement of OH by CH_3 or vice versa was seen in nicotinic acid (niacin) whose action is antagonized by 3-acetylpyridine [76]. The same relationship holds for thymine *(19)* (-CH_3) and isobarbituric acid *(20)* (-OH) [77]. Another comparison was made with indole-3- *(21)* and naphthalene-1-acetic and -acrylic acids *(22)* which exhibit similar heteroauxin properties but are antagonistic to tryptophan [78].

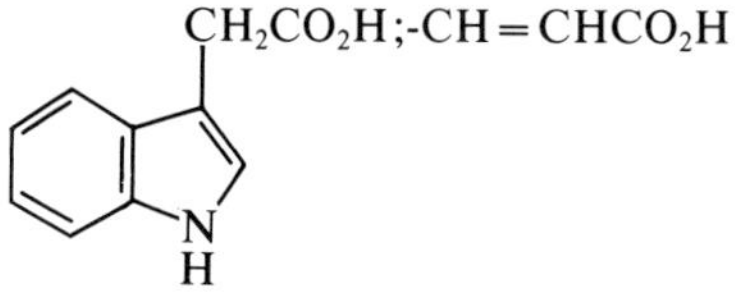

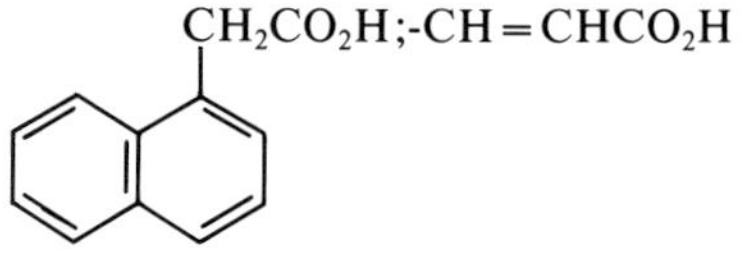

Amino alcohols derived from 5-methylacridine *(23)* and from phenanthrene *(24)* are low-grade experimental analgesics (79). 6-Aminonicotinic acid and *p*-aminobenzoic acid (-N= → -CH=) exhibit a similar antagonism to sulfanilamide [80], and adenine and aminobenz-imidazole *(25)* are also antagonists in some test systems [74]. The same type of bioisosterism is found in the pair, guanine, and 5-amino-7-oxo-1-v-triazolo(d)pyrimidine *(26)* which are antagonists [81], and in thiamine *(27)* and the antagonistic oxythiamine *(28)* [82].

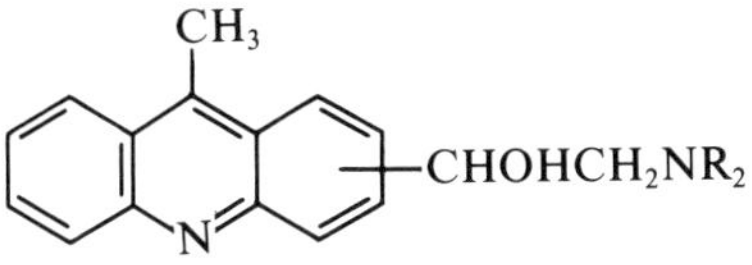

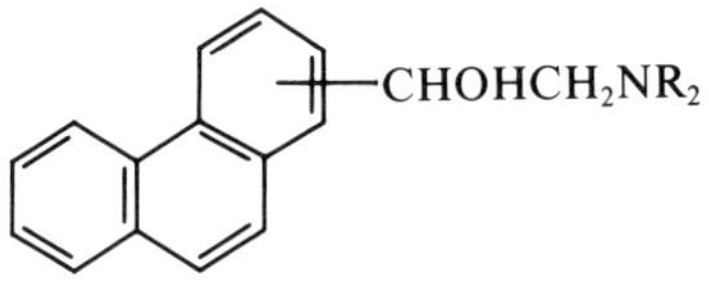

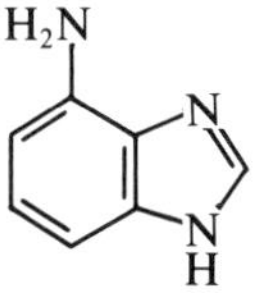

An ether oxygen → imino analogy lead to greatly diminished hemor-rhagic activity in the quinolone analog *30* of dicumarol *(29)* [83, 84]. Furan analogues of benzenoid compounds were studied [85] to illus-

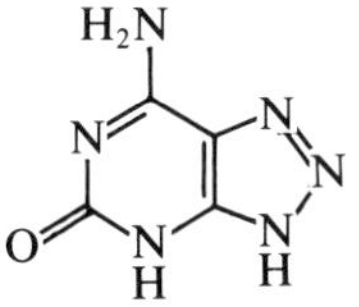

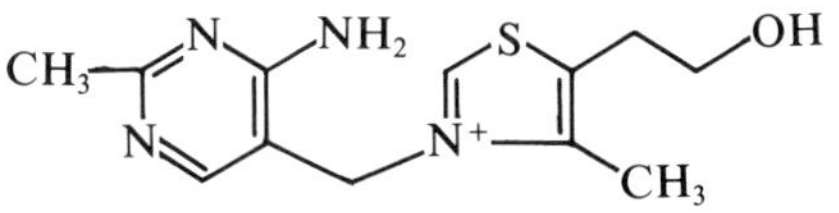

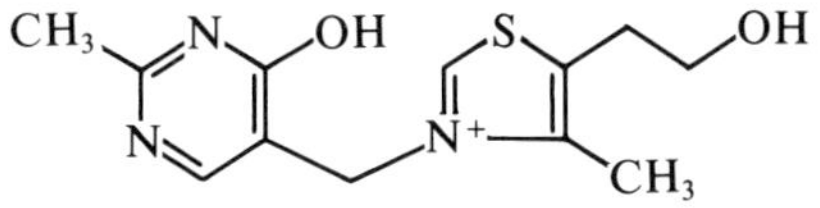

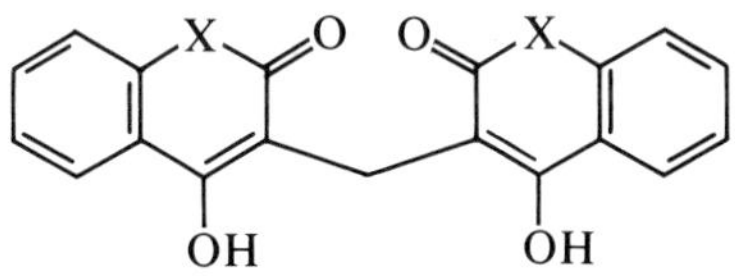

$$X = O: 29$$
$$X = NH: 30$$

trate -O- versus -CH=CH- isosterism. The pairs phenethylamine – 2-furylethylamine; N-methylaniline – 2-furyl-N-methylamine; and 2-methylamino-3-phenylpropanol – 2-methylamino-3-(2-furyl)propa-nol exhibited the same relative effect on the blood pressure. Cincho-phen *(31)* and 2-(2-furyl)-4-carboxyquinoline *(32)* behaved similarly in tests for analgesia and antipyresis and cocaine *(33)* and its furan an-alogue *34* acted similar in local anesthetic tests.

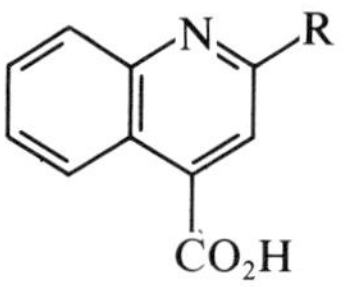

R = C₆H₅: **31**

R = 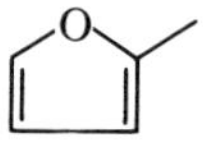 : **32**

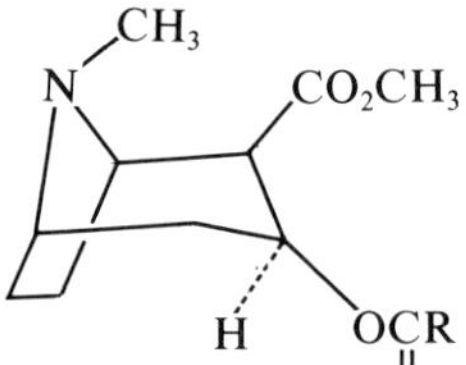

33: R = C₆H₅

34: R =

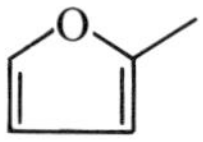

Local anesthetic tests were also compared for diethylaminoethyl esters of aromatic acids such as *p*-aminobenzoic acid and 2-furanoic acid, as well as 2-furylacrylic acid [86] because vinylogous conjugation of the carboxyl with an ethylenic or acetylenic linkage often increased local anesthetic potency [87]. All these analogies suggest the similarity of chemical and physical properties of true aromatic and pseudoaromatic systems. In their effect upon local anesthetic activity, the relative contribution of various nuclei appear to be as follows: $C_6H_5 >$ 2-pyrrolyl $>$ 2-thienyl $>$ 2-furyl, but there are exceptions to this sequence depending on the character of the acid and the tertiary amino group.

The most popular bioisostere of the phenyl group has been the thienyl radical, usually but not necessarily the 2-thienyl group because of the availability of thiophene-2-derivatives. 2-(2-Thienyl)-4-carboxyquinoline *(35)*, the thiophene isostere of cinchophen *(31)*, has similar analgesic and antiphlogistic properties [88] as *31* but it dyes the tissues of laboratory animals a deep purple. The thiophene bioisostere *36* of cocaine *(33)*, called an isologue by the authors [40], showed the same potent local anesthetic activity as cocaine in the rabbit eye test; the thio-

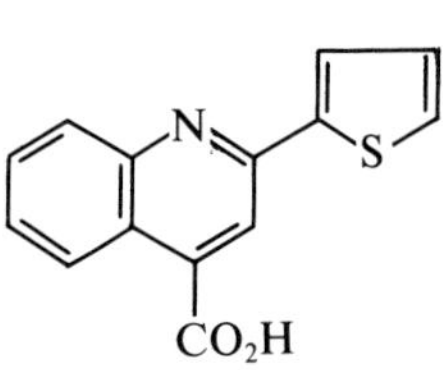

35

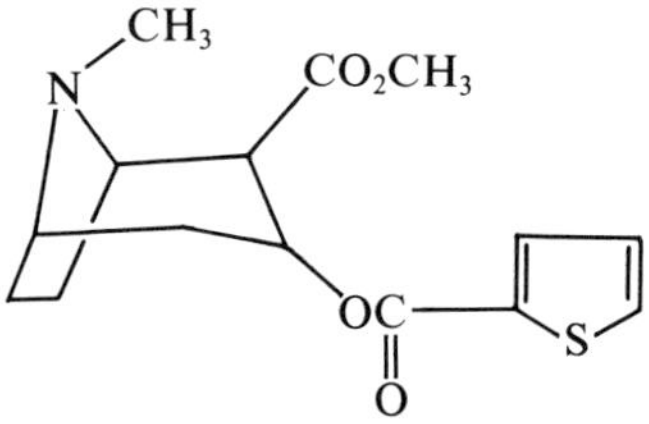

36

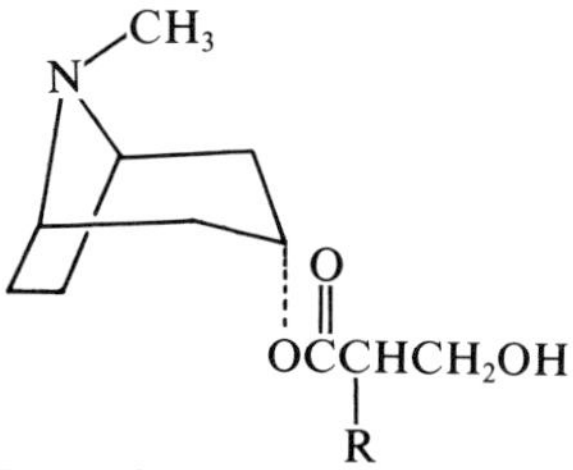

37: R = C₆H₅

38: R =

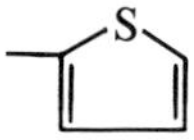

phene isostere *38* of atropine *(37)* was not tested biologically for lack of material [89]. Eucaine A and its thienyl bioisostere also behaved similarly [90]. By contrast, phenylalanine and 2-thienylalanine were antagonists in promoting the growth of yeast [91].

Diphenyliodonium sulfate *(38a)* inhibits the macrophage and endothelial cell nitric oxide synthase, and so does its di-2-thienyl bioisostere *38b* [91a].

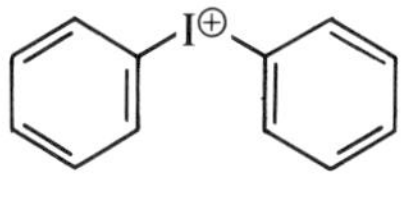

38 a 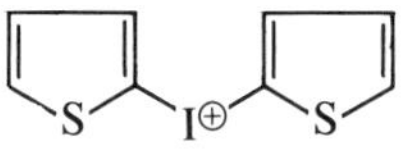   38 b

Of the many other thiophene analogues of phenyl-containing prototypes, a few are listed in Table II. Their biological action has been reported only as "similar".

Table II
Some classical thiophene isosteres with "similar" biological activities

Benzene isostere	Thiophene isostere	References
p-Aminobenzanilide	*p*-Amino-2-thenoylanilide	[30–32]
Benzoic Acid	Thiophene-2-carboxylic acid	[92, 93]
Amylocaine	Thiophene isostere	[90]
Phenacetin	Thiophene isostere	[90]
O-Benzoylquinine	O-(2-Thenoyl)quinine	[90]
Hippuric acid	2-Thenoylglycine	[93]
N-Ethylaniline	N-Ethyl-(2-thienyl)amine	[94]

The electronic aspect of benzene-thiophene isosterism is not restricted to medicinal chemistry. In nonlinear optical properties which are used in computer data storage and communication systems based on light instead of electricity, hyperpolarizability can be manipulated to increase the frequency of an infrared laser. The second hyperpolarizability, γ, involves interactions of these photons in materials. Fused ring structures such as the benzothiazole *39* in which Ar is phenyl in-

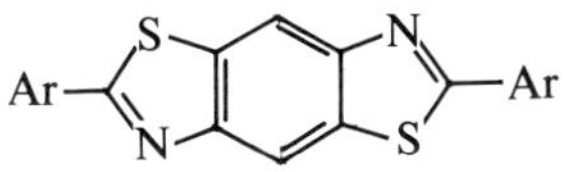

39: Ar = C_6H_5

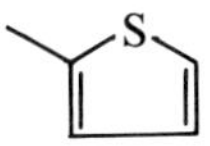

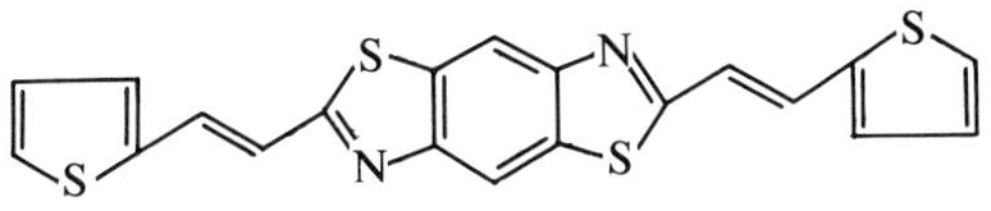

40

crease delocalizable π electrons. Exchange of phenyl for 2-thienyl further increases effective conjugation and electron density. Insertion of double bonds between the thiophene rings *(40)* and the central system further raises the number of conjugated π electrons [95].

Another series of classical bioisosteres involving the replacement of -CH=CH- by sulfur is found in the comparison of pyridine and thiazole. This has furnished a number of instructive examples as well as useful drugs. The synthesis of sulfathiazole *(41)*, a potent and well-tolerated antibacterial agent, was undertaken to improve upon the effective but much more toxic sulfapyridine *42* [96].

Table III
Some classical thiazole bioisosteres of pyridine derivatives

Sulfapyridine *(42)* 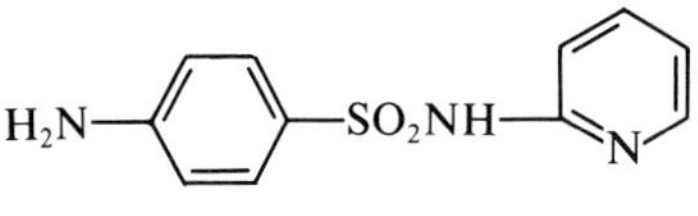	Sulfathiazole *(41)* 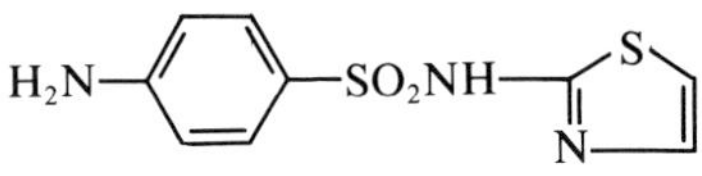	[96] Bacteriostatic

Nicotinamide (niacinamide)	Thiazole-4-carboxamide	[97]

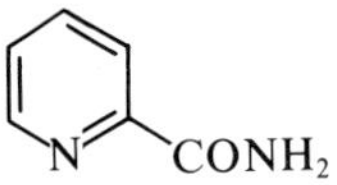

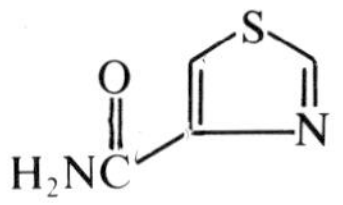

α-Picolinic acid	Thiazole-4-carboxylic acid	0.1 % activity [98]
Nikethamide 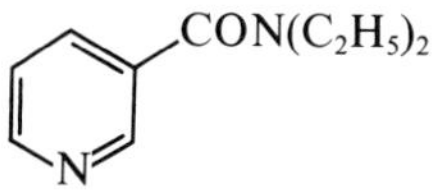	Thiazole-4-(N,N-diethyl)carbox-amide 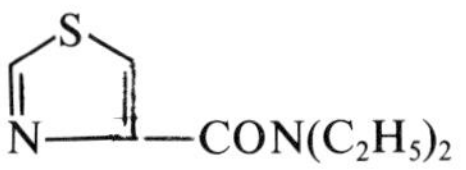	[99] Analeptic

Neopyrithiamine *(43)* 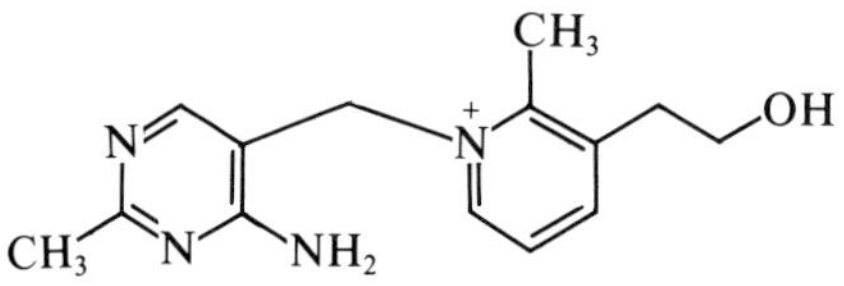	Thiamine *(27)* 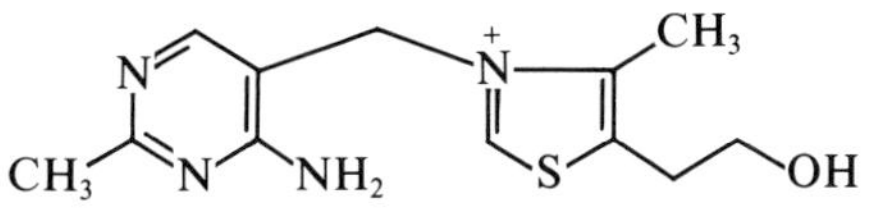	Antagonistic in several bacterial growth systems [98, 100–102]

Sulfur has also been regarded as a nonclassical isostere of the group, -CH$_2$-CH$_2$- (see Table IV).

Table IV
Bioisosteres in which sulfur replaces -CH$_2$CH$_2$-

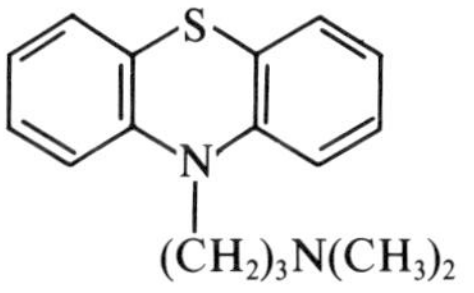	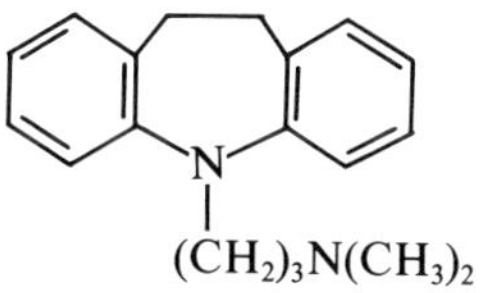	Analogous activity in several tests [103, 104]

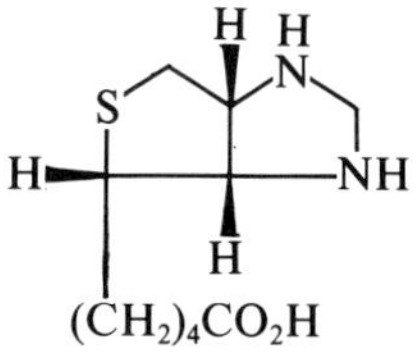

Promazine *(44)*   Imipramine *(45)*

Biotin *(46)*   Cyclohexane Analogue *(47)*   Antagonistic [105]

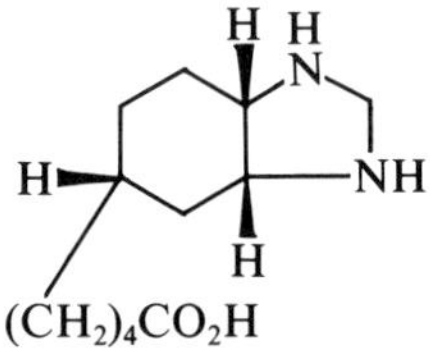

(CH$_2$)$_3$N(CH$_3$)$_2$ (CH$_2$)$_3$N(CH$_3$)$_2$

(CH$_2$)$_4$CO$_2$H   (CH$_2$)$_4$CO$_2$H

1.5.1   Bioisosterism involving O, NH, CH$_2$, S

Steric factors account for many of the differences and analogies when oxygen, sulfur, imino and methylene replace each other. The valence angles of these atoms and groups are similar, at least in uncrowded aliphatic compounds, in ether, secondary amine, hydrocarbon and dialkyl sulfide linkages. They are approximately $108° \pm 3°$ for -O-; $112° \pm 2°$ for -S-; and $111.5° \pm 3°$ for -CH$_2$- [106]. Ruling out connections of these atoms and groups to hydrogen (-OH, -SH, -NH$_2$, -CH$_3$), all other groups to which they are linked are larger and provide more shielding from other molecules which would compete for reactive sites. This effect, usually perceived as a means of preventing the approach of a damaging pathogen such as histamine or excessive concentrations of a neurohormone (e. g. epinephrine or acetylcholine) to an active site of an involved enzyme or receptor is seen in the structures of antihistaminics (histamine H$_1$ antagonists) *48* and *49* in which X can be any of the trivalent groups, -N<, -CH<, or -C=. Antihistaminic or anti-neurohormone activity can be fine-tuned by further bioisosteric variation of the Ar or ArCH$_2$ substituents such as C$_6$H$_5$,

$C_6H_5CH_2$, $C_6H_5CH(CH_3)$, pyridyl or other heterocyclic groups. Many of the classical blocking agents (H_1 receptor antagonists, and anticholinergics including blocking sedatives and anti-motion sickness drugs) have been conceived on this basis [107–109].

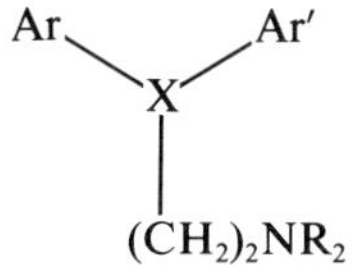

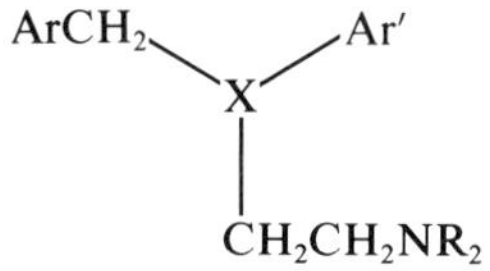

The two bulky blocking groups can be tied together by oxygen, sulfur, nitrogen, or carbon atoms or bridges. In such derivatives,

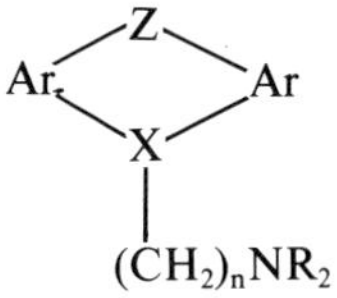

$Z = O$, S, NH, NR, CH_2, $CH=CH$ (classical sulfur isostere), CH_2CH_2, CH_2S, CH_2O, CH_2-NH etc.

CNS depressant activities become more pronounced. Promazine *(44)* derivatives with more or less electronegative ring substituents ($Y = Cl$: chlorpromazine; $Y = CF_3$: triflupromazine; $Y = SO_2CH_3$ with side chain

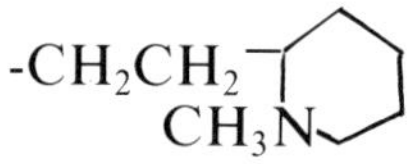

(sulforidazine)

are neuroleptics, while the bioisosteric drugs, imipramine *(45)* and amitriptyline *(50)* and many of their analogues are antidepressants. This transition to antidepressant properties has been attributed to the steric effect of the central seven-membered ring which tilts the two aromatic rings out of a planar conformation.

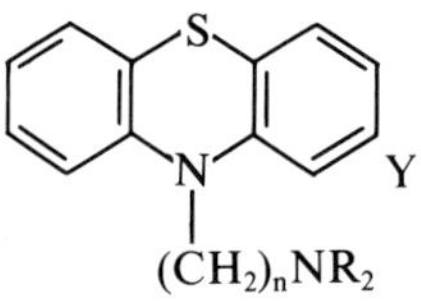

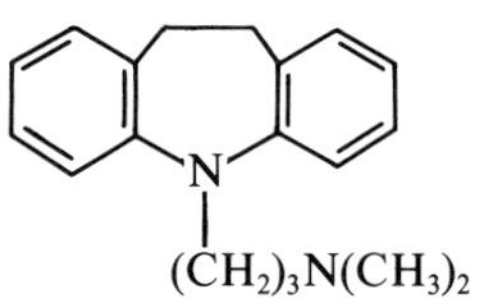

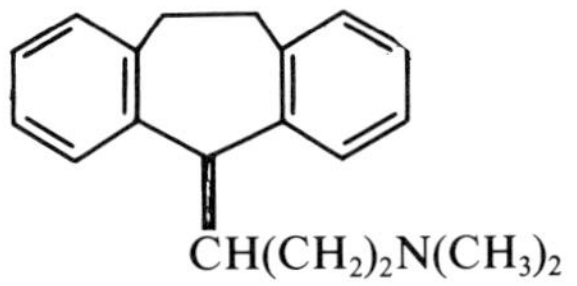

If the basic side chain of these compounds incorporates a dialkylaminoalkyl ester grouping such as $-CO_2(CH_2)_2NR_2$, the structures acquire more affinity to the receptor of the neurohormone, acetylcholine [$CH_3CO_2CH_2CH_2N^+(CH_3)_3$] and become candidates for anticholinergic (antispasmodic) properties. Again, the two blocking moieties may be separate as in adiphenine, *51*, or joined by a linkage as in carbofluorene aminoester, *52*, or by a heteroatom as in propantheline *(53)*.

In the design of basic derivatives of diphenylmethane, phenothiazine, dibenz[b,f]azepine, dibenzo[a,d]cycloheptene, fluorene, xanthene and similar systems, bioisosterism has played an initial important role to choose overall principles of structures that would furnish blocking compounds. The sheer number of hundreds of such compounds indicates that bioisosteric thinking takes a backseat to intuitive trials at molecular modification, and to the immense patience required to cull out a pharmacologically and toxicologically appropriate member of these series for therapeutic purposes.

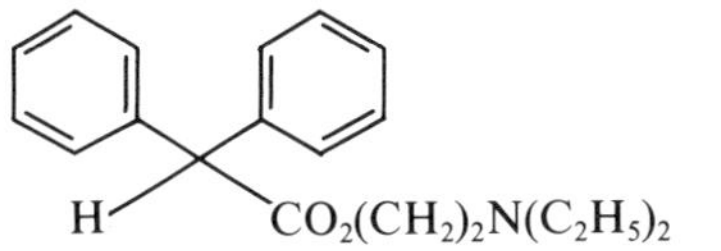

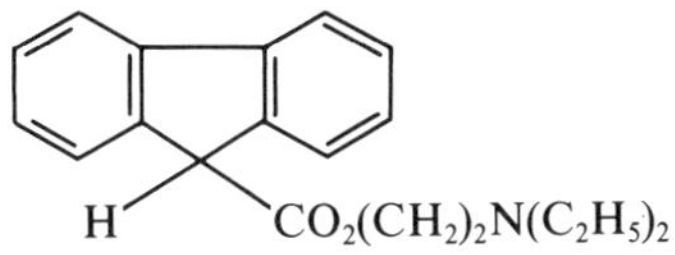

None of the antihistaminic H_1 receptor antagonists inhibited HCl secretion by the mast cells of the stomach which contributes to stomach and duodenal ulcers. Chemically, the antiallergic antihistaminics possessed blocking structures [48, 49] and not one of them resembled histamine or contained an imidazole moiety. When bioisosterism was invoked for imidazole derivatives, slow molecular modification of this heterocycle and opportunistic attachment of functional side chains laboriously led to the first H_2 receptor antagonists which are useful as antisecretory and antiulcer agents. The elegant story of the role of isosterism in elaborating their side chain will be detailed later, and so will the belated finding that the sacrosanct imidazole was finally not essential for high and useful activity.

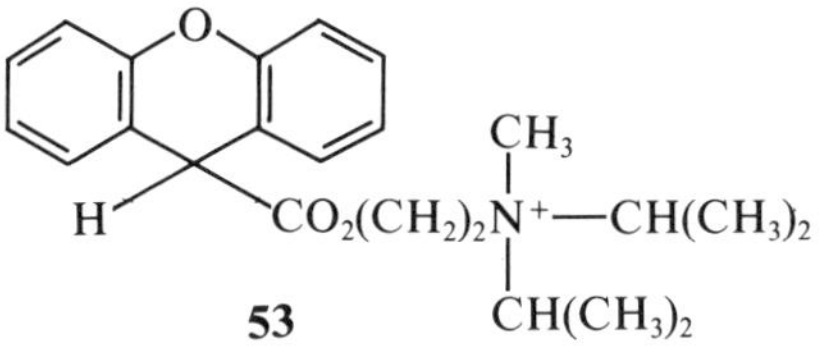

1.5.2   Esters, ketones, thioloesters, amides and thioamides

Bioisosterism in esters, ketones, amides (-COOR, -CO-R, -CONH-R), their sulfur analogues, and compounds containing reversed ester and amide groups (-OCOR, -NHCOR) has been observed in local anesthetics [ArCOO(CH$_2$)$_n$NR$_2$; ArCOS(CH$_2$)$_n$NR$_2$] and blocking agents such as anticholinergics [Ar$_2$CHCO-X-(CH$_2$)$_n$NR$_2$; X = O, S, NH]. Amide-type agents are often inferior to esters, but thioloesters (X = S) may be more potent, depending on the pharmacological test method used [110–112]. Decreased resistance to hydrolysis by unspecific esterases may cloud the evaluation of these results. More important are differences between barbiturates (54), thiobarbiturates (55), iminobarbiturates (56), and related ring systems which contain urea or thiourea

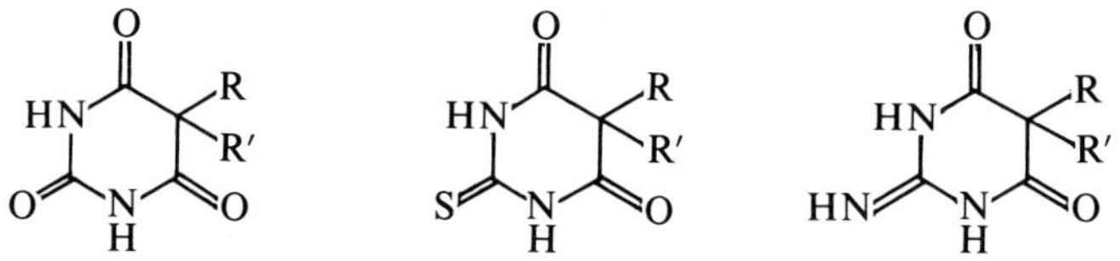

groupings. The thiourea-type compounds are often short-acting but more potent hypnotics and general anesthetics [113–115]. In H$_2$-receptor antagonists [116] containing thiourea moieties, the thiourea sulfur atom cannot be replaced by =NH, because the resulting guanidine derivatives are too basic to be bioisosteric with the thiourea derivatives. Activity returns readily if the basicity caused by the NH= analogues is weakened by electron-withdrawing groups, for instance, =NCN or =NNO$_2$ [117, 118]. Iminobarbiturates [58] corresponding to thiobarbiturates are similarly related; they were inactive [119], perhaps for the same reason, and moreover, they are too easily hydrolyzed.

Any biological differences of ester-type compounds in which the single-bonded oxygen atoms in R-O-R' or R-C(=O)-O-R' are replaced by -S- or -NH- may well be due to hydrolytic effects caused by the more polar properties of sulfur and imino linkages. Replacement of ester oxygens by methylene [R(C=O)OR'...R(C=O)CH$_2$R'] gives rise to ketones which are isosteric with esters in the classical sense. For instance, the propyl ketone 57 corresponding to meperidine (58) has about the same analgesic activity as the ethyl ester (58) drug [120].

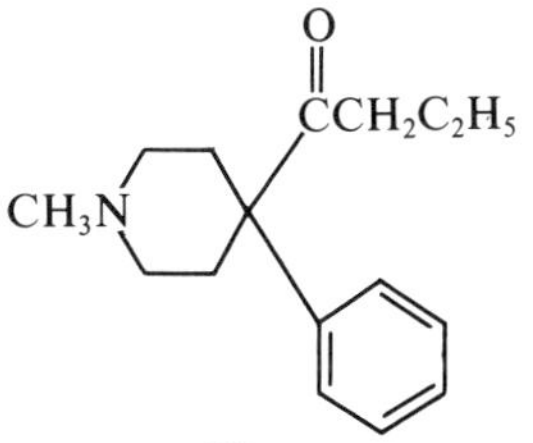

Extension of this ketone to branched and cyclic homologs weakens the analgesic properties but does not abolish it.

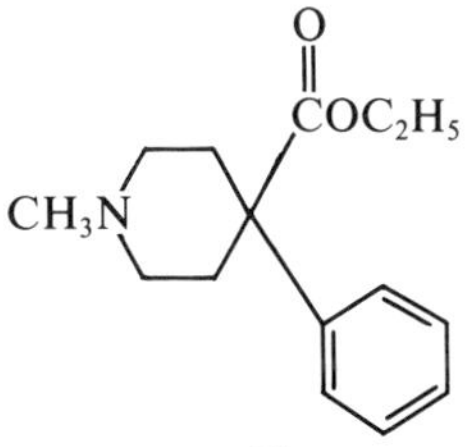

1.6   Transition from classical to nonclassical bioisosteres

One of the most disappointing aspects of even the time-honored methods as we see them in Grimm's hydride displacement rules [6–8] is the finding that instead of an analogue with similar biological activity, one has created an antagonist to one's prototype. Even in the simplest case of bioisosterism, that of Na^+ and K^+, one encounters biological antagonism. The explanation that the new compound has at least *some* effect on a given biological behavior provides little comfort for additional rational plans in molecular modification. To the medicinal chemist, the finding of antagonistic properties must await quantitative biological test results and forces him to start all over in his SAR projections. Of course, measurements of several physical properties can precede biological testing and permit some evaluation of probable bio-properties before such tests are performed. The almost universal observation of side effects in biological tests only confirms the need for animal experiments and the failure of even the most carefully planned mathematical calculations to meet the complexity of living, biosynthesizing and biodegrading animals.

Among steroidal hormones, minor structural alterations can produce a range of overlapping, agonistic, antagonistic or widely different biological consequences. Androgens never have an aromatic A-ring, estrogens always do, but otherwise their structures are not so different. Some of the cortical hormones exhibit some major or minor sex hormone activities, and androgens have long been subdivided into anabolic and non-anabolic types. Substitution of hydrogen by fluorine [121] or oxidation of secondary alcohol groups to carbonyl enhances some hormonal activities and suppresses others. Elimination of angular methyl groups and substitution by acetylenic groups at C-17 can change one hormonal activity into another (estrogen to progestational etc.). Most of these compounds are not isomers; should at least some of these structurally overall similar agents many of which act at related receptors be called bioisosteres? Such a claim would have to be supported by studies of the lipophilicity and other physical properties of paired series of steroid hormones.

1.6.1   Isosteric halogens

Fluorine differs from the other halogens by its smaller size which leans more towards the volume of hydrogen, and by its stable shorter bond to carbon. These properties have been taken advantage of in 9α-(or 12α)-fluorocortisols *(59)* which are several times as active in many respects as the parent hormones [121], but other modifications such as the introduction of methoxyl lead to the same results; yet fluorine and methoxy are not isosteric in the classical sense. The firm bond between fluorine and carbon also favors stability in trifluoromethyl compounds. Thus trifluoperazine *(60)* is a more potent neuroleptic than prochlorperazine *(61)* but the more pronounced electronegative

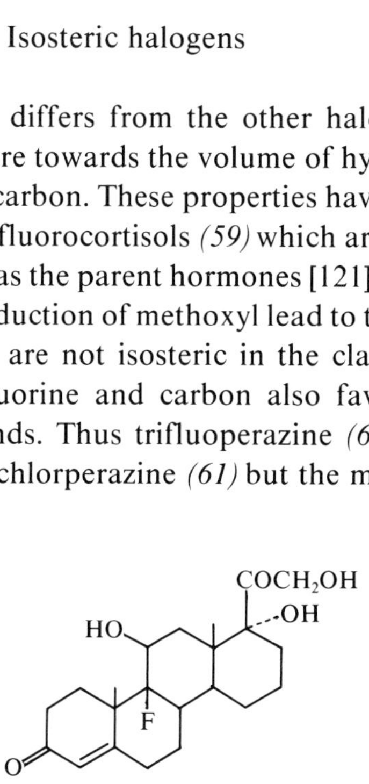

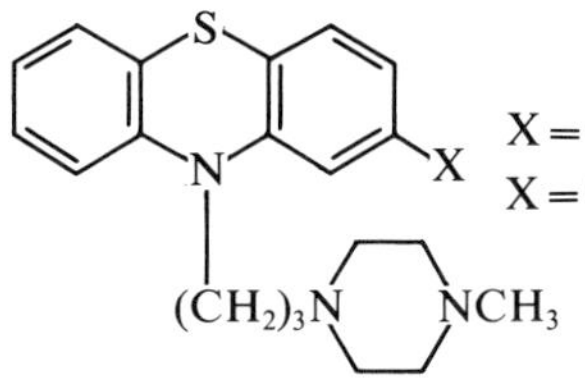

character of trifluoromethyl probably accounts principally for this difference. Other highly electronegative groups (NO_2, SO_2CH_3) share this tendency, while electron-donating groups such as methyl are dystherapeutic. In many cases CF_3 substitution yields compounds that are less toxic than compounds with other electronegative substituents, and this has influenced the choice of test drugs to be prepared.

The trifluoromethyl group has played a role in molecular modification of quinine analogs. The antimalarial alkaloid, quinine, is deactivated by metabolic oxidation at position 2 of the quinoline ring.

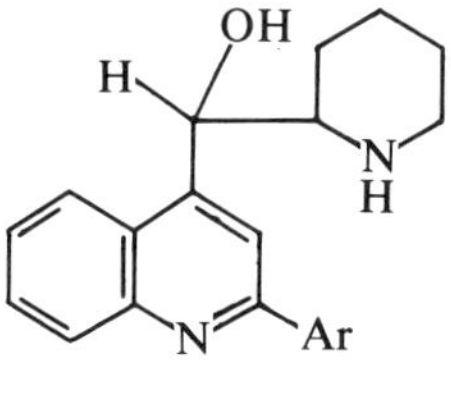

62 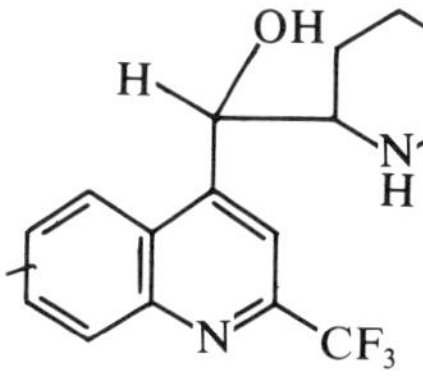   63 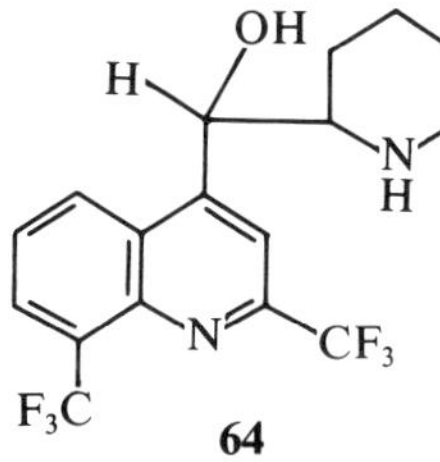   64

Blockade of this position by a variety of aromatic groups *(62)* regularly caused phototoxicity in the resulting derivatives and their analogues with a stripped-down piperidine ring [122]. It appeared possible that aryl substitution should be avoided and replaced by substitution with some other electron-rich but less conjugated structurally unrelated group. Trifluoromethyl was chosen as a test case *(63)* [123]. Although phototoxicity encountered in *62* was not eliminated completely, further substitution with CF_3 was undertaken because 3,6-bis(trifluoromethyl) substituted phenanthrene amino alcohols had shown a considerable increase in antimalarial activity over monotrifluoromethyl derivatives [124]. Empirical substitution in all benzenoid positions of the quinoline ring yielded the 2,8-bis (trifluoromethyl)quinoline piperidyl alcohol *64* (mefloquine) which has become an important antimalarial drug [125].

The relationship of fluorine, hydrogen, and other halogens is illustrated in a series of analogues of the contact insecticide, chlorophenothane (DDT) *(65)* in which the five chlorine atoms were systematically

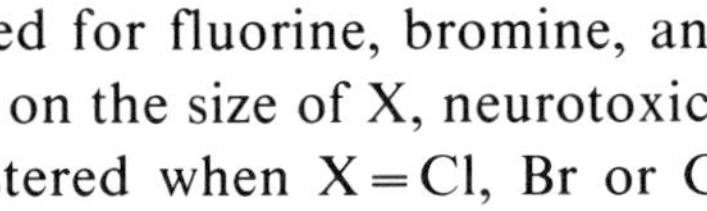

65
X = Y = Cl

exchanged for fluorine, bromine, and methyl. Here activity usually depends on the size of X, neurotoxic contact insecticidal activity being registered when $X = Cl$, Br or CH_3 with $Y = Cl$. No activity is found if $X = F$ or H, but if $Y = F$ and $X = Cl$, activity is comparable to $Y = Cl$ or Br. However, if $Y = F$ and $X = CH_3$, activity is lost [126], even though chlorine and methyl occupy comparable volumes [127]. This prediction is, however, confirmed in the bis(*p*-chlorophenyl)-*t*-bu-

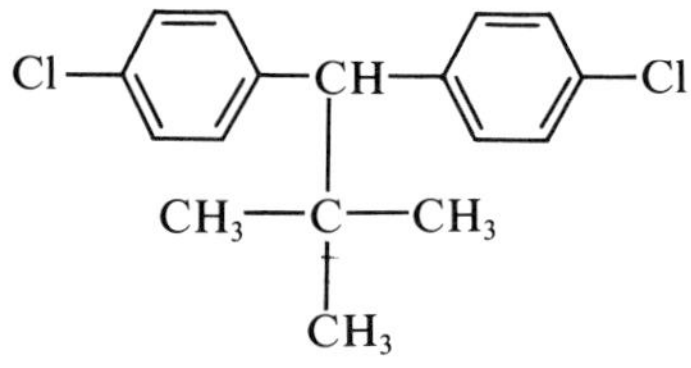

66

tylmethane analogue *66* which is as neurotoxic as chlorophenothane
(65). Possibly, steric factors are also involved, the trichloromethyl
group of *65* and the *t*-butyl group of *66* bending the two aromatic nuclei out of the tetrahedral angle one expects for diphenylmethane.
In the non-phenolic ring of thyronine analogues, 3,5-dichloro substitution of *L*-T$_3$ in lieu of iodine produces an appreciable thyromimetic
effect, and so does the 3,5-dimethyl derivative *(67)*. These substituents

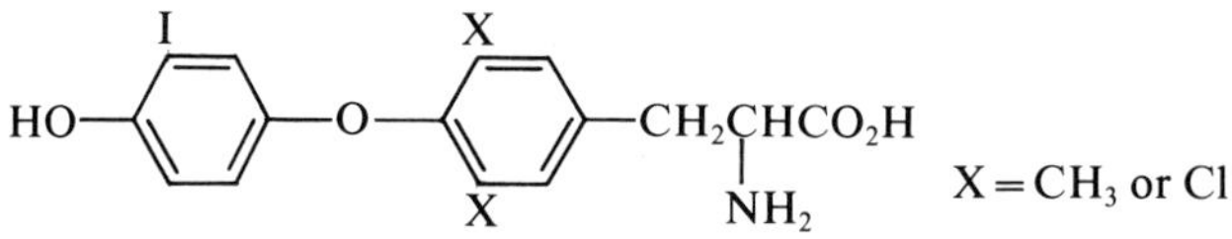

67

contribute to the hydrophobicity of the ring [128]. Binding free energy
values of the dimethyl analogue of *L*-T$_3$ and the dichloro analogue of
L-T$_4$ are almost identical [129]. It must be kept in mind, however, that
methyl groups can be oxidized metabolically, especially if they are attached to an aromatic ring. This may affect the half-life in tests *in vivo*.
The overall effects of fluorine substitution are hard to predict. Flur-
ethyl, bis(trifluoromethyl)ether, is a central stimulant with an action
similar to the initial phase of diethyl ether. In the replacement of the
o-chlorine atom in chlorazepam by fluorine, flurazepam *(68)* deepens
sedative-hypnotic activity [130]. On the other hand, while chloroform
(CHCl$_3$) is a general anesthetic, dichlorodifluoromethane (CCl$_2$F$_2$)

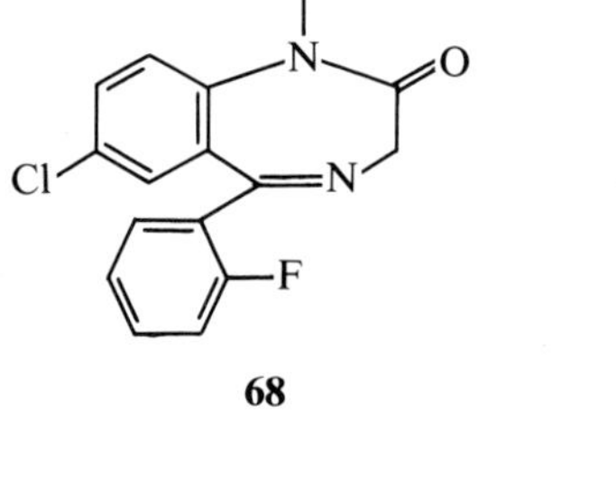

68

has little, if any, depressing or toxic properties. Here the lipophilic distribution may be the principal influence on activity.

3'-Azido-3'-deoxythymidine (AZT, zyvudine) *(69)* is a potent inhibitor of the replication of the human immunodeficiency virus (HIV) [131]. It is phosphorylated to the triphosphate which then inhibits the utilization of dTTP by reverse transcriptase and thereby prevents the elongation of viral DNA. Various 3'-azido nucleosides have been prepared and tested against HIV-1 in cell cultures; a few are listed in Chart 1. Of these modifications, AZT remained the most active drug. Trifluoromethyl substitution *(69 A)* that could be thought of as leading to a bioisostere, abolishes activity, whereas the halogen deriva-

Chart 1 [132]

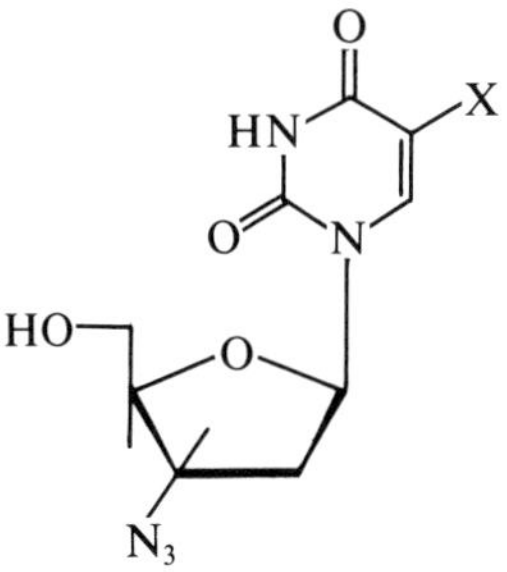

	X = H	X = OCH$_2$CH=CH$_2$ (70)
	CH$_3$ (69)	OCH$_2$C=CH
	CF$_3$ (69 A)	OCH$_2$CN
		SCH$_3$
	F, Br, I (69 B)	SCN
	OH	NH$_2$, NHCH$_3$
	OCH$_3$	N(CH$_3$)$_2$
	OC$_2$H$_5$	

tives (F, Br, I) *(69 B)* and the amino and hydroxyl compounds (other classical isosteres) retain significant antiviral potency. The allyl ether *70* analogue was highly active.

No clear relationship between antiviral activity and the electron-donating or electron-withdrawing capacities of the 5-substituents emerged from this study.

The replacement of chlorine by bromine in some drug structures generally, but not inevitably, deepens some biological actions, including toxicity. Bromide ion had been used as a calming sedative in the 19th century, and perhaps as a memory of this application some aliphatic bromo compounds such as diethylbromoacetyl-urea, $(C_2H_5)_2CBrCONHCONH_2$, and bromoisovalerylurea, $(CH_3)_2CHCHBrCONHCONH_2$, are still prescribed sporadically in some countries for this purpose. Chloral hydrate, $Cl_3CCH(OH)_2$, and chloroform are general anesthetics but the corresponding bromo compounds cannot be used. Here again, lipophilicity is the most important – at least the most widely studied – determinant in SAR. Force of inhibition of CNS enzymes may well shed more light on these questions. Thus, isosterism can be claimed for all the halogens but bioisosterism which postulates the similarity of biological properties cannot be predicted easily.

Two types of agents appear to depend on the presence of iodine in their molecules for useful activity. In the case of thyroid hormones, the several iodinated thyronines have not been rivalled by the corresponding bromo and chloro analogues. Enzymatic uptake of iodide and subsequent oxidative biosynthesis of the hormones is a process that has evolved over millions of years in aquatic and later in terrestrial animals. There is no reason to assume that other halogens could not participate in these natural reactions, but apparently this does not happen. That iodine is not unique in producing hormonal properties has been shown by synthesizing *D,L*-3,3'-diiodo-5-bromothyronine which increased the oxygen consumption of thyroidectomized rats and reduced the size of the thyroid gland in antigoiter tests [133]. *DL*-3,3',5-Triiodo-5'-fluorothyronine, an H...F isostere of triiodothyronine (T_3), shows about one-third the effect of thyroxine by the goiter prevention method [134].

The other case is that of organic iodinated radiopaque agents. Iodine, in organic linkage, endows compounds with a greater capacity for x-ray opaqueness than do the other halogens. Nevertheless, tetrabromophenolphthalein was used briefly in cholecystography until the more effective isomeric tetraiodo compounds could be prepared. Phenoltetrachlorophthalein has also been used in hepatography [135], and so has Rose Bengal, the disodium salt of tetraiodotetrachlorofluorescein *(71)*.

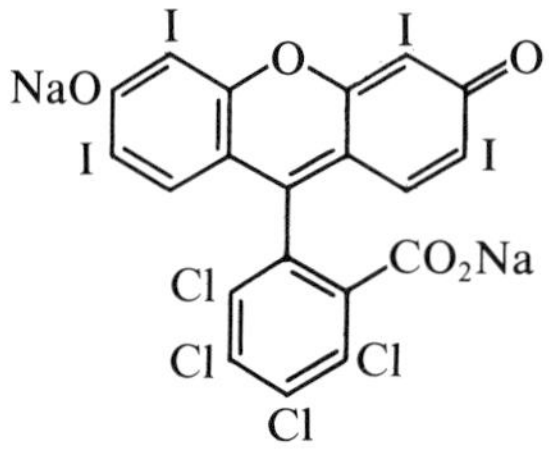

71

1.7.   Limits of bioisosterism

By the early 1960's, some uncertainties had surfaced in the explanation and applications of bioisosterism. One apparent shortcoming was that what seemed to be a solid rule in one series of structurally related compounds failed to work out in a series with different overall structural characteristics. In such cases one could not predict whether one would end up with an agonist, a mixed agonist – antagonist, or an antagonist. Ariens [136] and Korolkovas [137] tried to list those structural moieties which often turn an agonist into an antagonist. However, they did not include the possibility that the bioisosteric planning process, i.e. experiments to rationally design a drug structure, may have disturbed one of several parameters that had proved to be necessary for inducing a given biological activity. Such parameters include size and bond angles (shape), ability to form hydrogen bonds at active sites of enzymes or drug receptors, pK_a, chemical reactivity, hydrophilicity, lipophilicity (i.e. maintenance of the same or at least similar partition coefficients), and also the metabolic fate of the compounds to be prepared. There are limits concerning the number of these parameters that can be changed unpunished. Yet the hope for potential success in bioisosteric exchanges has intrigued many medicinal chemists, even if they or their physical chemistry colleagues have not measured all the constants and values involved. This has led to a silent understanding that at least in early research in a given structural series one might postpone adhering to the more rigid requirements of classical isosterism.

The reasons for this apparent self-deception are practical realities of daily work. No two manufacturers of automobiles, computers, breakfast cereals, swimwear and other necessities of the good life will copy every feature of their competitors. Instead, they will try to improve some aspects of the original product and delete, or at least play down, any point that had elicited justified criticism. In order to achieve these guidelines, the properties of the product to be modified would have to be analyzed and understood as far as the state of the art permits.

It is the same with medicinal agents. One will rarely seek to obtain a drug with completely identical properties but almost always try to improve potency and specificity and decrease side effects and toxicity. Bioisosterism provides descriptions of electronic, steric, lipophilic, and distribution characteristics of a compound, and these data help us to understand mechanisms of action and the role of a compound in producing measurable biological consequences. If the purpose of a research project is to come up with a drug that exhibits modifications of one or several properties and does not wholly match the model "lead" compound, then the description and definition of this "lead" compound will not suffice. At this point, human inventiveness and intuition and our gambling spirit as to which facet of the necessary properties we should change, will have to be brought into play. Experience in a structural field will be helpful in prompting our decision making. If we want to create a bioisosteric drug with some desirable changes, we will have to be aware of the fact that sooner or later we may step outside the limits of permissible classical bioisosteric alterations. As we transgress these limits we stand to lose activity altogether or sometimes, conjure up a totally new set of biological properties, some wanted, some undesirable, and usually baffling. The rules which delineate bioisosterism will point to compromise structures which may be just still acceptable as candidates. Such chemical structures are spoken of as non-classical bioisosteres. Their study and use has expanded steadily over the last several decades.

It will come as no surprise that reviewers of the subject of bioisosterism have given preference to either more biochemical or more physical aspects of the phenomenon [138, 139].

1.7.1   Interactions at receptor sites

One guideline how far we may venture in designing new drugs at the border of bioisosterism is provided by advances in our understanding of biochemical mechanisms at receptor sites. Receptors are glyco- and lipoproteins or, in some cases, nucleic acids. The protein receptors may be enzymes or membrane-spanning macropolypeptides. Active sites of enzymes are situated in the protein chains of these biocatalysts and are part of molecular bays formed by these chains. A drug or substrate has to fit more or less snuggly onto such harboring polypeptide bays and will try to make contact with the amino acid side chains or the amide groups of the peptide backbone. The side chains are SH groups, alcoholic and phenolic OH groups, amino and guanidino groups, carboxyls and carboxamide groups, and disulfide bridges which are partly responsible for the stereostructure of the enzyme.

Quite commonly, carbonyl and other groups of the enzyme's polypeptide chain attract drug molecules by way of hydrogen bonding. Since the angle of regions which permit hydrogen bonding can be as much as 60°, drug molecules differing considerably in atom-to-atom overlap but capable of hydrogen bonding may be attracted and bind to the same region of an enzyme protein. This type of combination will be favored if the approaching small molecule can assume a conformation complementary to the shape of the protein bay. In some cases, quite remote regions of the polypeptide will pass one atop of another, but at a distance that can be spanned by two or more hydrogen bonds of the drug molecule. In other cases, attractive van der Waals interactions or London dispersion forces will come into play between drug or substrate and polypeptide. If an enzyme contains a relatively small co-enzyme or cofactor moiety such as some vitamin or metal atom, a substrate or drug may react with these active portions by ionic or covalent interaction.

Similar conditions will affect recognition of foreign chemicals by trans-membrane receptor proteins. Here again, the usually heavily folded polypeptide chains will offer ample opportunity for attracting and ligating molecules that pass by in the circulation in search of a safely binding harbor. The need for steric fit cannot be overemphasized and emerges as the most important condition of bioisosteric requirements.

If a drug acts by intercalating between turns of the helix of a nucleic acid, steric fit to the available space in such turns will again be the precondition for intercalation. Hydrogen bonds plus van der Waals forces will be required to stabilize the hold of the polynucleotide onto the drug. These bonds may form with different groups of the polynucleotide and provide some latitude to details of the intruding drug molecule. That means, they will stretch the requirements of bioisosterism beyond classical limits.

1.7.2   Steric similarities

When distances between functional groups, and also molecular shapes are of prime importance to enable a compound to be recognized at a receptor, it becomes possible to interchange substituents more freely provided they are spatially compatible and have more or less similar bond angles. The insertion of -OCO- in lieu of -CH$_2$CH$_2$-

in the (weak) estrogens *72* and *73* is an example of such design [140, 141].

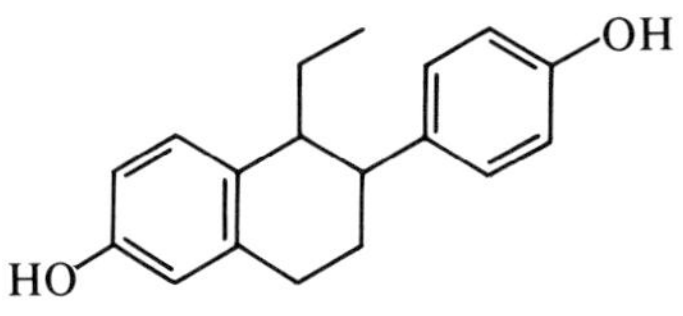

72 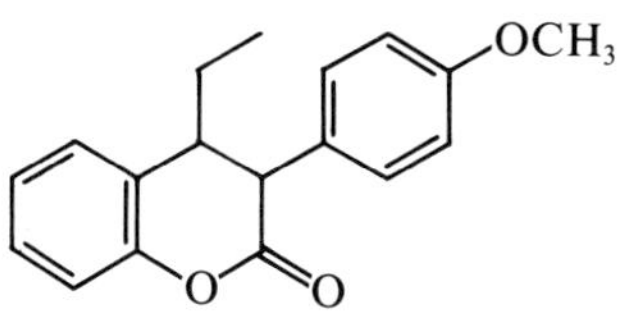   **73**

Another case of the replacement of -CH$_2$CH$_2$- by a lactone group is the comparison of 3,4-dihydro-2-methyl-1-naphthol *(74)* with the α, β-unsaturated lactone *75* [140]. The naphthol derivative has considerable vitamin K-type coagulant activity (in the range of 1 γ) probably because it can be oxidized to a naphthoquinone. The coumarin *75* has only very weak activity in the same test [142, 144].

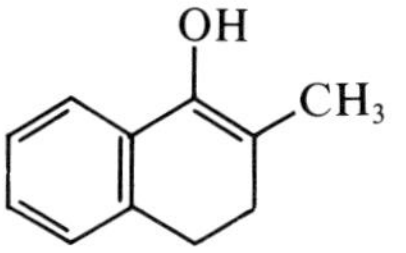

74 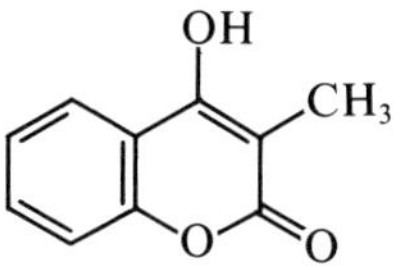   **75**

In another study of the significance of spatial analogy, the thyroid hormone, 3,3',5-triiodo-*L*-thyronine (T$_3$) *(76)* was modified. A large number of compounds in which the 3'-iodine atom was replaced by all kinds of saturated, unsaturated, small, large, hydroxyalkyl, carbonyl-containing and other functional groups were tested *in vitro* for hormone-receptor binding to intact nuclei, and *in vivo* thyromimetic activity. Analysis of these data using conformational and QSAR structure-affinity methods revealed that the 3'-substituent recognition site on the T$_3$ receptor is hydrophobic and limited in depth to the length of the natural iodine substituent, but sufficiently wide to accommodate a phenyl or cyclohexyl group. These two groups may therefore be

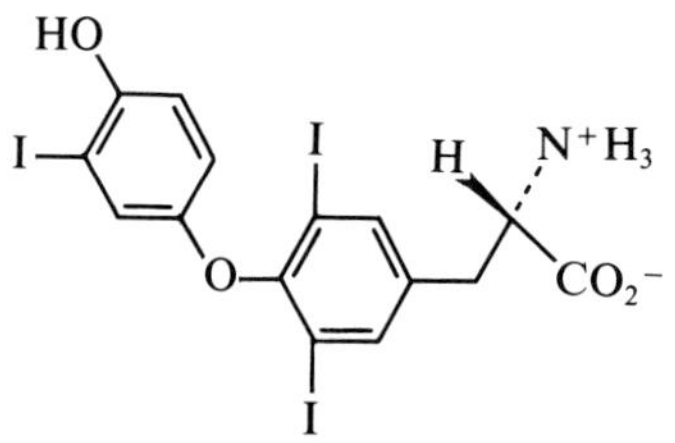

76

regarded as bioisosteric with iodine in this particular instance, but this suggestion could not be applied to unrelated situations with quite different receptor functions [143].

A flat hydrophobic surface at least 11 Å long, 4 – 5 Å wide, and approximately 2 Å above or below the plane of the aromatic ring has been calculated for the active site of phenylethanolamine N-methyltransferase (PNMT) (from bovine adrenals) whose catalytic properties are inhibited by conformationally defined analogues of amphetamine and phenylethanolamine. If the aromatic rings of the biphenyl systems *(77, 78)* are conformationally restricted by incorporation in

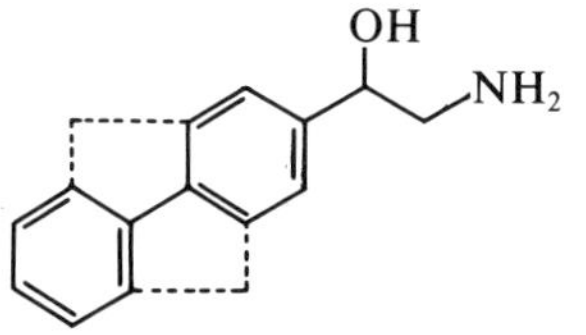

77 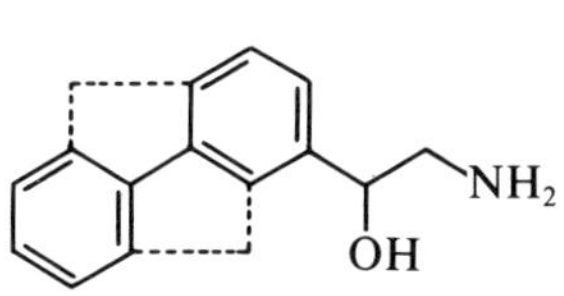   **78**

fluorene structures, dotted lines), the affinity for PNMT is enhanced. Thus, either the *p*- or *m*-biphenyl derivatives *(77, 78)* as well as the corresponding fluorenes may be regarded as bioisosteres in this enzyme system [144].

Potential bioisosteres of squalene *(79)* may be seen in some antifungal allylamines [145]. Squalene is a substrate of squalene epoxidase which is the first enzyme requiring molecular oxygen in the biosynthesis of

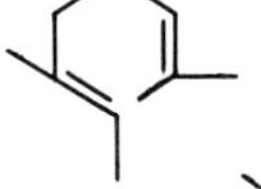

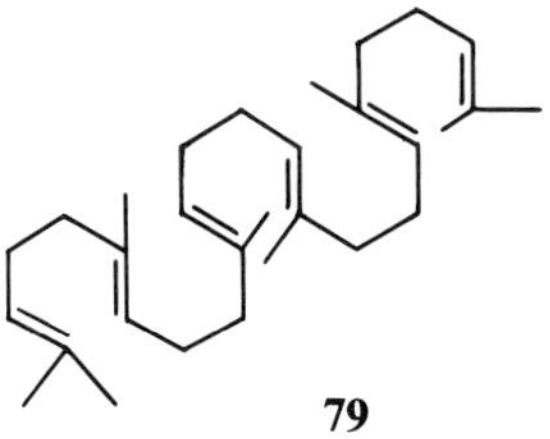

79 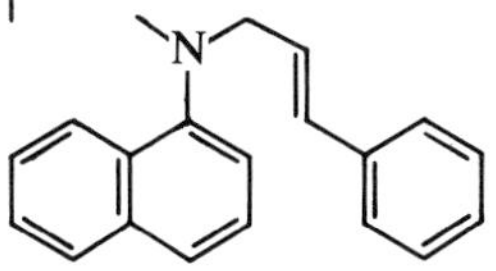   **80** 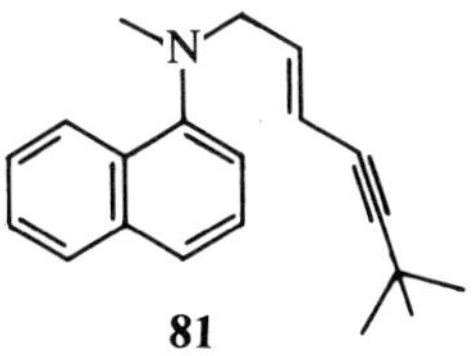   **81**

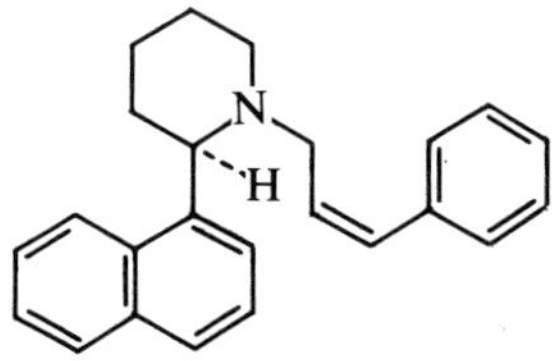

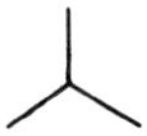

82

sterols. The N-1-naphthyl-N-allylamines *80* and *81*, and also the piperidino analogue *82* are specific inhibitors of squalene epoxidase and seem to exert their antimycotic activity by this mechanism. The formal similarity of squalene and these inhibitors lends credence to this interpretation. The acetylenic derivative *81* acts by noncompetitive kinetics at an inhibition constant of 3×10^{-8} M.

Thornber [138] has listed and referenced 32 variations of the central cyclopentane ring of the prostaglandins, some of which may be re-

Chart 2. Analogues of prostaglandins [138]

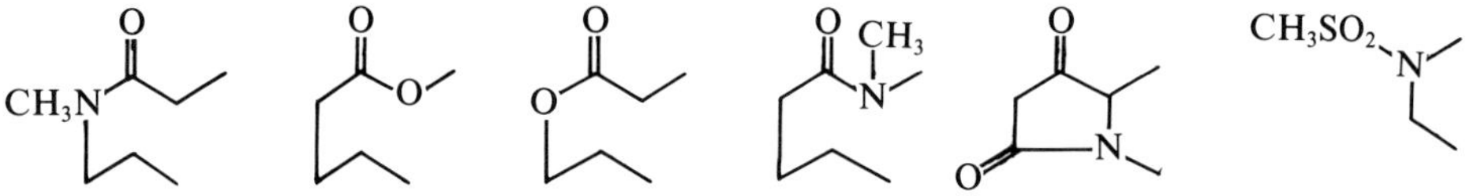

(146) (146) (146) (146) (147) (148)

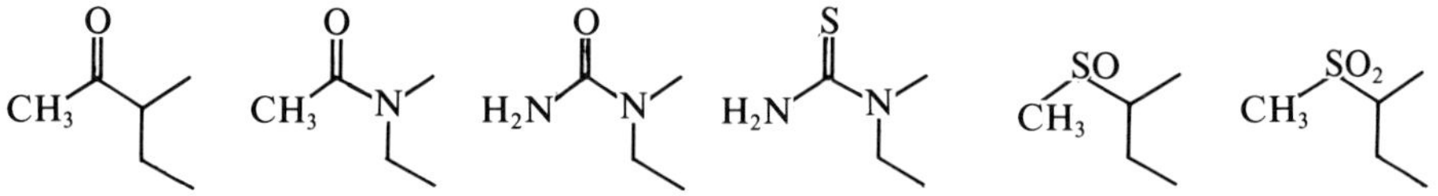

(149) (150) (150) (150) (151) (151)

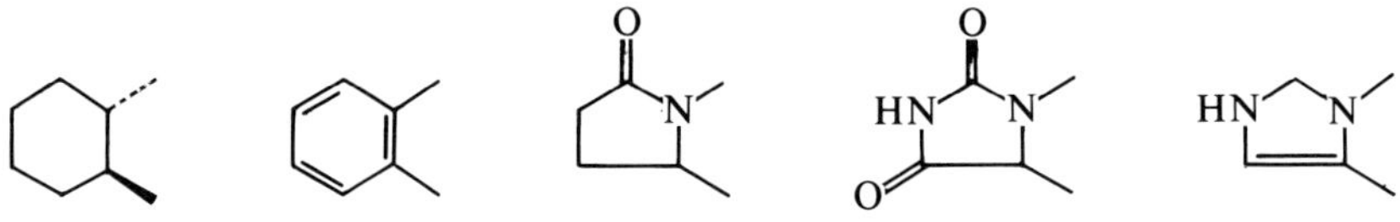

(152) (152) (153, 154, 155) (156) (156)

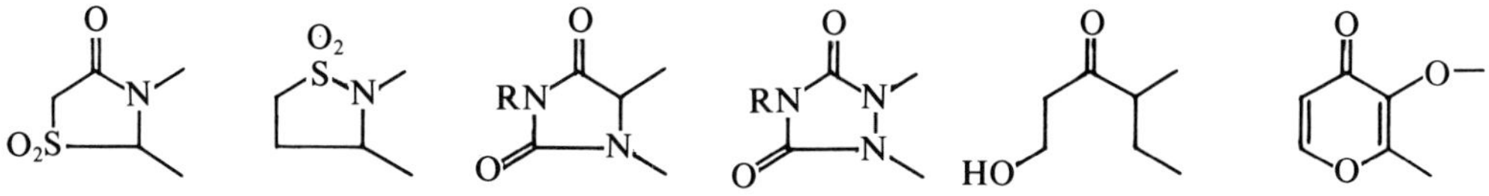

(156) (157) (158) (159) (160) (161)

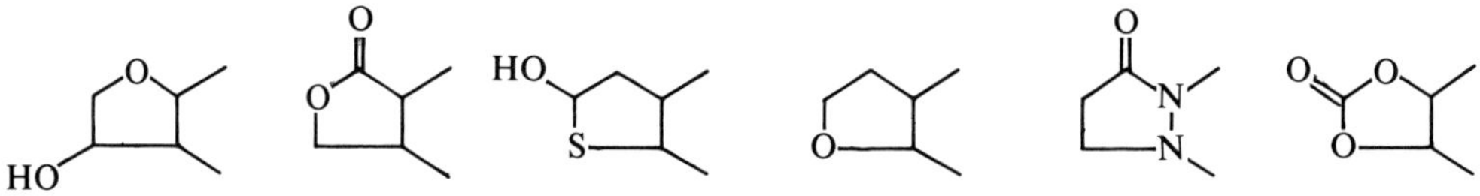

(162) (163) (164) (165) (166) (167)

garded as bioisosteres of the dihydroxycyclopentane and hydroxycyclopentanone structures of the natural hormones. Carbon has been replaced by oxygen and nitrogen, the keto group has given way to amide, ureide, sulfonamide, methylsulfoxide, methylsulfone and cyclic oxygen (tetrahydrofuran) and sulfur (tetrahydrothiophene) functions, and the cyclopentane ring has been expanded to cyclohexane, benzene, pyranone and related systems. These derivatives may be a source of information on how far nonclassical bioisosterism can be carried. In these derivatives, the groups listed (Chart 2) represent the turning point of the long unsaturated carboxylic acid chains of the prostaglandins.

Even a cursory survey of these groups which are to mimic or systematically alter the central cyclopentane ring of the natural prostaglandins suggests that shape and molecular volume are the decisive attributes of bioisosterism in this series barring polar differences. Similar conditions are found in a series of analogues of the potassium-sparing diuretic, amiloride (83). In this study the early application of ring equivalents in isosterism [4] has included hydrogen-bonded rings, specifically a hydrogen-bonded acylguanidine (84). By slightly shortening the distance between the amide oxygen and the guanidine nitrogen, the 3-aminooxa-2,4-diazole 85 was designed; it had very similar diu-

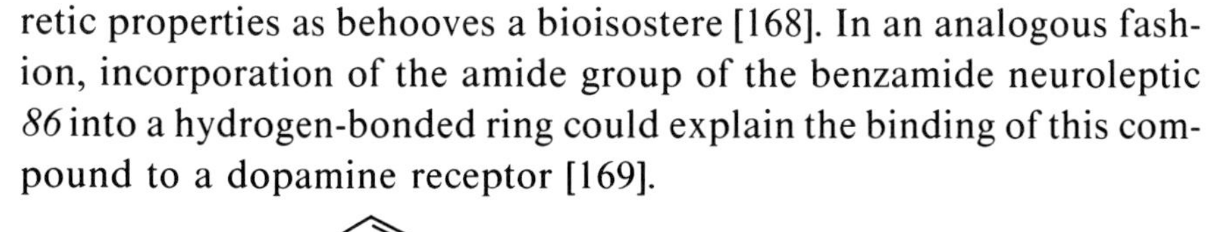

| 83 | 84 | 85 |

retic properties as behooves a bioisostere [168]. In an analogous fashion, incorporation of the amide group of the benzamide neuroleptic 86 into a hydrogen-bonded ring could explain the binding of this compound to a dopamine receptor [169].

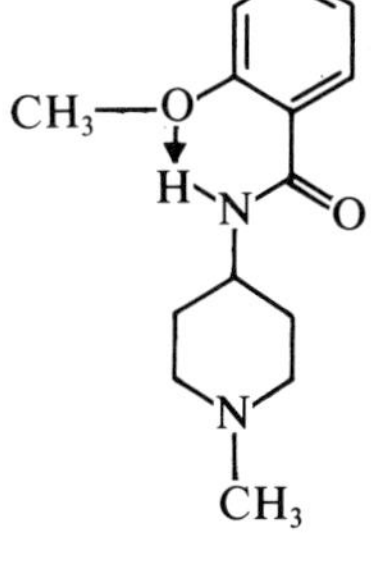

86

1.8   Non-classical bioisosteres of carbonyl-type structures
1.8.1   Carbonyl-type structures

This structural segment comprises ketones ($R_2C=O$), both saturated, enolic tautomers ($=C\text{-}OH$) and α, β-unsaturated carbonyl compounds [$=CH\text{-}C(=O)R$], carboxylic acids [$RC(=O)OH$], esters [$R\text{-}C(=O)OR$], amides [$R\text{-}C(=O)NHR'$], amidines [$R\text{-}C(=NH)NHR'$], guanidines [$R\text{-}NHC(=NH)NHR'$], and their cyclic and hetero analogues. Any of these groups can accept hydrogen bonds from receptor sites, or extend such bonds to macromolecular points. This happens also if the functions are inverted as in reversed esters [$-C(=O)OR$, $-O\text{-}C(=O)R$] which often exhibit almost identical biological properties. Hydrogen bonds can thus be diverted to neighboring positions. Bioisosteric incorporation of keto groups into heterocyclic arrangements is seen in oxazole analogues (89) [170] of the neuroleptics, benperidol (87) and haloperidol (88). Similar examples are encountered in bioisosteres (91) [171] of diuretic 4-acylphenoxyacetic acids (90).

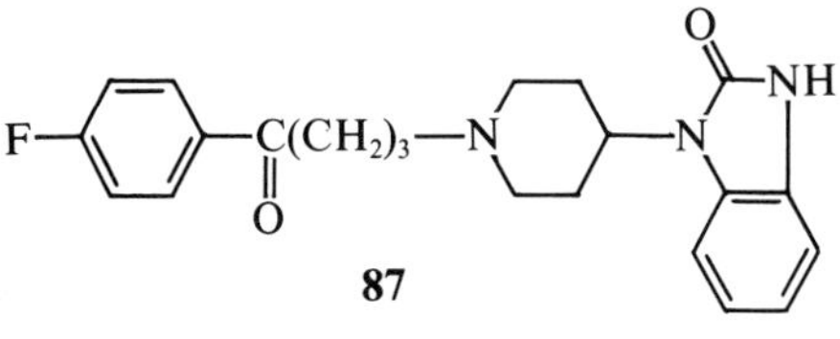

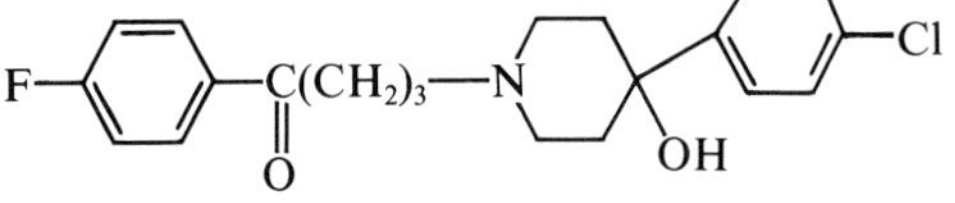

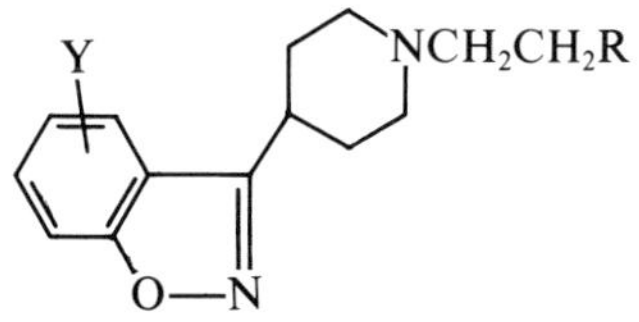

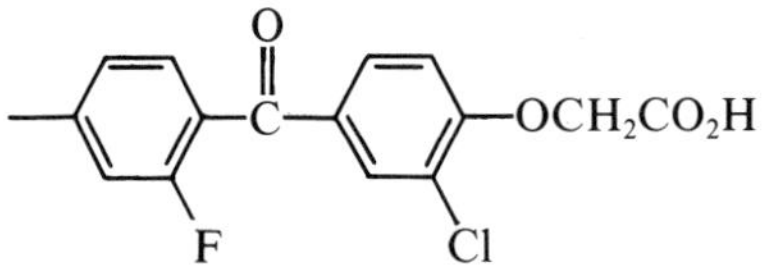

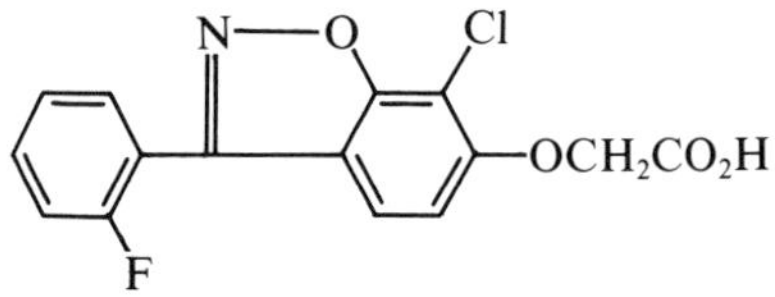

The keto carbonyl has been replaced by sulfoxide (> SO) and sulfone (> SO$_2$) *(93)* in methadone *(92);* the sulfone isostere *93* is slightly more active and less toxic than methadone [172, 173].

$(C_6H_5)_2$ > C-X-C$_2$H$_5$

|

CH$_2$CH(CH$_3$)N(CH$_3$)$_2$

X = CO: *92*

X = SO, SO$_2$: *93*

Similar exchanges have been studied for meperidine *(58)* [174, 175].

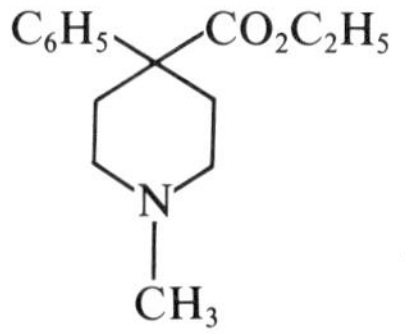

C$_6$H$_5$ CO$_2$C$_2$H$_5$	C$_6$H$_5$ COC$_3$H$_7$	C$_6$H$_5$ SO$_2$C$_2$H$_5$	C$_6$H$_5$ SO$_2$(CH$_2$)$_2$CH$_3$
N	N	N	N
CH$_3$	CH$_3$	CH$_3$	CH$_3$
58	**94**	**95**	**96**

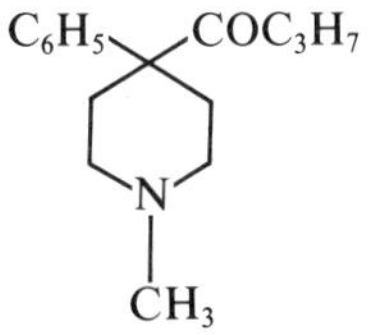

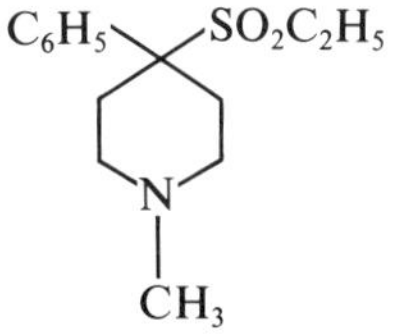

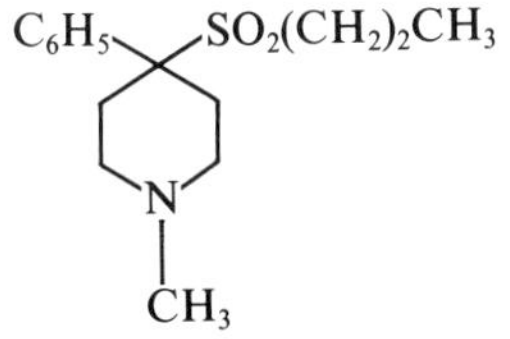

The ketone analogue, *94,* and sulfone derivatives *95* and *96,* are potent analgesics.

1.8.2   Sulfoxides and sulfones

Sulfoxides should resemble carbonyl compounds but they are more polar [41]. The sulfoxide, sulindac *(97),* is a nonsteroidal antiinflammatory arylacetic acid. The *p*-methylsulfinyl group causes the compound with this substituent to become much more soluble and to provide a center of metabolism to minimize the accumulation of any single metabolite in the kidney. Sulindac was developed in the course of molecular modification of the *p*-chlorobenzoyl indole derivative indomethacin *(98)* [176, 177]. The indene isostere *(99)* of indomethacin, a typical application of -C(=O)-N< → -CH=C< bioisosterism, had fewer CNS side effects. Considerable and laborious molecular modification led to sulindac *(97).* The active metabolite of *97* is its CH$_3$S- derivative. Bioisosterism of Cl and CH$_3$S had been observed in the indomethacin series. The indole → indene, and > N-C(O)- → > =CH- isosteric replacements could be anticipated, and the choice of a sulfoxide group to increase solubility was a logical plan. To complete the picture, the methylsulfonyl (CH$_3$SO$_2$) oxidation product is a metabolite of sulindac.

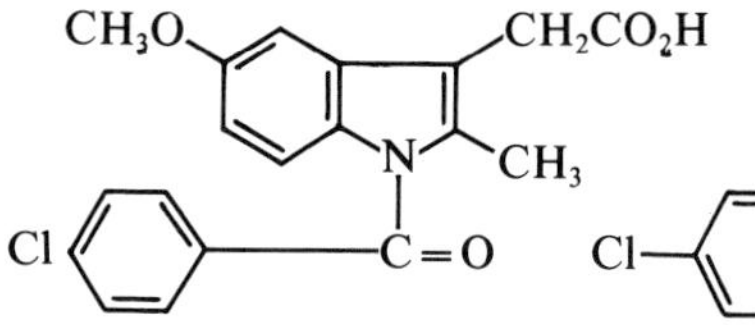

98 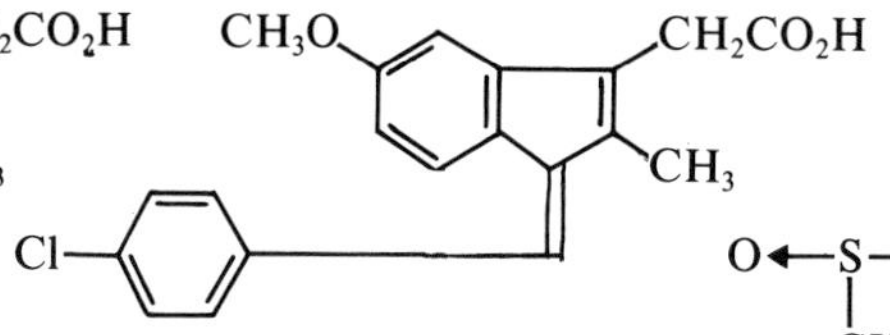   **99** 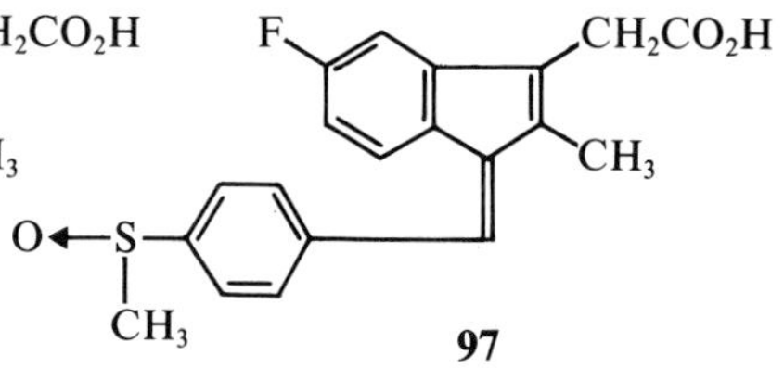   **97**

Another case of bioisosterism involving indole and carbocyclic systems is the pair, 2,4-dichlorophenoxyacetic acid (2,4-D), a herbicide, and 3-indoleacetic acid, a plant growth hormone (auxin). The herbicide is much more potent than 3-indoleacetic acid and more slowly degraded in plants. It accumulates in treated plants, causing them to grow much too rapidly. Thus young plant cells do not mature in a normal way. Parts of the plant's food-transporting vessels are plugged up by clusters of cells, inhibiting the movement of nutrients. 2,4-D is believed to damage plant respiration, cell division, hormone balance and protein synthesis.

Along with the extensive molecular modifications of the cyclopentanolone ring of the prostaglandins E_1 and E_2 listed in Chart 2, replacement of the 9-carbonyl by methylsulfoxide *(100)* and methylsulfone *(101)* has been recorded [178]. In addition, several derivatives incorporating the sulfoxide *(102)* [179] and sulfone groups [180] in the 5-membered ring have been prepared.

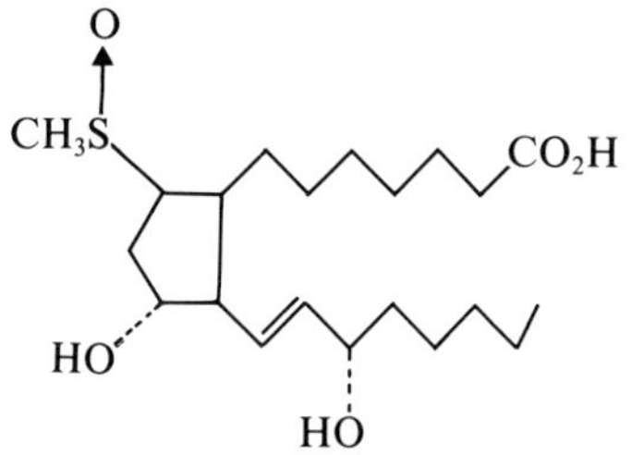

100 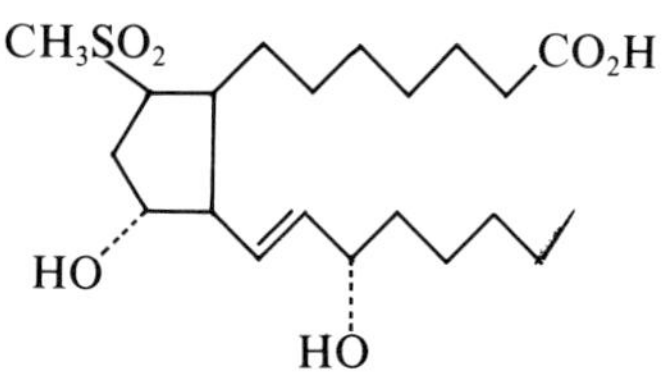   **101** 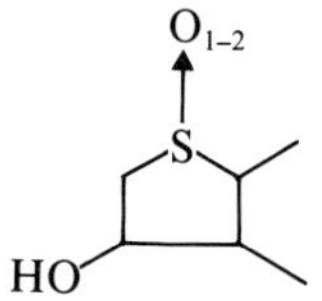   **102**

1.8.3   Reversal of functional groups

Reversal of the ester group of meperidine produces 1-methyl-4-phenyl-4-propionoxypiperidine (MPPT) *(103)* which is said to be five times more potent than meperidine in analgesic tests (181, 182). If too much heat is applied in the esterification of 1-methyl-4-phenyl-4-pip-

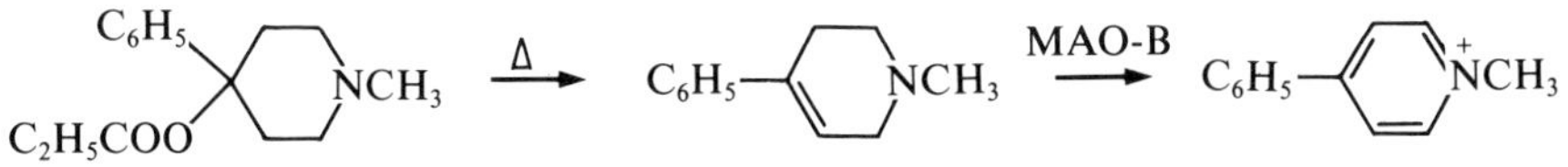

$$\underset{\mathbf{103}}{\underset{C_2H_5COO}{\overset{C_6H_5}{\bigtimes}}NCH_3} \quad \overset{\Delta}{\longrightarrow} \quad \underset{\mathbf{104}}{C_6H_5-\bigtimes NCH_3} \quad \overset{MAO\text{-}B}{\longrightarrow} \quad \underset{\mathbf{105}}{C_6H_5-\bigtimes \overset{+}{N}CH_3}$$

eridinol which yields *103*, propionic acid is eliminated *(104)* and this unsaturated compound can be dehydrogenated biochemically by the action of monoamine oxidase-B to 1-methyl-4-phenylpyridinium *(105*, MPP$^+$), a dangerous hallucinogenic neurotoxin referred to as a "designer drug". It also causes severe extrapyramidal symptoms.

Reversal of functional groups in cholinergic and anticholinergic agents also results in very similar activity in the respective pairs. The muscarinic betaine *106* and its isomer *107*, as well as the antispasmodic diphenylacetate ester *108* and its benzhydryl isomer *(109)* may serve as examples [183–185].

$$\underset{\mathbf{106}}{CH_3OCOCH_2N^+(CH_3)_3} \qquad\qquad \underset{\mathbf{107}}{CH_3COOCH_2N^+(CH_3)_3}$$

$$\underset{\mathbf{108}}{(C_6H_5)_2CHCOOCH_2CH_2N(CH_3)_2} \qquad \underset{\mathbf{109}}{(C_6H_5)_2CHOCOCH_2CH_2N(CH_3)_2}$$

Not all kinds of isomeric exchanges and reversals are permissible in structures that are related to certain adrenergic hormones. Thus, reversal of the alcoholic hydroxyl and the amino groups in the norepinephrine homologue *110*, a pressor agent, leads to loss of activity *(111)*[186, 187]. Perhaps the genetic memory of biochemical evolution overrides bioisosteric considerations.

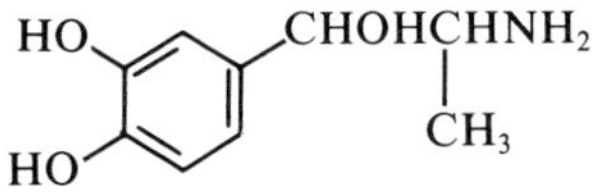

$$\underset{\mathbf{110}}{\underset{HO}{\overset{HO}{\bigcirc}}\overset{CHOHCHNH_2}{\underset{CH_3}{|}}} \qquad \underset{\mathbf{111}}{\underset{HO}{\overset{HO}{\bigcirc}}\overset{CH-CHOH}{\underset{NH_2 \ \ CH_3}{|\ \ \ \ |}}}$$

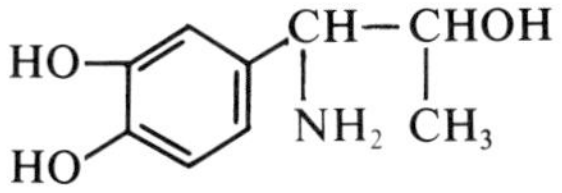

1.8.4   Deletion of oxygen

A ketonic analogue *(94)* of meperidine *(58)* has already been mentioned in connection with bioisosteric exchanges of CO with other electron-withdrawing groups. A lower homologue of *94*, with a *m*-phenolic hydroxyl group, is called ketobemidone *(112)* [188, 189]. It

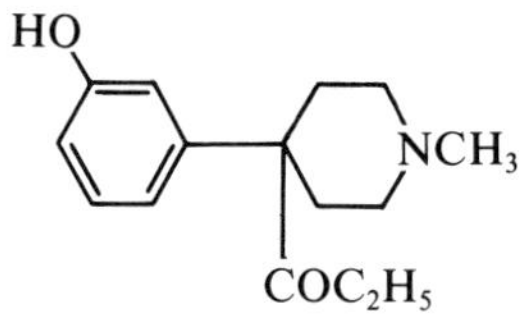

112

illustrates another suggestion that biological activity may be retained sometimes if an ether oxygen is deleted in nonclassical bioisosteres [190]. However, this is not a general rule and should be used with misgivings. A replacement of ether oxygen in esters and ethers by methylene as a spacer group offers a safer approach to the construction of bioisosteric compounds because at least the distance from other points in the molecule has been maintained in an -O-—→-CH$_2$- exchange. An example in which the deletion hypothesis failed is the removal of the ether oxygen in *D*-glucopyranose 6-deoxy-6-phosphonic acid *(113)* [191]. This did not cause inhibition of several enzymes which require glucose 6-phosphate for catalytic performance.

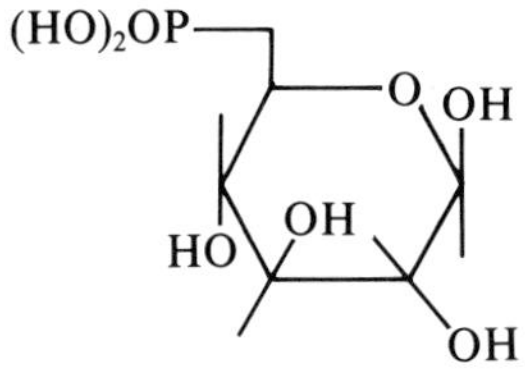

113

1.8.5   Bioisosterism of carboxylic acids

Some of the most clearcut bioisosteric relationships have been established for carboxylic acids. The carboxylate ion, RCO$_2^-$, resembles the sulfonamide ion, RSO$_2$N$^-$ [38]. This nonclassical isosterism explains the antagonism of *p*-aminobenzoic acid (PABA) and sulfanilamide [200, 201]. At a concentration of 3.03 X 10^{-4}M, sulfanilamide action is reversed by a molar concentration of 1.2–5.7 X 10^{-8} of PABA [200]. The distances between the two oxygen atoms of the sulfanilamide *(115)* and PABA *(114)* anions are virtually the same. Also, at phy-

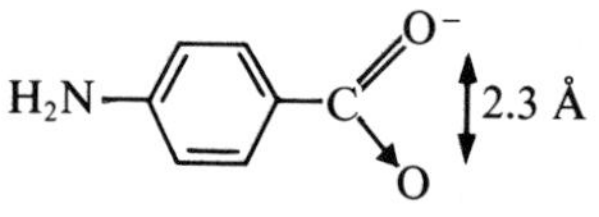

114 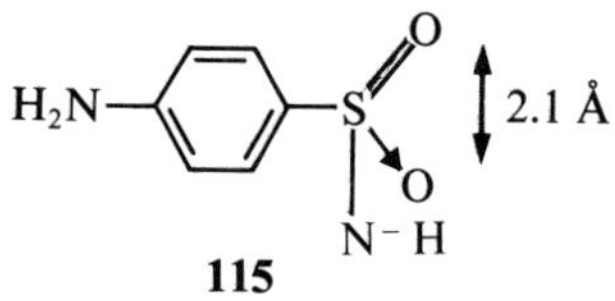   **115**

Table V (190)
Effects of Omissions and Replacements of Ether Oxygens on Biological Activities

Chemical Structure	Biological Test	X = O	X = CH$_2$	X absent	Ref.
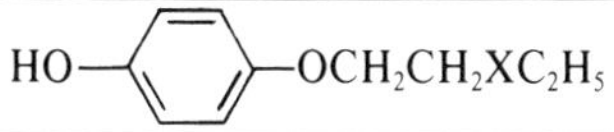 HO—⟨ ⟩—OCH$_2$CH$_2$XC$_2$H$_5$	Phenol Coefficient *Staph. aureus*	5	30	9	(192)
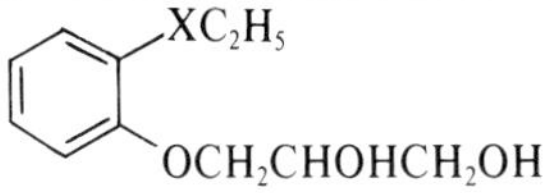 ⟨ ⟩ XC$_2$H$_5$ / OCH$_2$CHOHCH$_2$OH	ED$_{50}$ mg/kg for muscular paralysis	1.4	5.8	1.8	(193)
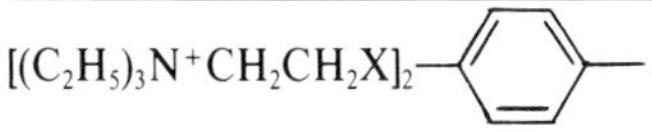 [(C$_2$H$_5$)$_3$N$^+$CH$_2$CH$_2$X]$_2$—⟨ ⟩—	Curaremimetic Activity	100%	0	100%	(194)
(CH$_3$)$_3$N$^+$CH$_2$CH$_2$]$_2$X	Ganglionic Blockade	10%	100%	33%	(195)
[(CH$_3$)$_3$N$^+$CH$_2$CH$_2$X]$_2$(CH$_2$)$_n$	Curaremimetic PD$_{50}$ micromoles/kg <u>n</u> = 1 <u>n</u> = 2 <u>n</u> = 3	91 50 0.3	1.5 0.25 0.01	60 61 0.25	(196)
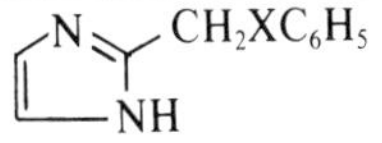 N⟩—CH$_2$XC$_6$H$_5$ / —NH	Effect on Blood Pressure	Pressor	Weak depressor	Strong depressor	(197)
C$_6$H$_5$XCH$_2$CH$_2$NH$_2$	Effect on Blood Pressure	Depressor	Weak depressor	Strong depressor	(198) (199)

siological pH the SO$_2$ group of the anion of sulfanilamide abstracts electrons from the nitrogen atom and thereby acquires a higher electron density than in the non-ionized state. Substituents which further attract electrons and strengthen the ionization of the sulfonamide ion have been shown to increase the bacteriostatic activity of sulfanilamide derivatives.

Bacteria which cannot biosynthesize tetrahydropteroylglutamic acid from available PABA will be inhibited by competition of SA at the step at which PABA is incorporated into the pteroylglutamate structure, and thereby lose the fundamental avenue to ribonucleic acid and hence to protein biosynthesis. Sulfanilamide must be present at concentrations higher than those of PABA to inhibit PABA incorporation. So great is the biochemical similarity of PABA and its antagonist that bacteria susceptible to SA can become resistant to this drug by acquiring the ability to synthesize unusually large amounts of PABA and thus overcome the inhibition of their reproduction.

Other acid functions such as phosphonic acids have also been studied as bioisosteres of carboxylic acids. Phosphanilic acid,

p-$H_2NC_6H_4PO(OH)_2$ [202], p-aminobenzenephosphonous acid, p-$H_2NC_6H_4P(OH)_2$ [203], and phosphanilamide, p-$H_2NC_6H_4PO(NH_2)_2$ [204], are bacteriostatic and the action of the two acids is antagonized by PABA [203–205]. Other phosphonic acids with useful biological activities include phosphonoacetic acid, $(HO)_2POCH_2CO_2H$, a bioisostere of malonic acid, and some of its carboxylate esters [206]. These compounds have antiherpes activity *in vivo* by inhibiting DNA polymerase induced by herpes and by cytomegalo viruses [207–210]. Another phosphonate-carboxylate analogy is that of the plant growth regulator, 2,4-dichlorophenoxyacetic acid (2,4-D) *(116)* and its monoethyl phosphonate bioisostere *(117)*. The latter has slight but appreciable auxin activity [211].

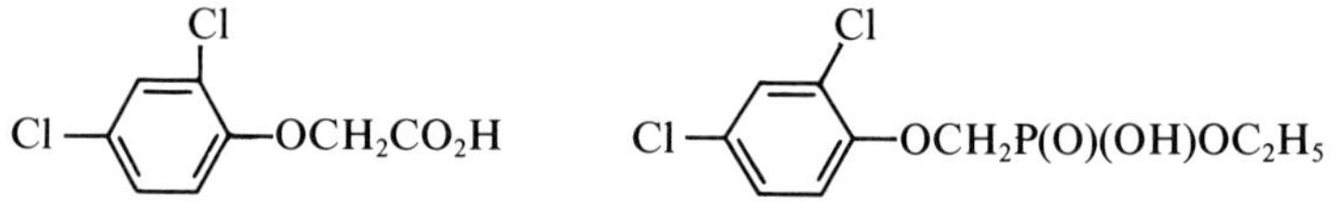

116   117

On the other hand, 3-pyridylphosphonic acid *(118)*, an analogue of niacin, did not inhibit the multiplication of *Lactobacillus arabinosus* which requires niacinamide, nor did it interfere with the incorporation of niacin into coenzymes or with the biosynthesis of niacin by two mycobacteria [212].

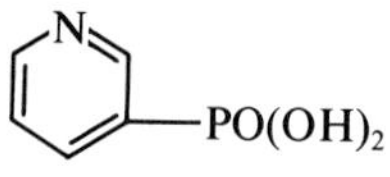

118

Unesterified phosphonic acids are more acidic than carboxylic acids and therefore monoesters can be expected to show a lower degree of acidity, approaching the range of carboxylic acids, i.e. to be more isoelectric. Phosphonate diesters may be more bioisosteric to β-diketones rather than to carboxylate esters. The antiherpetic arildone *(119)* has been compared to its diethyl phosphonate bioisostere *(120)* [213].

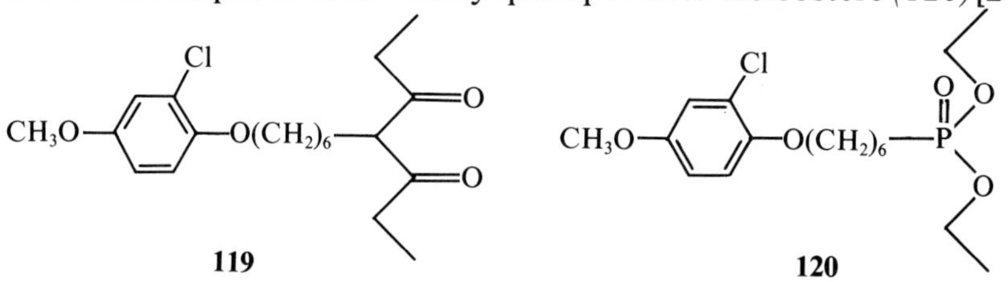

119   120

Phosphate ester groups as they occur in nucleotides cannot be re-placed successfully because nucleotides cannot enter cells but must be hydrolyzed to nucleosides which can penetrate cell walls and are then rephosphorylated intracellularly. The unique role of phosphate esters as agonists in many biochemical reactions has been detailed by West-heimer [214]. Analogues with ester groups other than phosphates will suffer the same fate and be converted to nucleotides inside the cell. However, a few hopeful variations have been recorded. Replacement of the terminal phosphate ester oxygen X of ATP (*121*, X = O) by NH, CF_2, CCl_2, CHF and CH_2 leads to an amide (X = NH) and

Adenine-$CH_2OP(O)(OH)$-O-$P(O)(OH)$-X-$P(O)(OH)_2$

121

to phosphonate-type compounds whose similarity to ATP decreases from NH to CH_2 [215]. The amide, AMP-PNP, is used widely in bio-chemical mechanistic studies.

In another nucleotide, a diphosphate ester was replaced synthetically by $OSO_2NHC(=O)O$- and the resulting bioisostere inhibited HSV-1 virus *in vitro* [216].

Platelet-activating factor (PAF-acether) *(122)* is a phospholipid medi-ator of anaphylaxis. Isosteric replacement of the phosphate ester by

CH_2-R
|
CH ~ $OCOCH_3$
|
CH_2-$OP(=O)O(CH_2)_2N^+(CH_3)_3$
|
O^-

R = $C_{18}H_{37}$ or $C_{16}H_{33}$

122

carboxylate ester groups *(123)* and also introduction of an ethyl ether group at C-2 *(124)* as well as changes in the ammoniumalkyl at C-3 *(125)* gave antagonists which provided 77–100 % protection against PAF-acether effects [217].

$CH_2OC_{18}H_{37}$
|
CH ~ $OCOCH_3$
|
$CH_2OCO(CH_2)_{2-4}N^+(CH_3)_3$
123

$CH_2OC_{18}H_{37}$
|
CH ~ OC_2H_5
|
$CH_2OCO(CH_2)_4N^+(CH_3)_3$
124

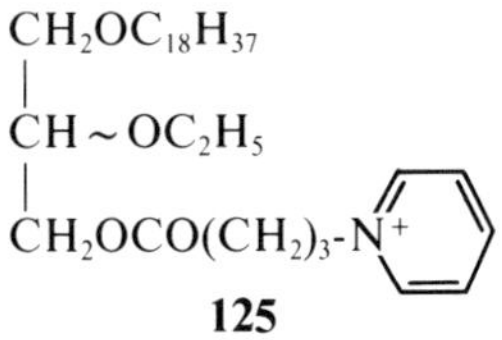

$CH_2OC_{18}H_{37}$
|
CH ~ OC_2H_5
|
$CH_2OCO(CH_2)_3$-N^+⟨⟩
125

Similarly, the carboxyl group of furosemide *(126)* can be replaced by SO_3H *(127)* without loss of diuretic activity [218]. GABA has been imitated in the gabaergic sulfonic acid, $H_2N(CH_2)_4SO_3H$ [223].

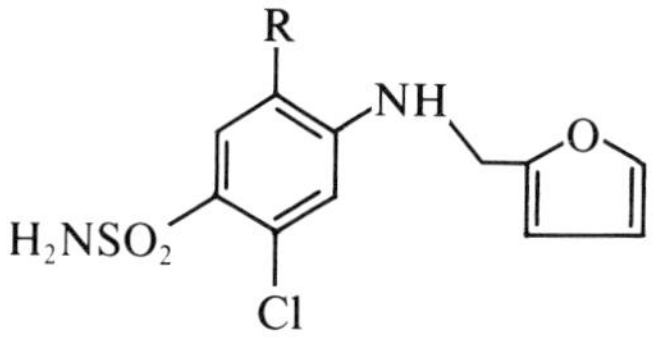

126: R = CO_2H
127: R = SO_3H

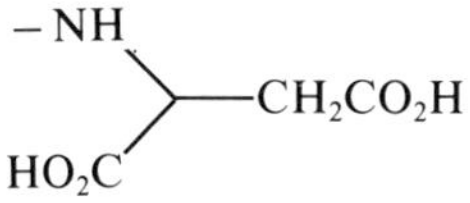

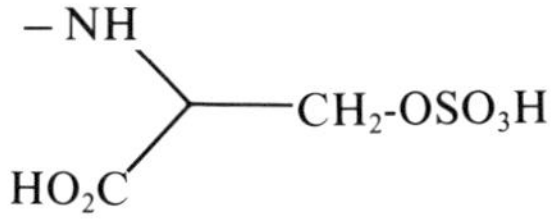

128

129

When the C-terminal aspartic acid residue *(128)* of gastrin was replaced by the electronically equivalent serine O-sulfate ester *(129)*, activity was retained [219]. In a number of enzyme systems, exchange of amino acid carboxyl for O-phosphate [220], phosphinate or phosphonate [221] or even for boronic acid groups [222] led to inhibitors of the catalytic activities.

Cyclic systems which contain the $-C\stackrel{}{\underset{XH}{}}$ arrangement can be classified as non-classical isosteres. Among them are especially tetrazoles *(130)* which resemble the corresponding carboxylic acids *(131)* in

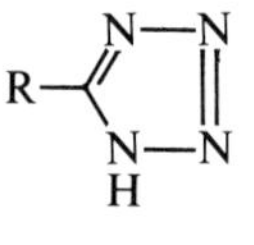

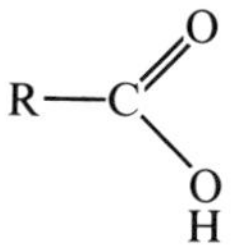

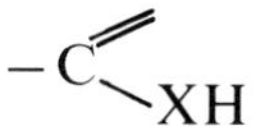

130   131

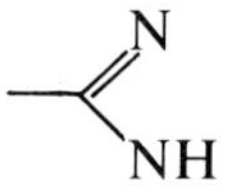

dissociation constants and can be interpreted as carboxylates in which -NH takes the place of -OH and in which the double and single bonds are stabilized by participating in the heteroring. One could even picture N_2 being discarded to unveil the isosteric moiety [224]. This system has also been extended by vinylogy, for example for GABA (γ-aminobutyric acid) analogues. The heterophen-

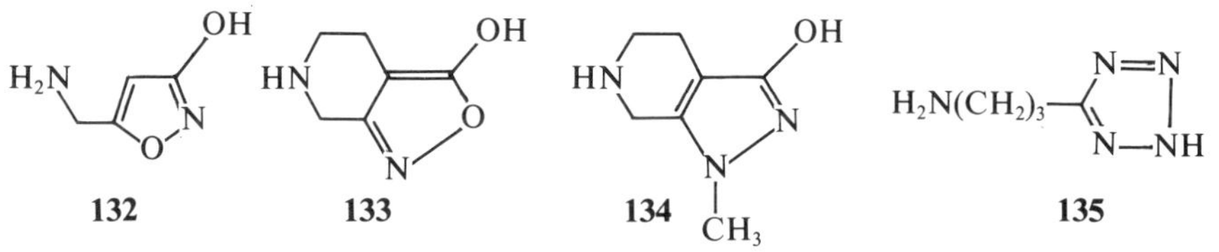

132   133   134   135

olic analogues *133* and *134* of the GABA agonist, muscimol *(132)*, have an acidity range of 3.0 *(133)* to 7.1 *(134)* and inhibit the binding of GABA to its receptor [225]. The tetrazole bioisostere *135* of GABA inhibited GABA transaminase [226]. In modifications of valproic acid *(136)* both the tetrazole *(137)* and 3,5-dioxo-1,2,4-oxadiazolidine *(138)* analogs inhibited SSA-DH [227]. On the other hand, branched analogues *(139)* where X is CH_2 or NH, were convulsants [228].

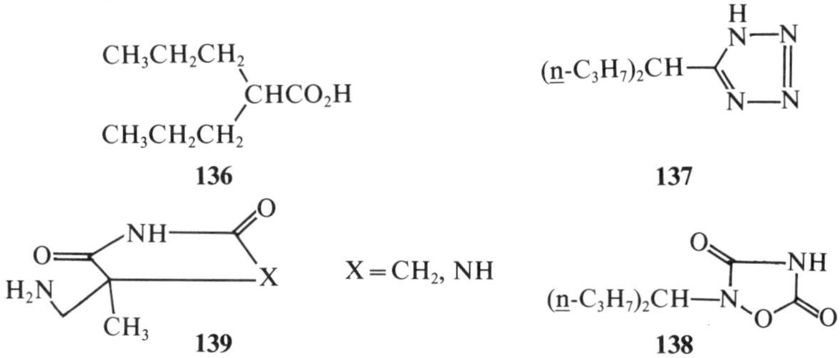

136   137

139   X = CH_2, NH   138

The inhibitory action on aromatic ring glycolic oxidase by the α, β-unsaturated α-hydroxy-γ-keto acid *140* and the 3-hydroxypyrroleine-2,5-dione *141* shows two partially superimposable compounds with the same biochemical behavior [229].

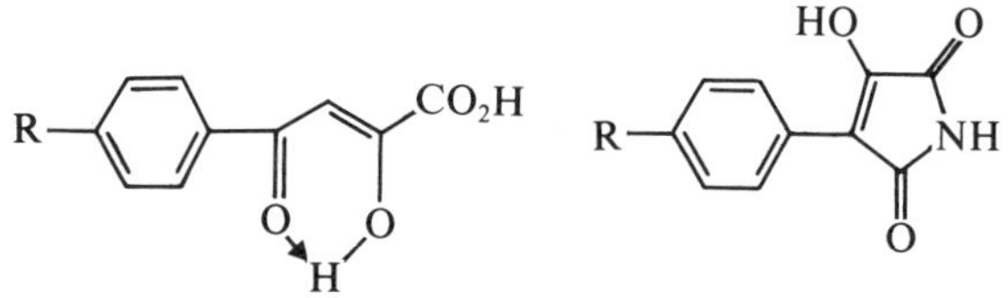

140   141

Not all replacements of carboxyl need to be actually or potentially acidic. The typically analgesic-antiinflammatory 2-arylpropionic acid, ketoprofen *(142)* can have its carboxyl exchanged by the basic morpholinomethylene group without loss of cyclooxygenase inhibitory activity *(143)* [230].

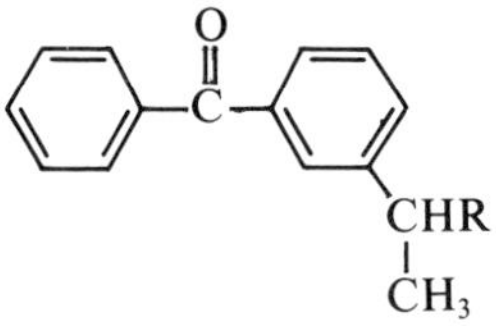

142: R = CO₂H

143: R = CH₂N⟩O

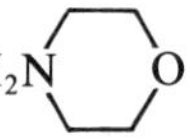

1.8.6   Amide and peptide bioisosteres

Bioisosteric changes of carboxamides follow most of the alterations studied with carboxylic acids. The group -C(=O)NH- permits such permutations as -SO₂NH-, -C(=S)NH-, -CH₂NH-, and reversal of such structural fragments as in -NH-CO- (procaine versus lidocaine-type amides), or insertion of a spacer ring such as phenylene in a process referred to as arenology. Other spacer groups are -CH=CH- and other conjugating systems. In recent years, such changes have assumed intriguing aspects for the bioisosteric treatment of peptides, polypeptide antibiotics, hormones, and even biocatalytic enzymes and antibodies [231–233]. Apart from disulfide bridges, the conformation of a peptide is affected by the side chains of the participating amino acids and by resulting hydrogen bonds which tie overlaying but sequentially separate portions of the peptide chain together. This leads to the globular rolling-up of most biologically involved peptides with their ring formation, bay-like structures and other architectural characteristics which lend biological specificity to these peptides.

It is therefore of interest to alter both the side chains and the backbone of the peptides and to investigate any biochemical changes that can be attributed to such modifications. Such compounds have been called peptidomimetics [234], and can be regarded as bioisosteres of peptides. They can be synthesized by solid-phase methods using bioisosteric bifunctional acids or unnatural, heterocyclic, or enantiomeric amino acids at proper intervals. For example, phenyllactic acid, $C_6H_5CH_2CHOHCO_2H$ (OH→ NH₂ exchange), will give rise to esters, -NHCHRCOOCH($CH_2C_6H_5$)CO₂H, which can then be used in additional peptide construction. Such isosteric peptidomimetics fulfill two functions. One is increased resistance to hydrolysis by peptidases, although this may be counterbalanced by a greater sensitivity to esterases in this example. But monofunctional carboxylic acids such as cinnamic acid ($C_6H_5CH = CHCO_2H$) can initiate a peptide chain at position 1 and gain resistance to peptidases.

The second function of bioisosteric peptides would be improved conformational complementarity at active sites of enzymes or receptors, which might facilitate docking of the peptide drug. This is still in early phases of investigation because the three-dimensional structures of only few active sites have been determined. Taking into account the exquisite specificity of antibodies, and the genetic availability of vast numbers of antibodies, peptide modification of antigens and antibodies should hold great promise.

1.8.7   Coordination isosteres [235]

Coordinating agents or chelating agents are formed from primary, secondary and tertiary amines, imines, oximes, thioethers, ketones and thioketones, alcohols, and other hydrogen-bond forming groups. Many natural biologically active materials, e. g. insulin, hemoglobin, myoglobin, chlorophyll, cobalamine, and many enzymes are chelates. They have many vital functions: catalysis of redox reactions, oxygen transport, the biosynthesis of proteins, proteolysis, CO_2 transport by carbonic anhydrase, reactions in which pyridoxal phosphate participates, etc. Chelating agents can destroy parasitic microbes by removing metal ions essential for microbial life (isoniazid, tetracycline), or they can withdraw harmful metal ions from tissues as seen in dimercaprol, penicillamine, and such sequestering agents as ethylenediaminetetracetic acid (EDTA). Compounds which enhance or antagonize these activities by affecting ligating ability can be regarded as coordination isosteres. Antibiotics of the valinomycin family which transport metal ions across membranes by enclosing them in macrocycles, and other complexes formed by synthetic molecular hosts [236] could be interpreted in this manner.

1.8.8   Phenols

Phenols are weak acids but their ionization is stepped up by the presence of electron-attracting groups. Phenolic compounds have been varied by substituting other weakly ionized groups for the phenolic hydroxyl. The most popular bioisosteric substituents are methanesulf-amide (CH$_3$SO$_2$NH-), hydroxymethyl (HOCH$_2$-) or hydroxyisopropyl [HOC(CH$_3$)$_2$-], various amide groups (-NHCHO, -NHCOCH$_3$, -NHCOC$_6$H$_5$) etc., methanesulfamidomethyl (CH$_3$SO$_2$NHCH$_2$-), di-methylaminosulfonamide, (CH$_3$)$_2$NSO$_2$NH-, and others with an ioniz-able proton next to, or near an aromatic ring. These groups should be not much larger than hydroxyl, they should have the same approx-imate acidity range, form hydrogen bonds and, on occasion, redox systems, in conjunction with a *p*-OH. To some extent, these require-ments are fulfilled by -NHCN and -CH(CN)$_2$ in which the electron-withdrawing nitrile groups increase protonation [224]. Examples of such drugs are R-albuterol *(144)*, a *β*-selective adrenergic bronchodi-lator [237], and the *β*-receptor stimulant, soterenol *(145)* [238].

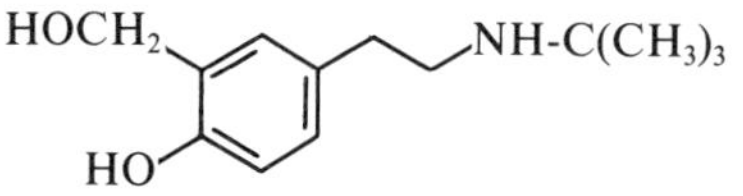

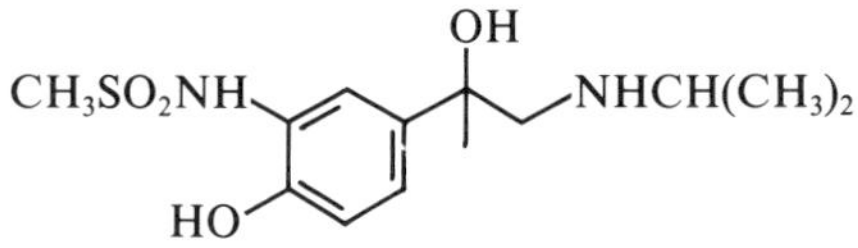

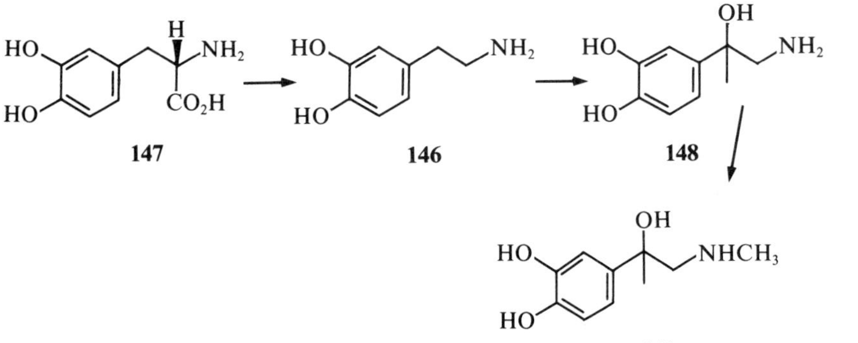

Catechols have been the targets of many attempts to place one or two other groups in their *o*-(OH)$_2$ positions. The reason for these experi-ments has been the potential oxidizability of catechols to *ortho* qui-nones, with a concomitant loss of their original biological purpose. Another reason is found in the frequent and annoying gastrointestinal side effects of catecholic drugs which limit their medicinal utility. Dopamine *(146)* is the neurohormone responsible for normal motor activity. It is formed in the corpus striatum in the brain by decarboxy-lation of *L*-dopa *(147)* under the influence of aromatic *L*-amino acid decarboxylase. The same biosynthesis occurs also in peripheral tissues, especially in the kidney. Dopamine is an intermediate in the biosynthesis of norepinephrine *(148)* and thereby also of epinephrine *(149)*. The pK_a values of dopamine are 9.06, 10.60 and 12.05. Its log *P* in 1-octanol buffer at pH 7.4 is -2.36.

Only agonists and antagonists of the catecholamines will be contemplated here which have, in the widest sense, a bioisosteric relationship to the natural prototype structures. Compounds which, by virtue of divergent mechanisms, act as agonists or antagonists of catecholamines will be excluded because their chemical relationship is tenuous. At least two dopamine receptors, DA_1 and DA_2 receptors, are being distinguished. Among antagonists to these receptors, there are several neuroleptics of the phenothiazine and butyrophenone types [239],

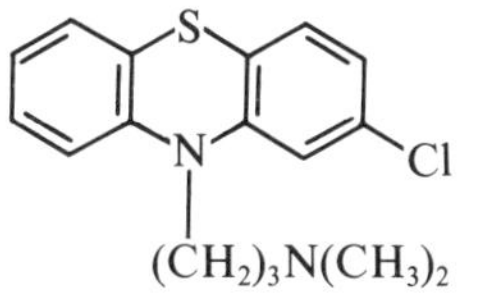

150 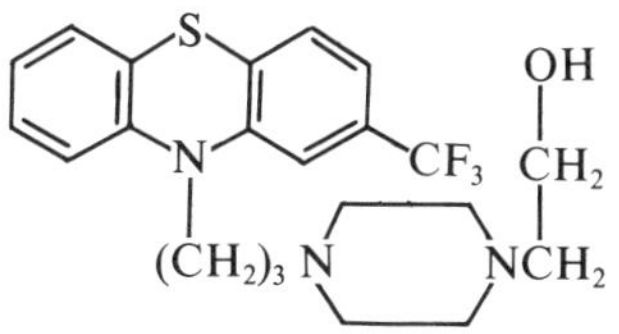   **151** 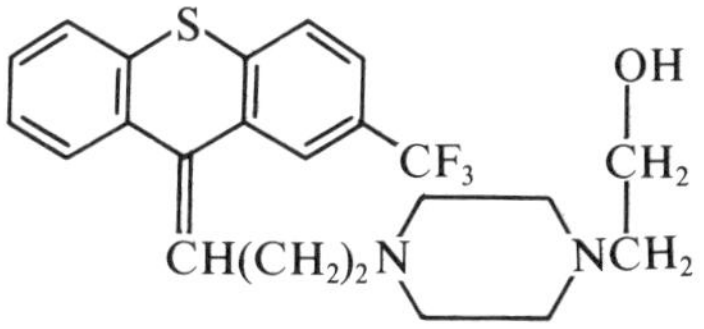   **152**

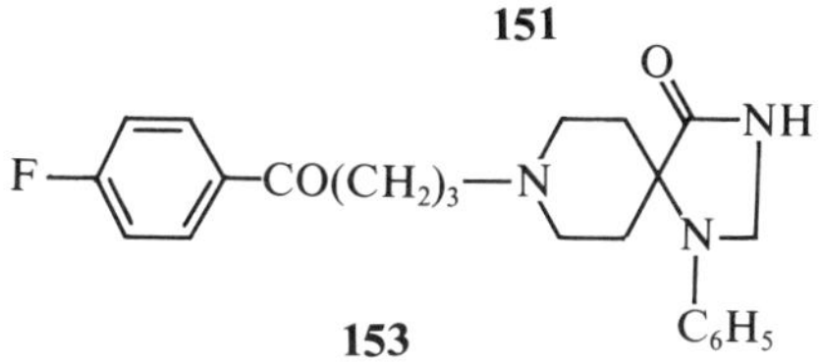

153

among them chlorpromazine *(150)*, fluphenazine *(151)*, and the thioxanthene, *cis-α*-flupenthixol *(152)* as well as butyrophenone neuroleptics such as haloperidol *(88)* and spiperone *(153)*. It has been suggested that the N.......N chains of the phenothiazine neuroleptics can span the HO......NH distance of dopamine and thus induce receptor blockade. The same could be true for the C=O......N stretch of butyrophenones but this picture of bioisosterism has remained unclear. The available data on central and peripheral adrenergic neurotransmitters and their autocoid receptors have been reviewed [240].

The antiarrhythmic drug, moricizine *(154)* apparently defies bioisosterism. This phenothiazine derivative contains a nuclear carbamate substituent but otherwise does not differ too widely from phenothiazine neuroleptics. However, its biological activity is different. It slows the initial bursts of electrical firing in Purkinje fiber cells and speeds

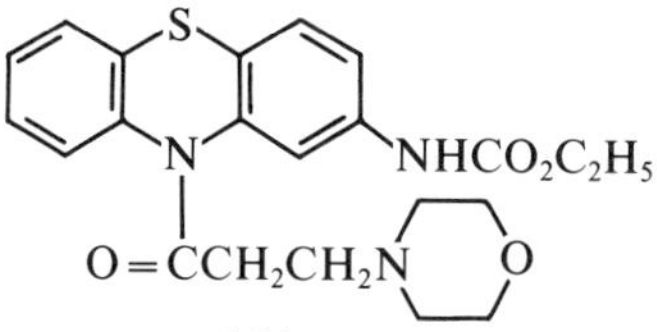

154

up the re-setting of the cells for re-firing. This is valuable in suppressing ventricular arrhythmias.

The structure of catechol *(155)* itself can be replaced by analogous heterocycles in various derivatives *(156, 157, 158, 159)* [138]. All these compounds share the ability to chelate metal atoms and to form hydrogen-bonded second rings; the benzimidazole *156* imitates this by way of a covalent ring structure. Such ring potentials are not restricted

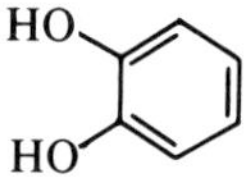

155 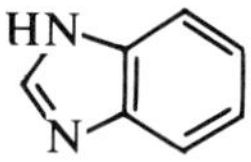   **156** 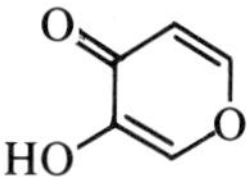   **157** 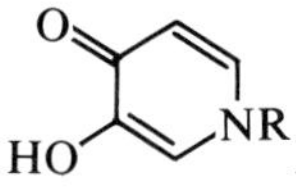   **158** 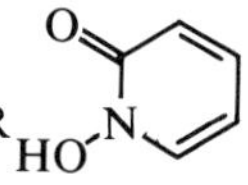   **159**

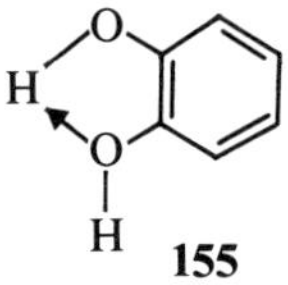

155 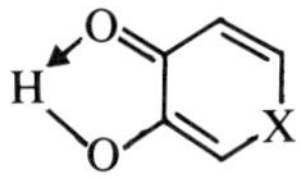   **157, 158** 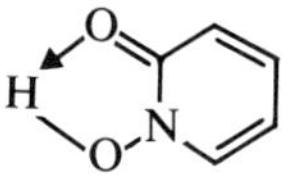   **159**

to aromatic catechol analogues. The β-adrenergic blocking agent, nadolol *(160)*, contains an alicyclic diol arrangement.

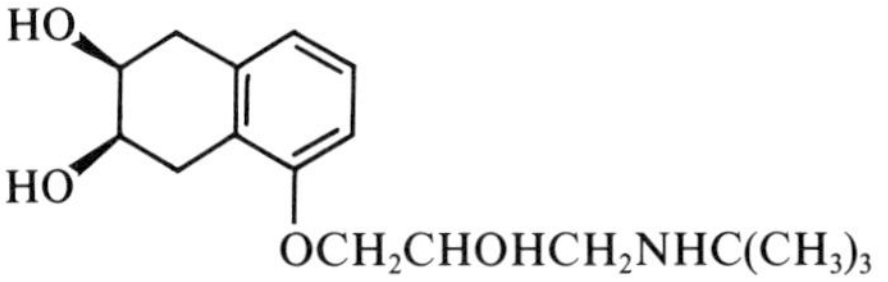

OCH₂CHOHCH₂NHC(CH₃)₃

160

The interplay of medicinal chemistry and pharmacology has been particularly fruitful in the study of catecholamine receptors, of agonists and antagonists of these multiple receptor systems, the delineation of SAR and bioisosteres, and the discovery of new medicinal agents of adequate specificity. One of the structural characteristics that has held up well in these investigations is the steric restriction of the -C-C-N chain by incorporating it in inflexible rings. This is shown best in apomorphine *(161)*, the most widely studied standard of dopamine agonists. Some more or less related analogues in which some of the phenolic hydroxyls have been transferred to cyclic imino functions include pergolide *(162)* in which the rigid -C-C-N group has the same conformation as in apomorphine [241]. Many other bioisosteric variations with the same conformational rigidity are cited in reference [138], p. 569.

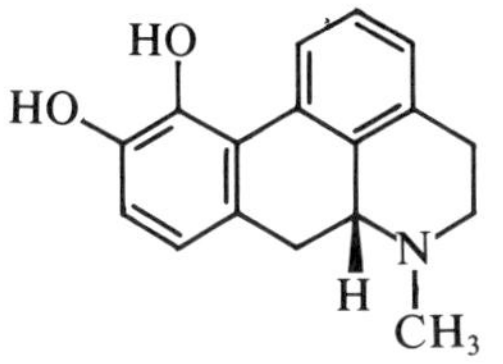

161 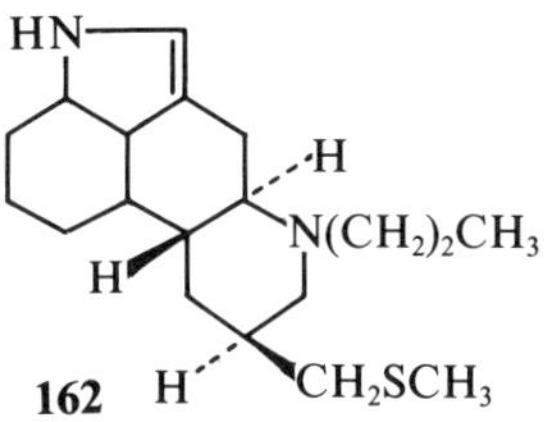   **162**

The ring compounds, 2-amino-6,7-dihydroxytetralin *(163)* (242, 243), 2-amino-4,5-dihydroxyindanes *(164)* [244], 6-amino-1,2-dihydroxy-benzocycloheptene *(165)* [245], (+)*trans* N-propyloctahydrobenzo (*f*)hydroxy-oxaquinoline *(166)* [246], ergoline *(167)*, 4-aminobenz[c, d]indole *(168)* [247], fenoldopam *(169)* [244, 247], nomifensin *(170)* [244], and [1R, 3S] 7-aminomethyl-5,6-dihydroxy-3-phenylisochroman *(171)*[248] illustrate additional cases of conformational similarity in the catecholamine series.

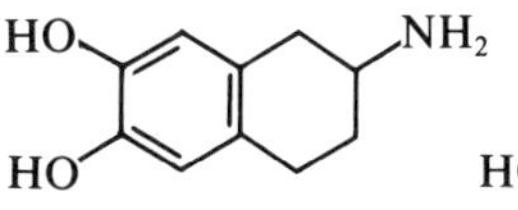

163 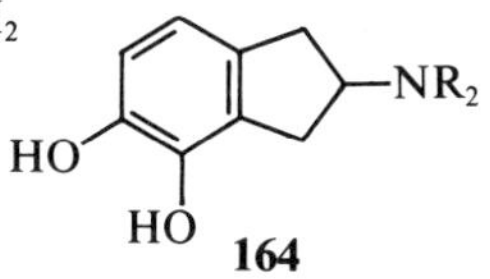   **164** 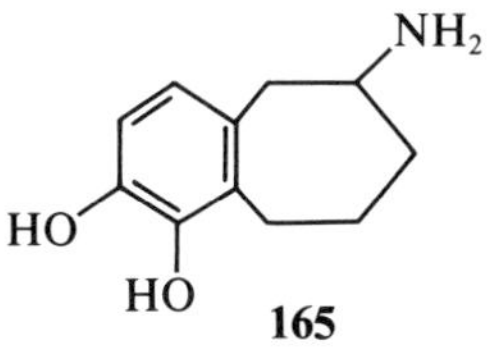   **165**

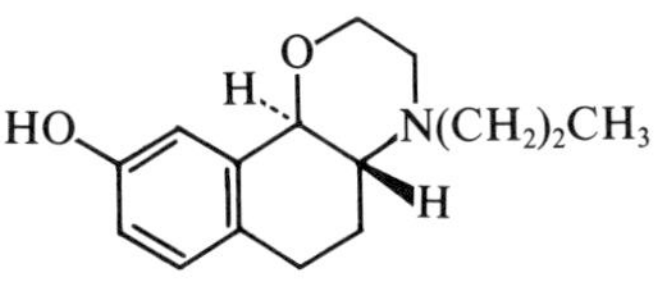

166 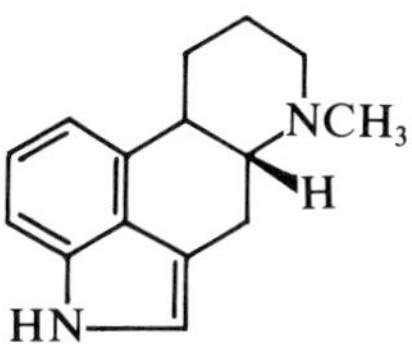   **167** 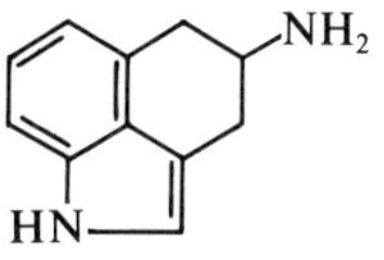   **168**

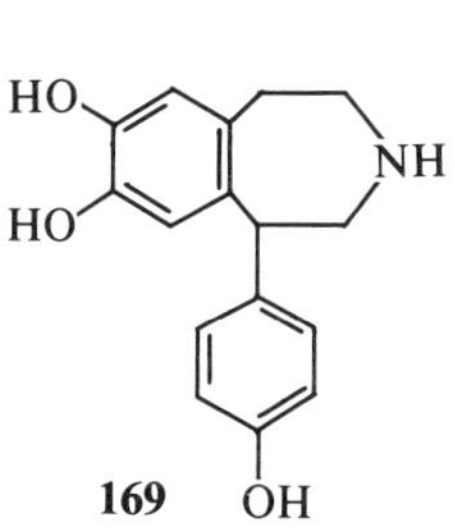

169 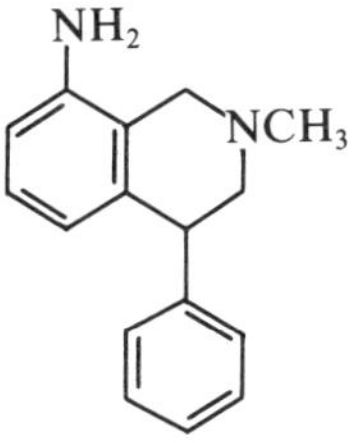   170 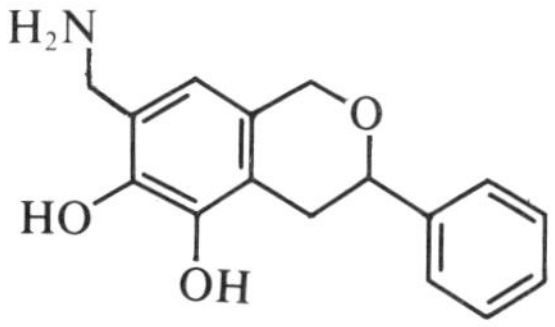   171

In ganglionic blocking agents an old procedure to increase biological activity has been the doubling of functional groups and connecting them through a "spacer" chain as in hexamethonium (172), decamethonium (173), their homologs and sulfonium bioisosteres. In the dopamine series, such "bissing" resulted in the selection of the unsymmetrical dopexamine (174) as a selective dopamine₁ receptor and adrenoceptor antagonist [249, 250].

$(H_3C)_3N^+$-$(CH_2)_n$-$N^+(CH_3)_3$

n = 6: 172

n = 10: 173

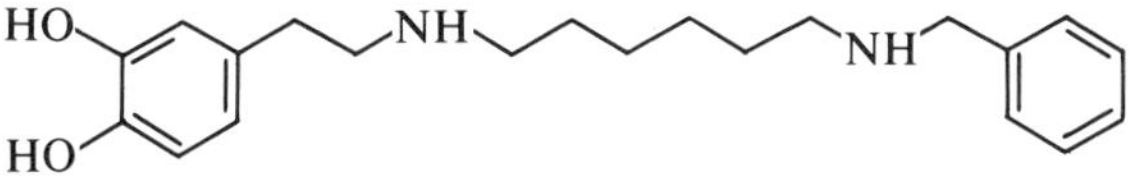

174

As seen in these examples, the phenolic hydroxyls are not required for dopaminergic activity. However, in all compounds that are active at dopamine receptors, the nitrogen atom must be protonated.

1.8.9   Divalent and sulfonium sulfur

The charged nitrogen of dopaminergic compounds can be replaced by permanently charged sulfur (175, 176, 177) with retention of activity

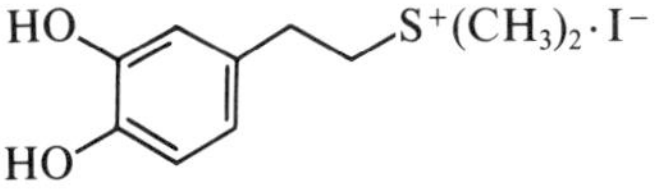

175 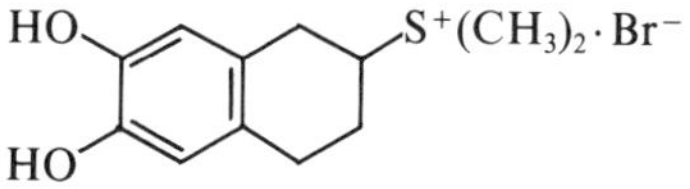   176

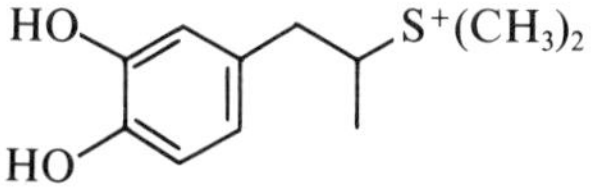

177

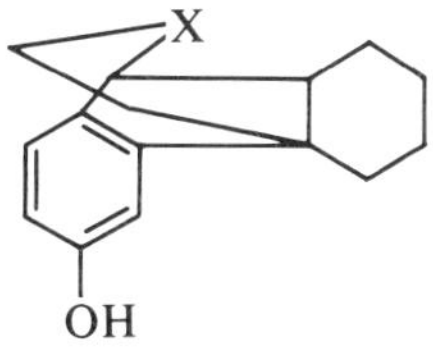

X = NCH$_3$: **179**
X = S$^+$CH$_3$: **178**

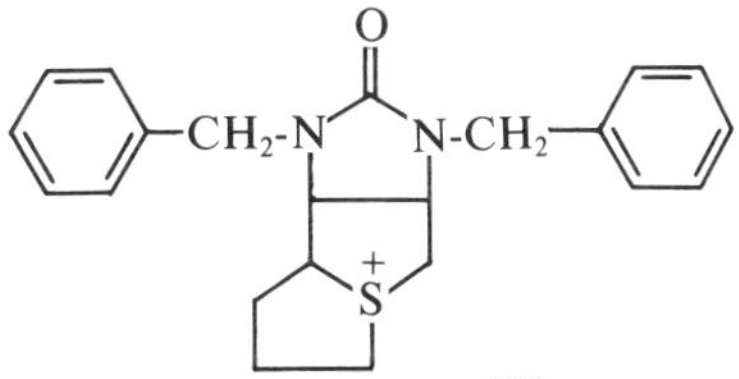

180

[248, 251]. The sulfonium bioisostere *178* of the potent analgesic, isole-vorphanol *(179)* has also been prepared and tested [252].

Ganglionic blocking agents traditionally contain ammonium ions but sulfonium achieves the same activity in trimethaphan *(180)* [253].

Divalent sulfur has been used repeatedly to replace oxygen and methylene (-CH$_2$-), and two-carbon bridges can also be exchanged for thioether groups bioisosterically. This is seen in the relationship of imipramine *(45)* to promazine *(44)* and in the tetrahydrofuran and tetrahydrothiophene rings of ring-A modified androgens *(181)*[254]. Other groups such as >NCN *(182)* can take the place of sulfur.

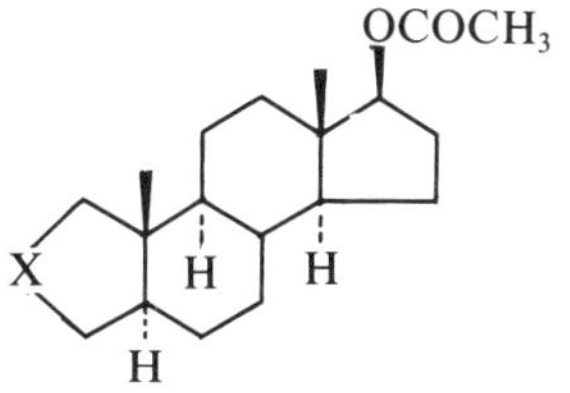

181: X = O,S 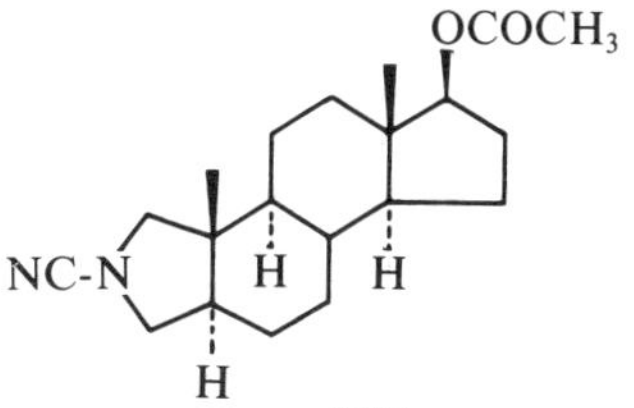   **182**

It is the steric, rather than the electronic, properties of the oxygen or sulfur ring atoms that are the determinants of pharmacological activity. In aza steroids the basic nitrogen often gives rise to biologically inactive compounds either by virtue of its high electron density or by formation of a cationic center. These effects are cancelled out in the cyanoazo derivative *182,* which is truly bioisosteric with the thia compound *181;* its androgenic activity is only slightly weaker than that of *181* (X = S).

Replacement of methylene by divalent sulfur (thioether) has been probed extensively in histamine H$_2$ receptor antagonists. These researches have been reviewed comprehensively [255]. Starting with the premise that such inhibitors should have a component containing imidazole like histamine *(183)* itself, some likely derivatives with modified side chains *(184, 185)* were examined. These side chains were to bind to the receptors more strongly than histamine and for this purpose were equipped with a guanidine group *(184)* [256] or its thiourea isostere in place of the amino group of histamine.

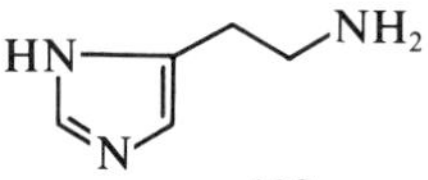

$$HN\text{—}\underset{N}{\overset{}{\boxed{}}}\text{—}CH_2CH_2\text{—}NH_2$$

183

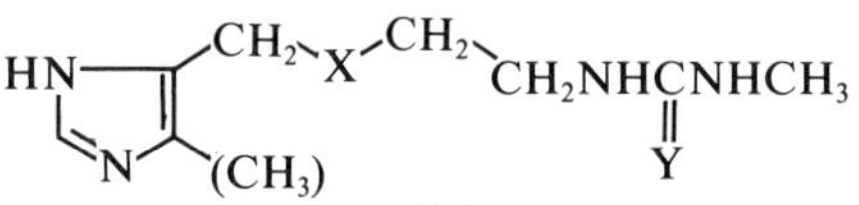

$$HN\text{—}\underset{N}{\overset{CH_2\diagdown X\diagup CH_2\diagdown}{\boxed{}}}_{(CH_3)}CH_2NH\underset{Y}{\overset{\parallel}{C}}NHCH_3 \qquad HN\text{—}\underset{N}{\overset{CH_2\diagdown X\diagup CH_2\diagdown}{\boxed{}}}_{(CH_3)}CH_2NH\underset{S}{\overset{\parallel}{C}}NHCH_3$$

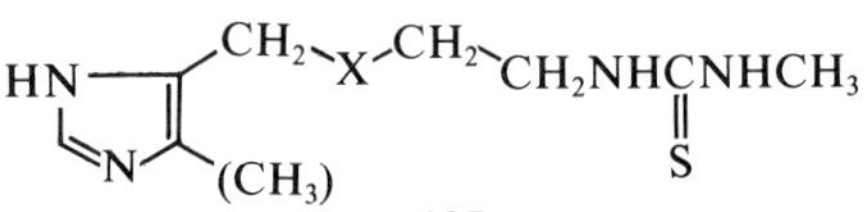

184   **185**
X = CH₂   X = CH₂, O, S
Y = NH

Even in these carefully planned modifications some 200 structural analogues were prepared and tested before burimamide *(186)* was chosen for clinical trials. The 4-carbon side chain was selected because systematic molecular modifications revealed that potency increased when the side chain was lengthened. Burimamide was not potent enough in the clinic and further modifications were contemplated. At this point it was remembered that in another series, that of β-adrenergic receptor inhibitors, interspersion of the traditional adrenergic side chain, ArCHOHCH₂NHR, by oxymethylene, ArOCH₂CHOHCH₂NHR, had led to highly active inhibitors such as propranolol *(187)*.

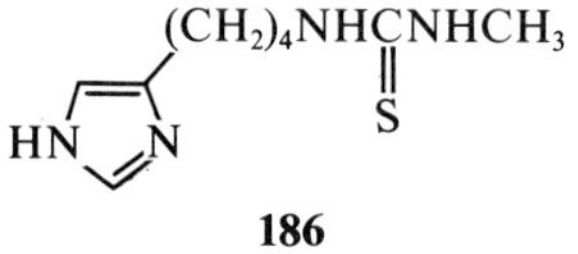

$$\underset{HN\diagdown N}{\overset{(CH_2)_4NH\underset{S}{\overset{\parallel}{C}}NHCH_3}{\boxed{}}} \qquad \underset{HN\diagdown N}{\overset{H_3C\qquad CH_2SCH_2CH_2NH\underset{S}{\overset{\parallel}{C}}NHCH_3}{\boxed{}}}$$

186 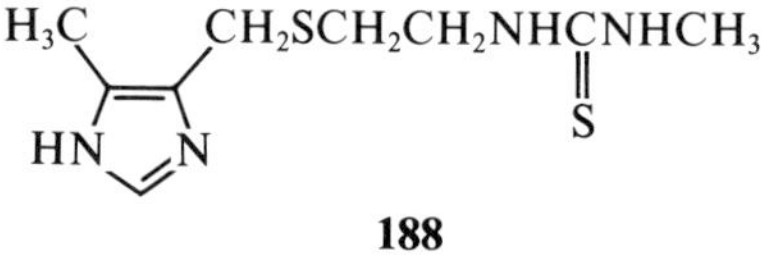   **188**

$$\overset{OCH_2\text{-}CHOHCH_2NHCH(CH_3)_2}{\boxed{}}$$

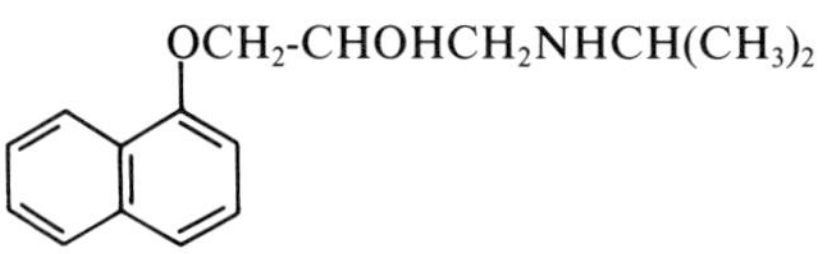

187

A similar change of the -(CH₂)₄NHC(=Y)NHR chain was applied to an isosteric replacement of a methylene by oxygen, and then by sulfur which furnished more potent derivatives (metiamide, *188*). This again produced some unacceptable clinical side effects which were attributed to the thiourea group. A guanidine group was tried, especially with electron-withdrawing substituents such as NH-C-($=$NCN)-NHR and NH-C-($=$NNO$_2$)-NHR; the group $=$CHNO$_2$ was also examined. In separate experiments the classical isosterism of thiourea and cyanoguanidine was established by comparing their proton dissociation (weakly amphoteric), polarity (dipole moments), partition log P between octanol and water, solubility characteristics, and planar geometry measurements [255, p. 387]. On the basis of these encouraging data, the cyanoguanidine derivative, cimetidine *(189)* was developed as an antiulcer drug.

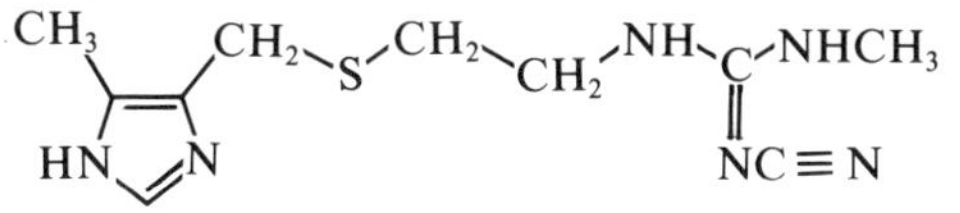

189

Subsequently, the need for a C-methyl-substituted imidazole moiety, originally thought de rigeur, had to be abandoned when H$_2$ receptor antagonism was discovered in compounds with other ring systems, for example, isothiazole, thiazole, oxazole, pyridine, furan and even benzene. In all these cases, ether or thioether-containing side chains with basic functions weakened by electron-withdrawing groups are optimal, and in the furan and benzene analogues the nitrogen functionality can be exocyclic. The four drugs *(190–193)* are used in medicine but represent only hundreds of analogues synthesized during their development. They are ranitidine *(190)*, famotidine *(191)*, nizatidine *(192)*, and roxatidine *(193)*. Roxatidine *(193)* is an example of

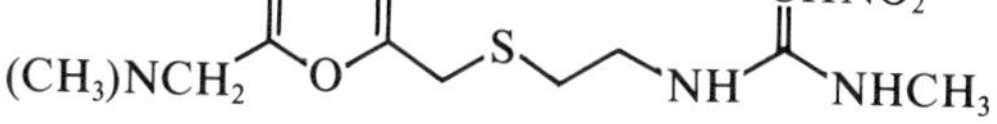

190

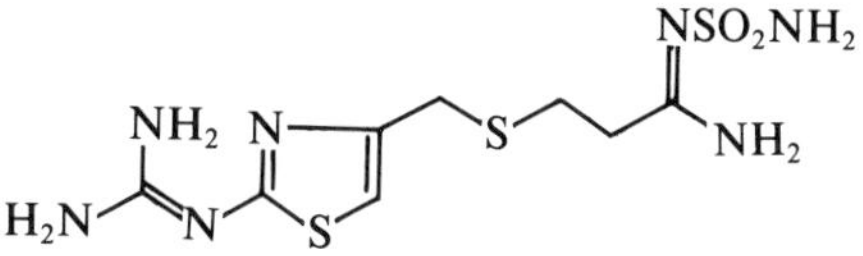

191

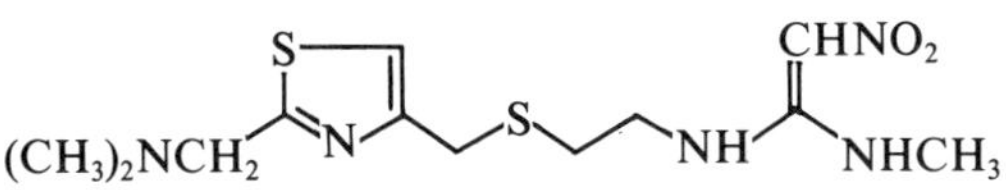

192

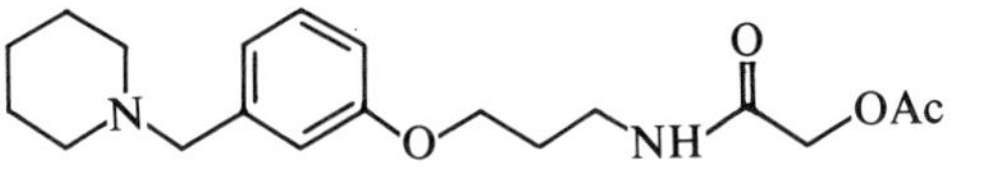

193

bioisosterism of *192*. The benzene ring carries a methylpiperidino group, and the phenoxy-attached side chain contains an amide group of acetyl glycolate.

1.8.10   Methine-nitrogen

Bioisosteres (agonists as well as antagonists) have been found in many ring systems in which $-CH=$ is exchanged for $-N=$. That is the relationship of benzene and pyridine, but also of pyridine and diazines, triazines and similar aromatic heterocycles. The ring nitrogen atoms strongly attract electrons which have to be furnished by the aromatically shared ring electrons and, if possible, by substituents such as $-NH_2$, $-OH$, $-OCH_3$, halogens, etc. This localization of electrons progressively weakens the aromatic character and that in turn will be manifest in changes in biological properties that depend on ring-substituent tautomerism.

One such property of altered reactivity may underlie the ability of certain sulfanilamides to withstand metabolic attack. Two isomeric dimethoxypyrimidyl sulfanilamides, sulfadimethoxine *(199)* and sulfadoxine *(200)*, remain antibacterially active for 60–100 hours before they are metabolized or excreted. Since the detoxifying removal of many other sulfanilamides is initiated by N^4-acetylation, steric hindrance cannot be invoked for these two drugs but rather an effect propagated through the aminopyrimidine system must be involved in the longevity of the compounds [257–259]. Sulfadimethoxine is acetylated to about 10 %, excreted intact to about 15 %, and is principally conjugated as the glucuronide [260].

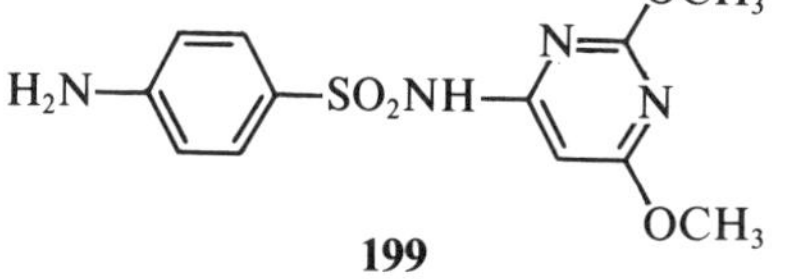

199

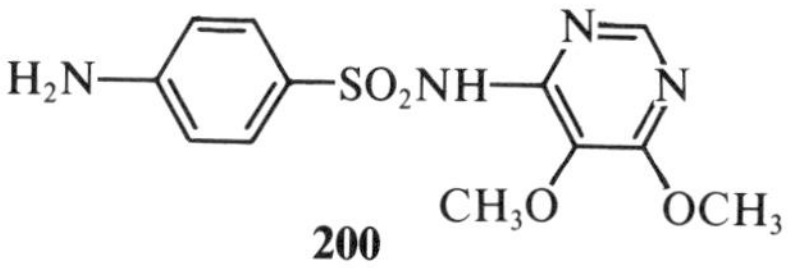

200

In a series of bioisosteres of 5-hydroxytryptophan, the 1,2-oxazine analogue *201* weakly inhibited 5-hydroxytryptophan decarboxylase. In

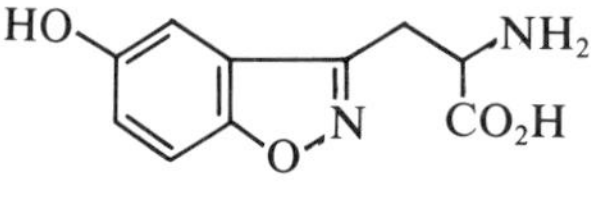

201

classical isosteres of 5-hydroxytryptamine (5-HT, serotonin) the in-
dole-imino group was shown to be essential for several biochemical
properties. Replacement of the cyclic NH by CH_2 inhibited the oxidation of 5-HT and norepinephrine by the enzyme, ceruloplasmin. Exchange of NH for oxygen caused only inhibition of 5-HT oxidation,
and the benzothiophene isostere (S for NH) was quite inactive [262].

1.8.11   Amino – hydroxyl isosteres

The hydroxyl and amino groups are in column 4 of Grimm's Table
and should be classical isosteres. They are both electron donors and
both orient primarily *ortho-para* in aromatic rings. In heterocyclic systems containing electron-donating atoms such as N, C-OH will tau-
tomerize to $C=O$ *(194)* while amino nitrogen will remain largely in
the C-NH_2 state *(195)*. On the other hand, nitrogen (-N, -NH_2, -NHR,
-NR_2) forms hydrogen bonds and coordinates metal ions more easily
than oxygen (-O-, -OH, -OR); this ability decreases if bulky substituents crowd the N or O atoms, but may be important biochemically in
the existence of coordination isosteres [218].

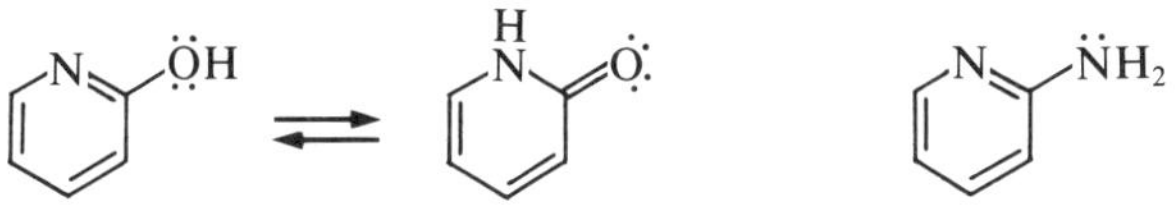

194   **195**

The alcoholic hydroxyl dissociates less than the phenolic hydroxyl,
and the aromatic amino group is less basic than its aliphatic counterpart. Nevertheless, phenol and many of its homologs destroy microbes and proteinogenous tissues, whereas aniline is a relatively non-
descript, perhaps mutagenic base. On the whole, OH and NH_2, or OR
and NR_2 analogues are more often bioantagonistic than bioisosteric in
a positive sense. Aminopterin *(197)* and by extension methotrexate
(198) are powerful antagonists of pteroylglutamic (folic) acid *(196)*
and interfere with the role of folate in nucleoside synthesis,

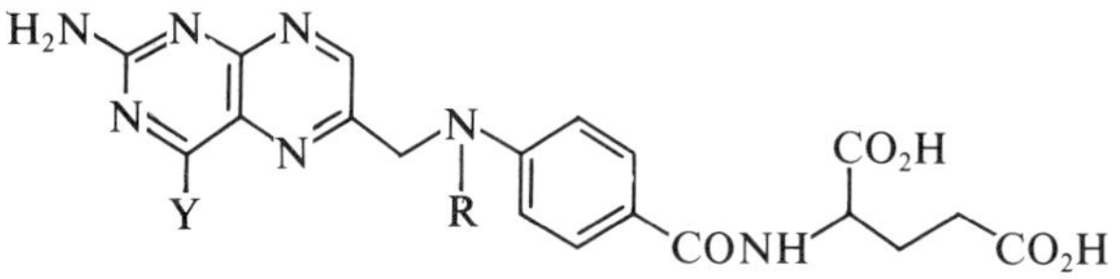

196: Y = OH, R = H
197: Y = NH_2, R = H
198: Y = NH_2, R = CH_3

1.9   Other nitrogen isosteres
1.9.1   Cyclic nitrogen compounds

Pyridine is sometimes compared to nitrobenzene in chemical substitution characteristics because electrons of both rings are drawn away, causing positions 2, 4 und 6 to be more electron-deficient than the *meta* 3- and 5-positions. An application to bioisosterism can be seen in the comparison of N,N-diethyl-3-nitrobenzamide *(199)* and nikethamide *(200)*. These two amides have similar analeptic properties [263] while N,N-diethyl-*p*-nitrobenzamide is inactive.

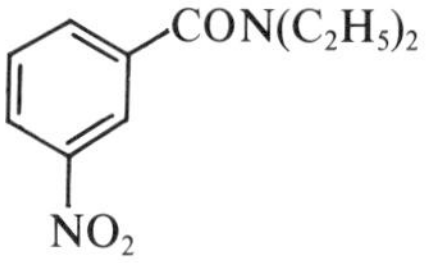

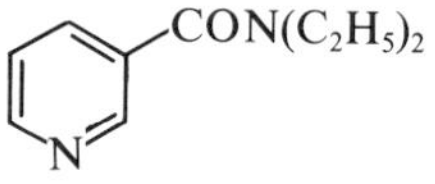

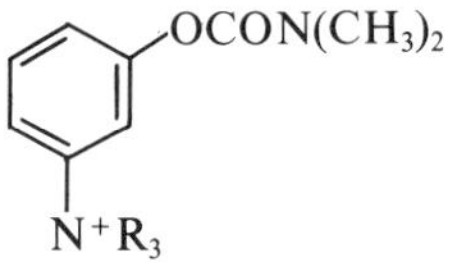

If the pyridinium nitrogen is quaternized, the resulting compounds *(202)* resemble the corresponding anilinium ions *(201)* in cholinergic properties [264, 265].

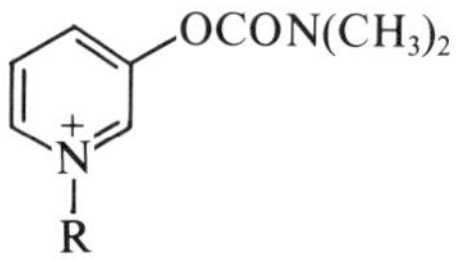

Ring size may be less important if other molecular distances become more significant. In a comparison of the cardiotonic agents, *203* and *204*, pyridine is equated with imidazole. Imazodan *(203)* is a dihydro-

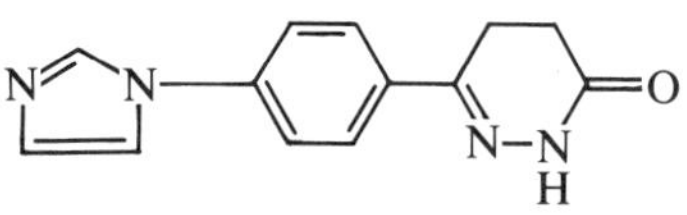

pyridazinone carrying a hydrogen bond acceptor site (an imidazole nitrogen) three atoms removed from the benzene ring; the *p*-(3-pyridyl)phenyldihydropyridazinone *204* possesses a nitrogen (in the pyridine ring) at the same distance but the molecular framework through

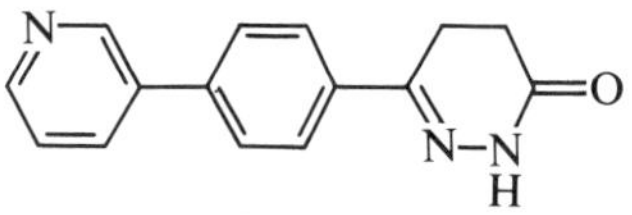

which it is connected (-N=CH-C-) versus that of *203* (-N=CH-N-) has been altered. Both compounds exhibit a high degree of inotropic activity [266]. Bioisosterism of imidazole and pyridine has also been noted in the development of thromboxane synthetase inhibitors [267–269].

The comparison of pyridine and aniline carries over to some arsenical drugs. Oxophenarsine *(205)* and its pyridine analogue *(206)* are both

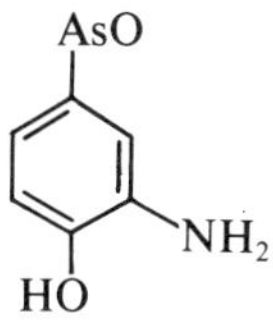

205 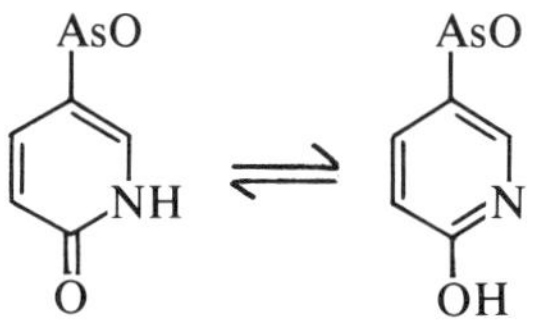   **206** 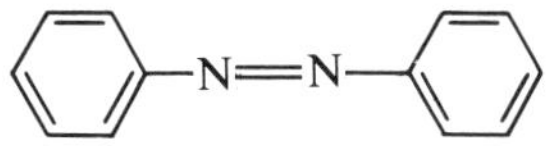   **209**

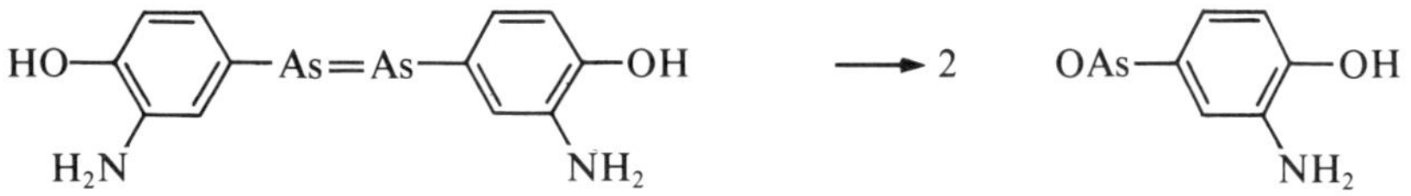

207   **208**

treponecidal [41, 270, 271]. It is not clear, however, whether this analogy is to be explained by electronic factors or by the presence of the arsenoxy group.

Arsenic is a classical bioisostere of nitrogen. Arsenoxides are usually spirocheticidal, and many nitroso compounds, especially nitrosoureas, inhibit the multiplication of malignant cells. On the other hand, many azo dyestuffs are carcinogens while arsenic isosteres such as arsphenamine *(207)* are spirocheticidal. However, this activity is probably due to their metabolic oxidation products, the arsenoxides *(208)*. Azobenzene itself *(209)* kills ascarides and is used to keep greenhouses free of these nematodes.

Nitroimidazoles such as metronidazole *(210)* and nitrofurans are drugs of value in the treatment of several protozoal diseases as well of infections due to anaerobic bacteria. Reduction of the nitro group is obligatory for the emergence of therapeutic activity. Obviously, reduction of the nitro group to NH_2 proceeds stepwise, and it may be surmised that intermediate reduction products such as the corresponding nitroso derivatives *(211)* should be closer to the end products of the reduction sequence *(212)*. Using *Escherichia coli* strain SR 58 whose defective DNA repair system makes it sensitive to metronidazole, it has been found indeed that the nitroso compounds are

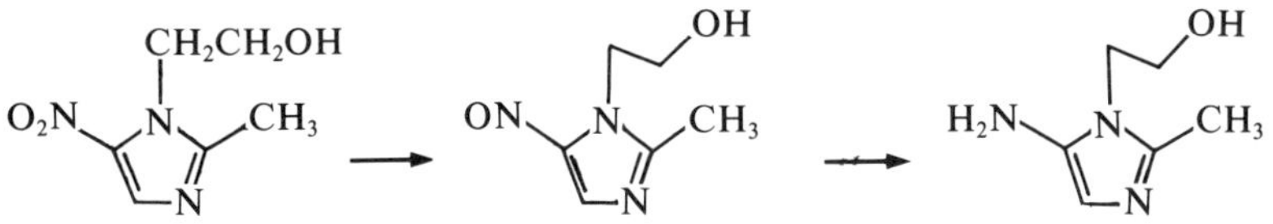

210   **211**   **212**

significantly more bactericidal than the corresponding nitro derivatives [272], perhaps due to the ability of the mutant to reduce *211* to
212.

The great interest created by the therapeutic success of *L*-dopa as a
pro-drug for dopamine in the treatment of Parkinsonism stimulated
searches for dopa isosteres that might have fewer of the limiting side
effects of dopa. Among such analogues were hydroxypyridine and
pyridinequinoid-type compounds *(213, 214, 215)* with aminoprop-
ionic acid chains attached to isomeric positions of the ring [273–276].

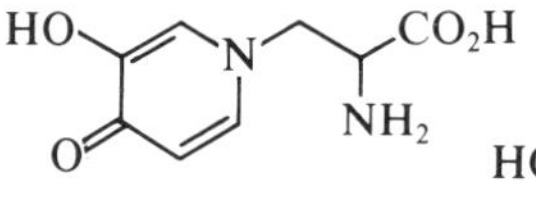

213	**216**	**217**

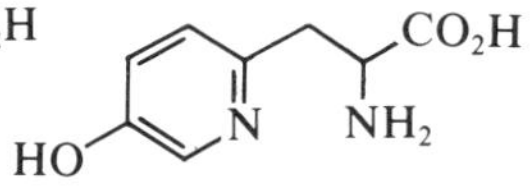

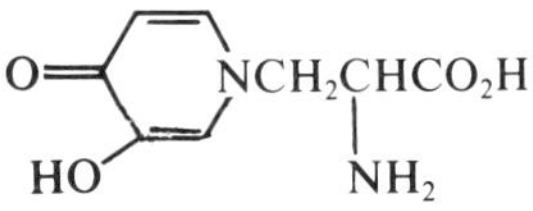

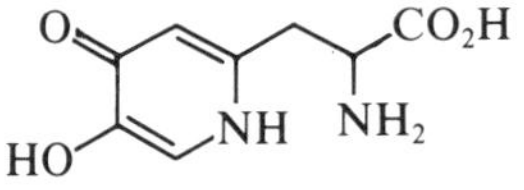

214	**215**

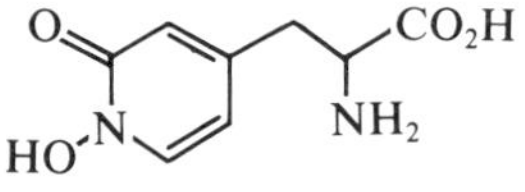

The tyrosine analogue *216* is a natural product obtained from *Streptomyces* species [274]. Mimosine (leucenol, *217*) is an amino acid [273]
found in the seeds and foliage of legume genera *Mimosa* and *Leucena*
[277]. It causes loss of hair growth in mice [278].

A hydroxypyridine ring has been constructed for a bioisostere *(218)* of
adrenergic hormone agonists [243].

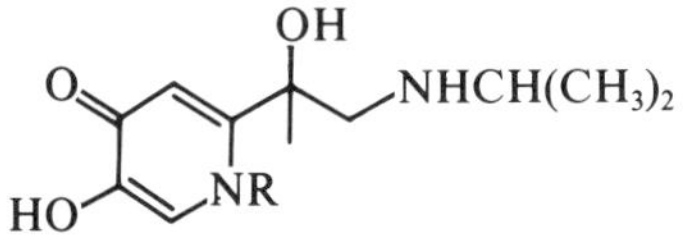

218	**219**

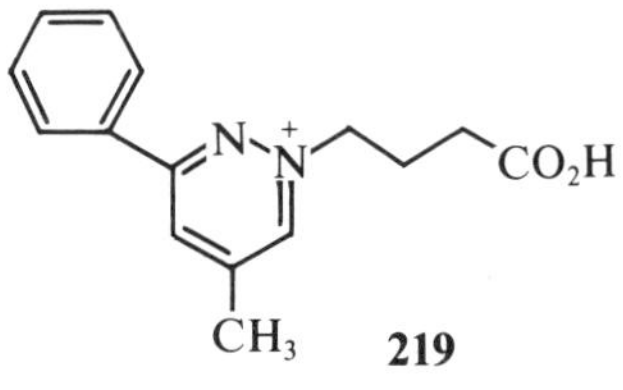

Introduction of a second nitrogen in pyridine leads to isomeric diazines. Among early diazine drugs were sulfonamides which carried a
diazine ring, substituted or non-substituted, on the sulfonamide
group. In other series of bioactive diazines was *219* in which a substituted pyridazinium ion took the place of ammonium in a GABA
chain. This compound is a GABA agonist [279].

The most widely studied diazines are the pyrimidines and their con-

densed-ring companions, the purines, which constitute the basic portions of nucleotides. Many analogues of the nucleic acid constituents
are bioisosteric antagonists of enzymes in natural nucleoside and nucleotide chemistry. See section 2.1.

The mesoionic pyridazine analogue *221* of 3-deazauridine *(220)* exhibits antibacterial properties [280] but here the phenolic OH has also
been altered.

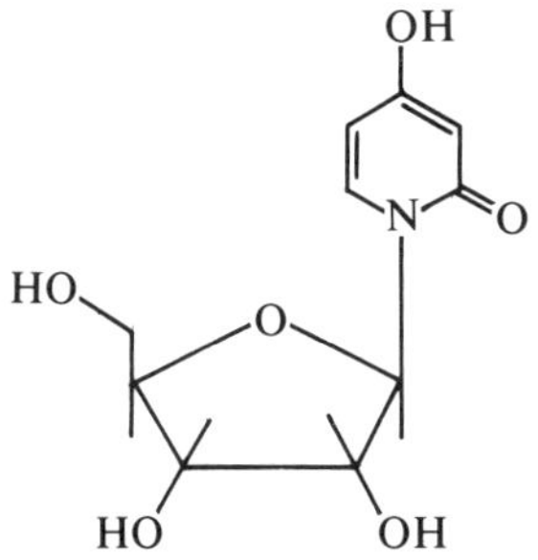

220 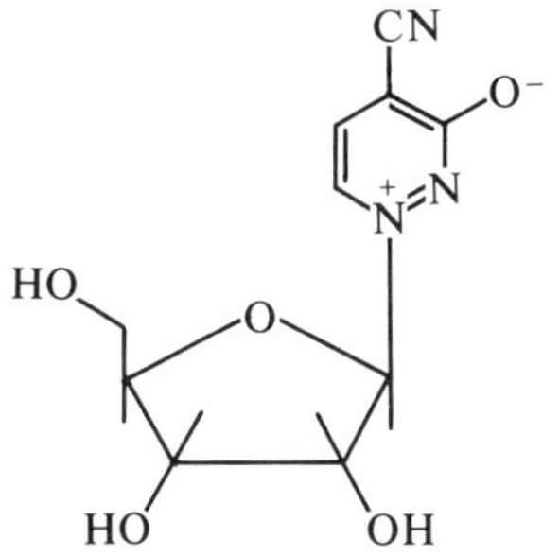   **221**

This particular change (OH to CN) was ineffective when the amide
carbonyl was maintained in the pyridone ring ($> N\text{-}CO\text{-}$) or changed
to $> N\text{-}CH =$ [281]. Other replacements of carbonyl by $> C = C(CN)_2$
and $-CH(CN)-$ bear some similarity to the 3-deazauridine case [282].
Additional changes involved replacement of the ring-CO by SO, SO_2,
or even by CHCN. This latter change is exemplified in the neuroleptic
piperidinoindoles *222* and *223* [283].

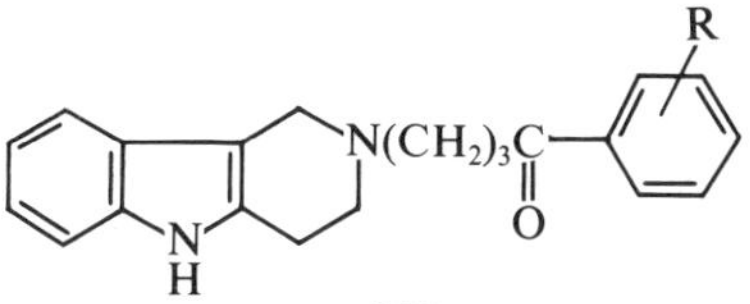

222 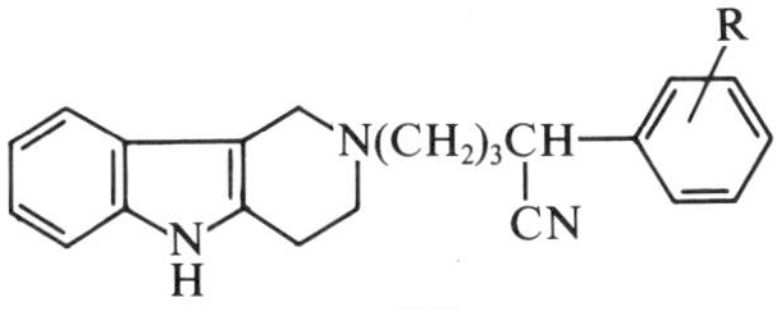   **223**

Vasodilatory activity has been found in benzofuryl phenyl ketones
and sulfones with basic side chains *(224)* [284–286] and in the ni-
trophenyl-substituted dihydropyridines *225* and *226* [287, 288].

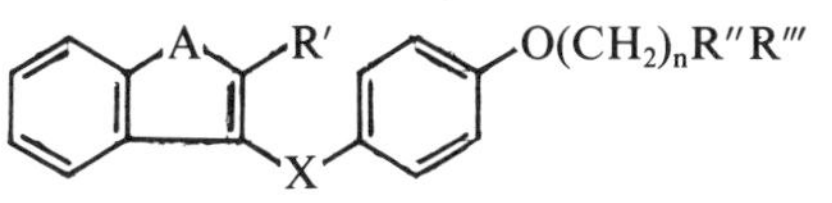

A = O or S	X = SO$_2$	(284)
A = O	X = CO	(285)
A = S	X = CO	(286)

224

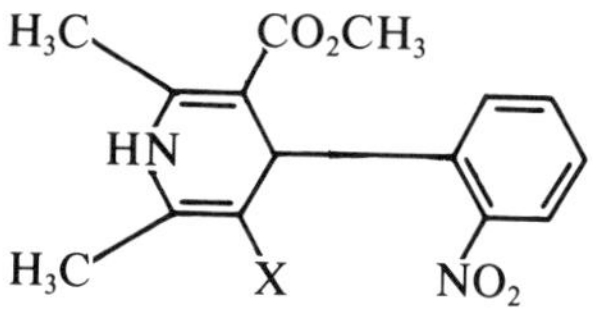

X = COOCH$_3$: **225**

X = SO$_2$CH$_3$: **226**

Similarly, the benzamide function of the hypoglycemic sulfonylurea drug, glyburide *(227)* could be replaced by sulfonamide *(228)*[289] but the carboxylic acid *229* also had similar antihyperglycemic activity [290]. This suggests a bioisosteric relationship of SO$_2$NHCO and COOH groups.

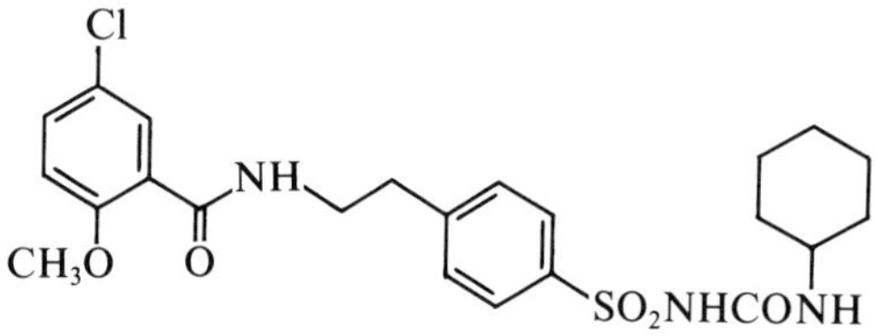

227

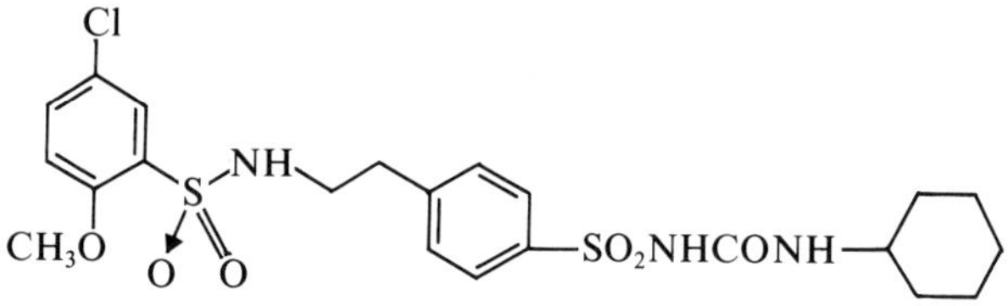

228

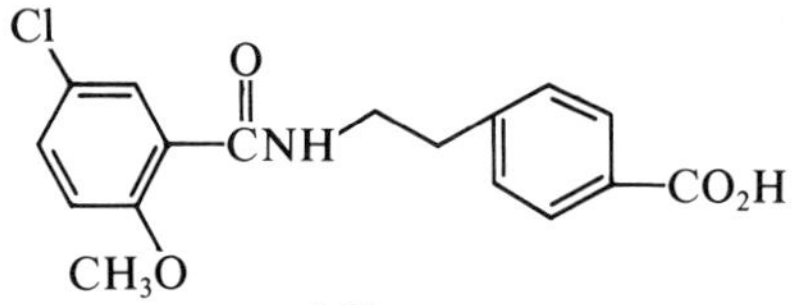

229

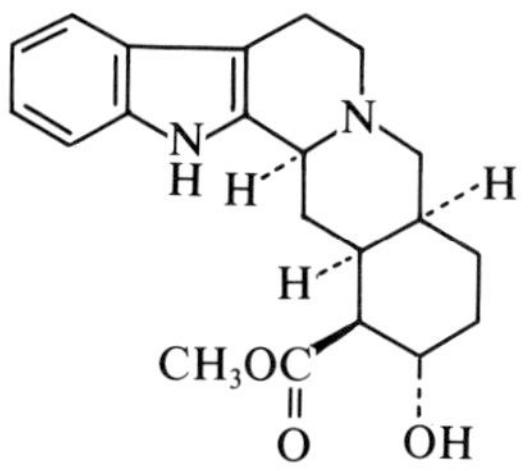

230

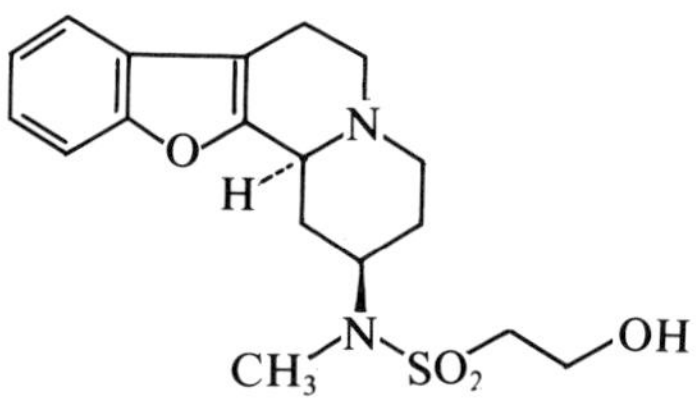

231

Farther afield is the replacement of the ester group of α-yohimbine (rauwolscine, *230*) by a sulfonamide in which the 17-hydroxyl of the alkaloid has been translocated into a side chain. The sulfonamide analogue *231* is an enantioselective α_2-adrenoreceptor antagonist but there were too many changes in the ring skeleton to assert defendable bioisosterism [291].

2   Metabolite analogues

Metabolites are chemicals needed or discarded by cells in the course of their metabolism. Some of them are biosynthesized by a cell from available chemicals, while others that cannot be produced in this manner have to be furnished by cellular nutrients from the environment. The chemistry, biochemistry and physiological significance of many metabolites has been reviewed repeatedly in monographs on amino acids, carbohydrates, hormones, lipids, nucleotides, steroids, vitamins and other essential and non-essential substances that play a role in the chemical support and chemical reactions which we call cellular life. All these materials represent prototype structures which can be altered by chemical reactions within the organism, or by experimentation in the laboratory. If the reaction products support or enhance the biochemical transformations of the metabolites, they are agonists of such biochemical missions. Other reaction products, whether obtained from metabolic events or by laboratory chemistry, slow down, halt or even reverse reactions of the metabolites; they are metabolite antagonists (antimetabolites). Both agonists and antagonists, regardless of their source, often but not always, are structurally related to the metabolites; if so, they are metabolite analogues. Some representative metabolite analogues will be assembled in this section. Some others have already been mentioned on the preceding pages.

The often complex biochemical relationship of metabolite and metabolite analogue requires a knowledge of the behavior at enzymatic sites and of the reactions of these reagents. For this purpose, some structural similarity will be needed. Emil Fischer compared the relationship of the reactions of metabolite and metabolite analogue to the relationship of a key to a keyhole. This rather static picture is improved in a more adaptable analogy of a glove and a hand. This allows for flexibility of reactions and for steric changes involving reagents and reaction sites. Even so, the structural segments of reagents fitting the reaction site "glove" will have to be highly similar. Segments adjacent to the structurally demanding sites can be much more varied, and therefore the differences between metabolite and metabolite analogue will be more pronounced in groups near but not in the pharmacophoric core of these agents. Bioisosterism will be most visible in those parts of the molecule which need to be as similar as possible in a metabolite and its analogue. Differences between such analogues will have to be placed in adjacent sections of the molecules. This idea has been promoted by Baker [282].

2.1   Nucleoside base isosteres

Biosisosteric replacements have been applied in every structural series of metabolites. Classical bioisosterism has been most successful in designing antagonists to metabolites in therapeutic areas where toxic metabolites of infectious and invasive cells have to be counteracted. Antimicrobial (antibacterial, antiprotozoal, antiviral) antimetabolites, and chemotherapeutic antitumor agents have been of great interest to medicinal chemists. Even the best planned molecular modifications in these series demand further systematic variations to cull out pharmacologically suitable members of widely spaced analogues. One such systematic search has been crowned by a Nobel prize [293].

The purine derivatives, adenine and guanine, and the pyrimidines, cytosine, thymine and uracil, form the basic components of the nucleic acids. In rapidly dividing cells, they must be resynthesized continually to replenish the supply of chemicals for the new cell nuclei. Adenine *(232)* contains an amino group, guanine *(233)* a tautomerizable hydroxyl and an amino group, and uracil *(234)* has two tautomerizable oxo groups. Thymine *(235)* carries a methyl function, and cytosine *(236)* an amino and a tautomerizable oxo group. These bases participate in many enzymic reactions in the form of their nucleosides (ribosides) or deoxynucleosides (2'-deoxyribosides) and the mono-, di-, or triphosphate esters, the nucleotides or 2'-deoxynucleotides.

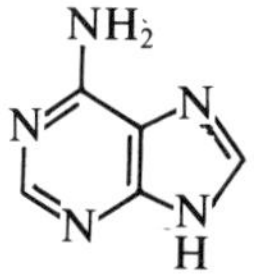

232 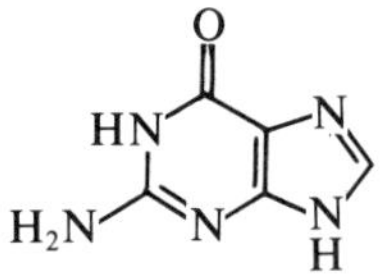   233 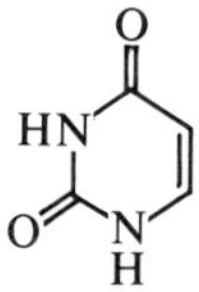   234 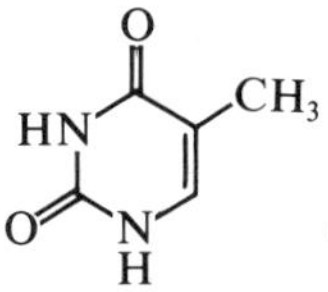   235 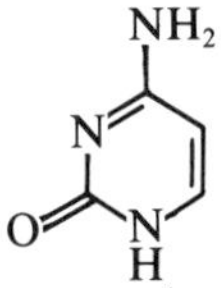   236

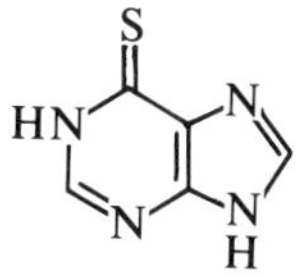

These NH_2 and tautomeric OH groups are amenable to bioisosteric replacement by halogens or SH; the reactive 5-hydrogen of uracil which normally can be biomethylated is an isostere of small halogens. Work on metabolite analogues of nucleoside bases started in the 1940's when the impact of isosterism was popular, and in short order the first wave of bioisosteric metabolite analogues was prepared and tested. They were 6-mercaptopurine (6-MP) *(237)* and its 2-amino and hydroxy derivatives, 5-halogenouracils *(238)* and especially 5-fluorouracil (5-FU) *(239)*. The complicated biochemistry of these compounds had to be unravelled and the enzymes they inhibited identified. 6-MP *(237)* and 5-FU *(239)* have become useful as antitumor drugs.

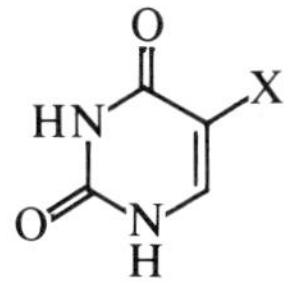

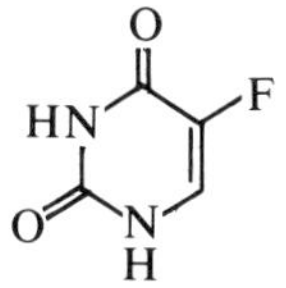

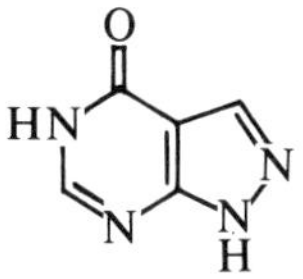

Another step in applying classical bioisosteric modifications to the purine and pyrimidine bases was to replace -CH= by -N=, -N= by -CH=, and -O- and -S-. Virtually every ring position has been subjected to such changes, and a few of these modifications have made it to clinical use. An example of the -CH=→-N= exchange is allopurinol *(240)* which inhibits the oxidation of hypoxanthine to uric acid and, since urate deposits in the joints are the cause of gout, can be used in this condition.

The relationship of allopurinol to uric acid biosynthesis illustrates some of the conditions imposed on metabolites of bioisosteres of purine and pyrimidine bases [294–296]. Hypoxanthine *(241)* is oxidized to xanthine (2,6-dioxopurine) *(242)* by the enzyme, xanthine oxidase, and xanthine is further oxidized to uric acid (2,6,8-trioxopurine, *243*). Allopurinol *(240)* can also be oxidized at its 2-position by the same enzyme, but its nitrogen at position 8 slows down recognition by the enzyme, and the initial oxidation to the isostere *244* of xanthine *(242)* is slow. Although allopurinol is thus a substrate of xanthine oxidase, albeit a poor one, it binds to the enzyme more tightly than hypoxanthine and thereby inhibits its oxidation. The next step, the oxidation of xanthine to uric acid, cannot be duplicated for the isosteric 2,4-dioxopyrazolopyrimidine *244* since this compound has N in place of CH at position 8 (purine numbering); *244* is therefore no longer a substrate but

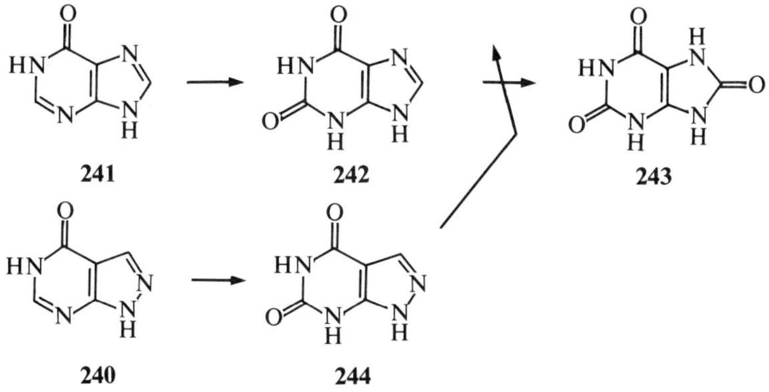

241   242   243

240   244

because of its stronger complexation with the enzyme, becomes an inhibitor of the oxidation of xanthine, i.e. an antimetabolite.

Another example of positive bioisosterism as compared to metabolite antagonism is the replacement of the methyl group of thymidine *(245)* in the form of its triphosphate nucleotide, by halogen.

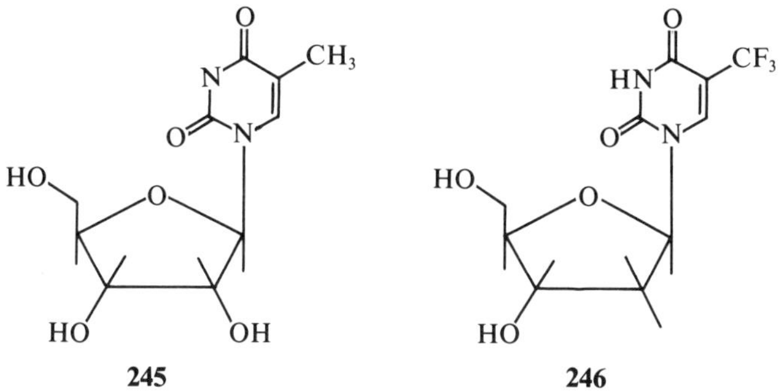

245   246

Thymidine triphosphate is a substrate of DNA polymerase. Replacement of the 5-methyl group by (the equivoluminous) chlorine atom, or the larger bromine or iodine atoms, furnishes analogues which increasingly lose the ability to substitute as substrates for the enzyme. At the end of this sequence, 5-iodouracil *(238,* X = I) (as the 2'-deoxynucleoside or nucleotide) whose iodine atom replaces CH_3, can no longer bind to DNA polymerase as a substrate but it is an inhibitor of the enzyme. It has antiviral activity in the topical therapy of ocular herpes diseases [297]. 5-Fluorouracil *(239)* [298, 299] is best interpreted as a bioisostere of uracil *(234)* since the fluorine atom has a van der Waals radius of 1.35 Å compared to hydrogen with a radius of 1.2 Å. It is a selective cancer chemotherapeutic drug, best in the form of its 2'-deoxynucleoside. Normal cells readily degrade 5-FU while cancer cells cannot reduce and thereby detoxify it [300].

5-Trifluoromethyl-2-deoxyuridine *(246)* is an isostere of 2-deoxythymidine with fluorine substituting for the methyl hydrogens. It is useful as a topical agent for herpes zoster-infected eyes, especially in cases resistant to iodouridine [301].

The most important therapeutic advances with purine and pyrimidine bioisosteres and metabolite antagonists have been made through increased selectivity for isozymes of invasive and malignant cells. The biochemical paths followed to bring selectivity to fruition may be found in reviews by Elion and by Montgomery et al. [293, 300].

Antiviral chemotherapy proceeded hesitantly as a sequel to cancer chemotherapy. Almost all antitumor agents were tested against experimental virus infections *in vitro* in infected egg membranes and in laboratory animals. When antiviral testing methods were firmly established, screening was extented to many structurally divergent chemicals. Within the discussion of bioisosterism, nucleoside analogues with altered carbohydrate moieties deserve attention.

The nucleic acids of viruses are similar to those of normal host cells. Ribotides are present in ribonucleic acids and therefore in RNA viruses. 2′-Deoxyribotides are found in 2′-deoxyribonucleic acids (DNA) and consequently in DNA viruses. Adenoviruses, Herpes 1 and 2, smallpox, vaccinia and polyoma viruses are DNA viruses. Many other viruses are RNA viruses, among them those that cause influenza, mumps, Newcastle disease, measles, distemper, polio, rabies, infectious bronchitis, yellow fever, encephalitis, rubella, some leukemias, and many other infections [302].

With the difference in the chemistry of RNA and DNA viruses concentrated in the carbohydrate moieties of their nucleic acids, bioisosteric changes of these moieties have been undertaken. The first modifications were made with carbohydrates isomeric with ribose, then with other sugar moieties that featured, if possible, furanose rings. Thus, 1-*β*-*D*-arabinofuranosylcytosine (cytarabine, Ara-C, *247*) was synthesized [303–305]. It can be applied in herpes zoster and other herpes infections and also as an antitumor agent.

Similarly, 9-*β*-*D*-arabinofuranosyladenine (vidarabine, Ara-A, *248*) was introduced. It can also be of value in herpes infections of the eye, brain and skin. Both these compounds contain arabinose rings, and inhibit the conversion of ribo- to deoxyribonucleotides.

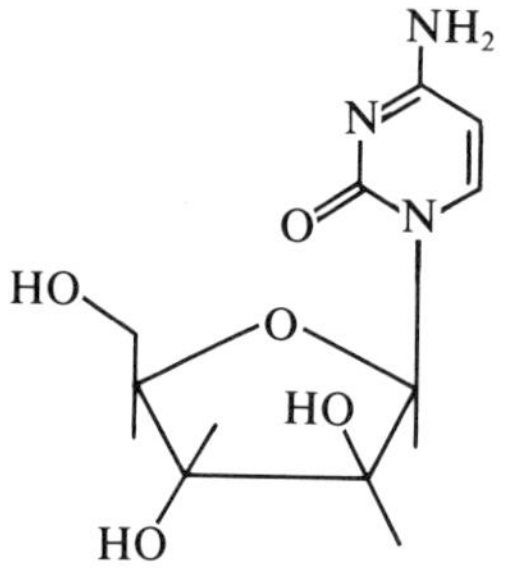

247 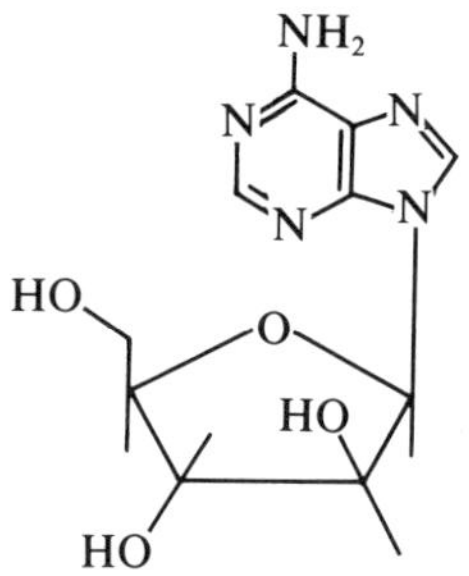   248

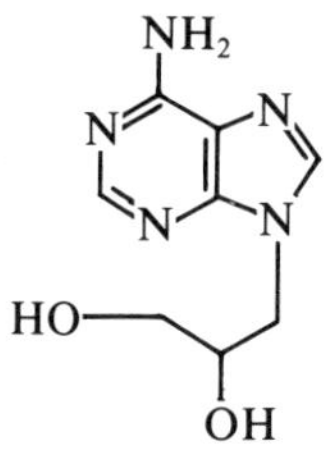

249 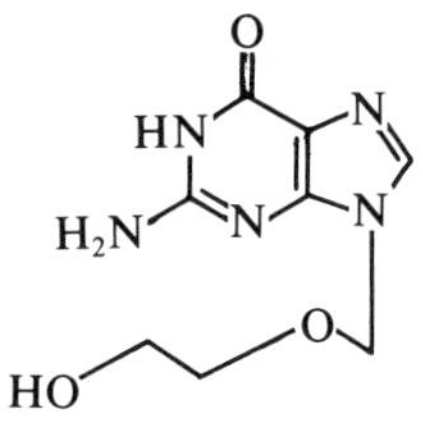   250

The next step was to probe whether a carbohydrate group was necessary for biological activity and enzyme binding. Instead of the glycosidic rings, aliphatic groups with two to five carbon atom chains
(HOCH$_2$CHOHCH$_2$-, in (S)-9-(2,3-dihydroxypropyl)adenine, 249), or
ether group-containing chains to simulate the oxygen bridge of ribo-
side groups (HOCH$_2$CH$_2$-O-CH$_2$-, in 9-(2-hydroxyethoxymethyl) guanine, acycloguanosine, acyclovir, 250) [306] were designed bioisosterically. Acyclovir (250) has become the drug of choice for the control of
herpes infections [307–309].

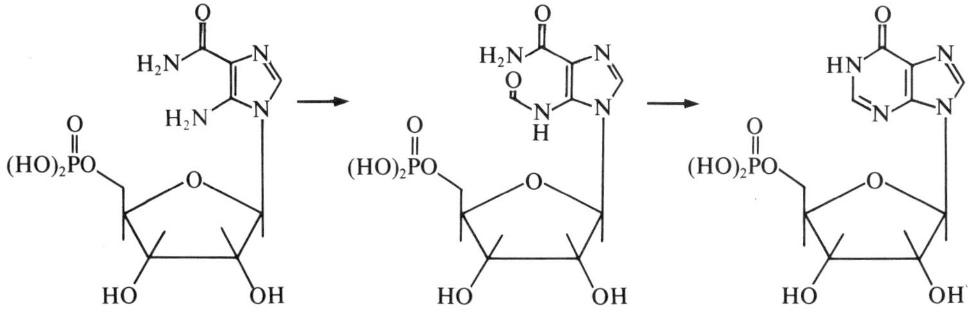

251   252   253

Since the biosynthesis of purine nucleotides *(253)* proceeds through
1-β-*D*-ribofuranosylphosphate)-5-aminoimidazole-4-carboxamide
(251), the missing carbonyl group for *252* being furnished by formyl-
tetrahydrofolate, the imidazole ring of *251* and *252* was modified
($=C<\longrightarrow=N$- replacement) in ribavirin *(254)* [310, 311], which inhibits herpes 1 and 2, vaccinia, influenza, parainfluenza, rhino and certain RNA tumor viruses *in vitro* and *in vivo.*

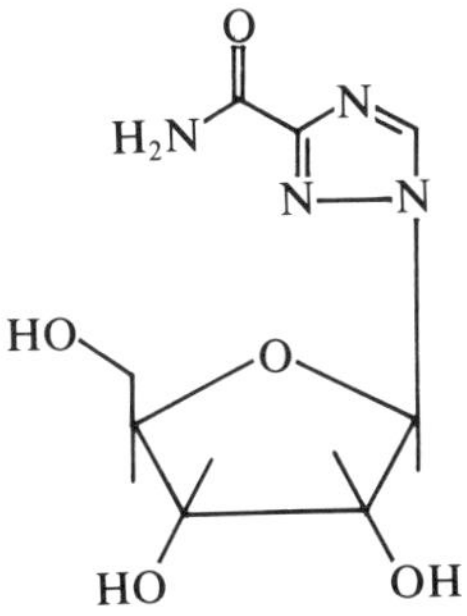

254

Many other bioisosteric replacements based on purines or their biosynthetic precursors have been reported, for example, a derivative of
the imidazole amide *251* in which the 5-amino group was exchanged
for fluorine *(255)* or other halogens [312].
Alternately, the pyrimidine portion of the purine nucleosides was
stripped of one nitrogen and functional groups, in 3-β-*D*-ribofurano-
sylimidazole [4,5-*b*] pyridine *(256)* [313, 314] which showed activity
against parainfluenza virus. A similar deazapyrimidine analogue
(221) has already been described.

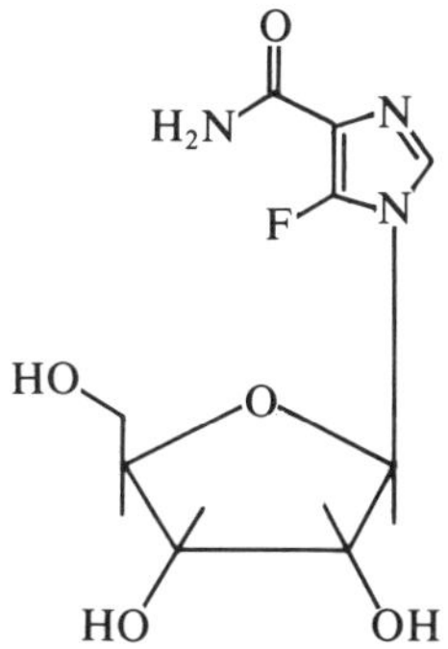

255 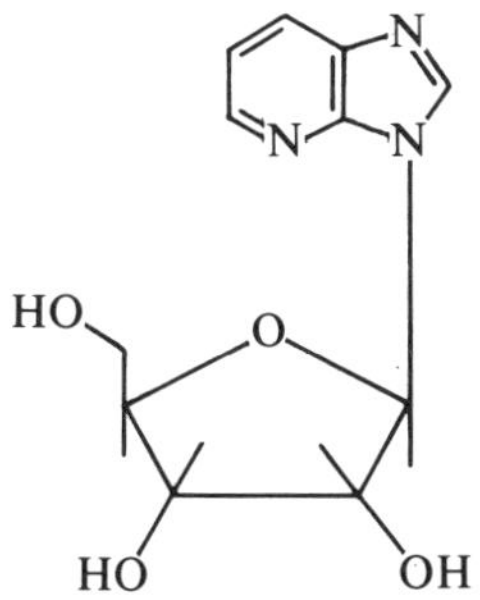   **256**

With the exception of the hydroxyalkyl-chain derivatives of nucleosides, with their principally anti-herpes activities *(249, 250)* and of zyvudine *(69)* and its congeners, almost all the analogues described here are classical bioisosteres of their prototypes. Non-classical changes with their more far-reaching modifications have not yet been contemplated widely. With interest in antiviral and antitumor drugs at a high level in view of the epidemic HIV infection (AIDS), non-classical bioisosteres will undoubtedly be investigated.

Metabolite analogues, especially metabolite antagonists, have been encountered in many structurally and functionally divergent types of compounds. Some of them, such as analogues of several B-vitamins and amino acids are mentioned in Baker's review [292]. Many others, arranged by structure rather than function, may be found in this review.

References

1   M. D. Hollenberg, J. Med. Chem., *33*, 1275 (1990).
2   J. Moir, J. Chem. Min. Soc. S. A., *98*, 335 (1909).
3   J. Moir, Chem. News, *124*, 105, 118, 133, 149 (1922).
4   O. Hinsberg, J. Prakt. Chem., *93*, 302 (1916); *94*, 179 (1916).
5   W. Hückel, Z. Elektrochem., *27*, 305 (1921).
6   H. G. Grimm, Z. Elektrochem., *31*, 474 (1925); *34*, 430 (1928).
7   H. G. Grimm, Angew. Chem., *42*, 367 (1929); *47*, 53, 594 (1934).
8   H. G. Grimm, Naturwissenschaften, *17*, 535, 559 (1929).
9   R. S. Mulliken, Chem. Rev., *9*, 347 (1931).
10   I. Langmuir, J. Am. Chem. Soc., *41*, 868, 1543 (1919).
11   K. S. Murty, Current Sci., *5*, 424 (1937); Chem. Abstr., *31*, 4644 (1937).
12   W. A. Hare and E. Mack, J. Am. Chem. Soc., *54*, 4272 (1932).
13   A. O. Rankin, Nature (London), *107*, 203 (1921).
14   A. W. C. Menzies, Nature (London), *107*, 331 (1921).
15   L. Birckenbach and K. Huttner, Chem. Ber., *62*, 153 (1929).
16   L. Birckenbach and K. Huttner, Z. anorg. u. allgem. Chem., *190*, 38 (1930).
17   W. Hieber, K. Ries, and G. Bader, Z. anorg. u. allgem. Chem., *190*, 215 (1930).
18   S. Goldschmidt, Chem. Ber., *60*, 1263 (1927).
19   G. N. Copley, Chem. Industry, *59*, 675 (1940).
20   H. G. Grimm, M. Gunther, and H. Titus, Z. physik. Chem., *B14*, 169 (1931).
21   H. Erlenmeyer and E. Berger, Biochem. Z., *252*, 22 (1932).
22   H. Erlenmeyer and M. Leo, Helv. Chim. Acta, *16*, 897 (1933).
23   H. Erlenmeyer, Z. physik. Chem., *B27*, 404 (1934).
24   H. Erlenmeyer and M. Leo, Helv. Chim. Acta, *15*, 1171 (1932).
25   L. Birckenbach, K. Huttner, and W. Stein, Chem. Ber., *62*, 2065 (1929).
26   L. Birckenbach and K. Kellermann, Chem. Ber., *58*, 786, 2177 (1925).
27   L. Birckenbach and M. Linhard, Chem. Ber., *62*, 2261 (1929); *63*, 2528, 2544 (1930).
28   K. Landsteiner, Naturwissenschaften, *18*, 653 (1930).

29   H. Erlenmeyer, E. Berger, and M. Leo, Helv. Chim. Acta, *16*, 733 (1933).

30   H. Erlenmeyer and E. Berger, Biochem. Z., *262*, 196 (1933).

31   H. Erlenmeyer and M. Leo, Helv. Chim. Acta, *26*, 733 (1943).

32   H. Erlenmeyer, Biochem. Z., *252*, 22 (1932).

33   H. Erlenmeyer, Bull. soc. chim. biol., *30*, 792 (1948).

34   W. Steinkopf and G. Lützkendorf, Ann. Chem., *403*, 45 (1914).

35   Sir R. Robinson and W. M. Todd, J. Chem. Soc., 1743 (1939).

36   L. Birckenbach and K. Kellermann, Z. anorg. u. allgem. Chem., *190*, 1 (1930); Naturwissenschaften, *18*, 530 (1930).

37   H. Erlenmeyer, A. G. Epprecht, and H. v. Meyenburg, Helv. Chim. Acta, *20*, 310 (1937).

38   P. H. Bell and R. O. Roblin, Jr., J. Am. Chem. Soc., *64*, 2903 (1942).

39   E. Preiswerk and H. Erlenmeyer, Helv. Chim. Acta, *17*, 329 (1934).

40   W. Steinkopf and W. Ohse, Ann. Chem., *437*, 14 (1924).

41   H. L. Friedman, Symposium on Chemical-Biological Correlation, Nat. Acad. Sci. Natl. Research Council, publ. No. 206, Washington, D. C., 1951, p. 295.

42   C. Hansch, Intra-Science Rept., *8*, 17 (1973).

43   Ref. 42, p. 23.

44   V. Schatz, in: Medicinal Chemistry, 2nd edn. A. Burger, Ed., Interscience, New York, 1960. Chap. 8, p. 72.

45   A. Burger, in: Medicinal Chemistry, 3rd edn. A. Burger, Ed., Wiley Interscience, New York, 1970. Chap. 6, p. 64.

46   A. Burger, Pharmaceutica Acta Helv., *38*, 705 (1963).

47   T. Fujita, J. Isawa, and C. Hansch, J. Am. Chem. Soc., *86*, 5175 (1964).

48   C. Hansch, in: Drug Design., E. J. Ariens, Ed. Academic Press, New York 1971. Vol. I, Chap. 2, p. 271.

49   C. Hansch and W. J. Dunn III, J. Pharm. Sci., *61*, 1 (1952).

50   A. Leo, J. Isawa, and D. Elkins, Chem. Rev., *71*, 525 (1971).

51   C. Hansch and T. J. Fujita, J. Am. Chem. Soc., *86*, 1616 (1964).

52   C. Hansch, J. Med. Chem., *19*, 1 (1976).

53   C. Hansch and A. J. Leo, Substituent Constants for Correlation Analysis in Chemistry and Biology. Wiley, New York 1979.

54   P. G. Schultz, R. E. Lerner, and S. J. Benkovic, Chem. Eng. News, May 28, 1990, p. 26.

55   M. E. Wolff and A. McPherson, Nature (London), *345*, 365 (1990).

56   H. Levitan and J. L. Barker, Science, *176*, 1423 (1972).

57   J. G. Topliss, J. Med. Chem., *15*, 1006 (1972); *20*, 463 (1977).

58   C. Hansch, S. D. Rockwell, P. Y. C. Jow, A. Leo, and E. E. Steller, J. Med. Chem., *20*, 304 (1977).

59   C. Hansch, A. Leo, S. H. Unger, Ki hwan Kim, D. Nikaitoni, and E. J. Lien, J. Med. Chem., *16*, 1207 (1973).

60   S. M. Free and J. W. Wilson, J. Med. Chem., *7*, 395 (1964).

61   Y. C. Martin, J. Med. Chem., *24*, 229 (1981).

62   Y. C. Martin, Quantitative Drug Design. A Critical Introduction. Marcel Dekker, New York 1978, p. 329.

63   H. Kubinyi, in: Comprehensive Medicinal Chemistry, C. Hansch, editorial chairman. Vol IV. C. A. Ramsden Ed. Pergamon, Oxford 1990, pp. 589–643.

64   A. Crum Brown and T. R. Fraser, Trans. Roy. Soc. Edinburgh, *25 (I)*, 151.

65   H. H. Meyer, Arch. Exp. Pathol. Pharmakol., *42*, 109 (1899).

66   E. Overton, Studien über die Narkose, Fischer, Jena 1901.

67   T. C. Bruice, N. Kharasch, and R. J. Winzler, Arch. Biochem. Biophys., *62*, 305 (1956).

68   T. Fujita and T. Ban, J. Med. Chem., *14*, 148 (1971).

69 M. S. Tute, in: Comprehensive Medicinal Chemistry, C. Hansch, Editorial Chairman. Vol. IV, C. A. Ramsden, Ed., Pergamon, Oxford, 1990. pp. 1–31.

70 J. K. Seydel, J. Med. Chem., *14*, 724 (1971).

71 S. W. Dietrich, R. N. Smith, S. Brendler, and C. Hansch, Archs. Biochem. Biophys., *194*, 612 (1979).

72 C. Hansch, S. W. Dietrich, and R. N. Smith, Chem. Biol. Pteridines, Proc. 6th Int. Symposium, 1978, 425 (1979).

73 B. S. Pitzele, A. E. Moorman, G. W. Gullikson, D. Albin, R. C. Bianchi, P. Palicharla, E. L. Sanguinetti, and D. E. Walters, J. Med. Chem., *31*, 138 (1988).

74 H. Erlenmeyer and E. Willi, Helv. Chim. Acta, *18*, 740 (1935).

75 G. Orestano, Arch. ital. sci. farmacol., *8*, 353 (1939); Chem. Abstr. *39*, 1926 (1945).

76 D. W. Woolley, J. Biol. Chem., *154*, 31 (1944). (-NH-.....-CH = CH-).

77 G. H. Hitchings, E. A. Falco, and M. B. Sherwood, Science, *102*, 252 (1945).

78 H. Bloch and H. Erlenmeyer, Helv. Chim. Acta, *25*, 694, 1062 (1942).

79 L. Ruberg and L. F. Small, J. Am. Chem. Soc., *60*, 1591 (1938).

80 A. R. Martin, F. L. Rose, and G. Swain, Nature (London), 154, 639 (1944).

81 R. O. Roblin, J. O. Lampen, J. P. English, Q. P. Cole, and J. R. Vaughn, J. Am. Chem. Soc., *67*, 290 (1945).

82 M. Sodak and L. R. Cerecedo, J. Am. Chem. Soc., *66*, 1988 (1944).

83 K. Link, Harvey Lectures, 1944.

84 P. Meunier, C. Mentzer, N. Ph. Buu-Hoi, and P. Cagniant, Bull. soc. chim. biol., *25*, 384 (1943).

85 H. Erlenmeyer and M. Simon, Helv. Chim. Acta, *24*, 1210 (1941).

86 H. Gilman and R. M. Pickens, J. Am. Chem. Soc., *47*, 245 (1925).

87 O. Kamm, J. Am. Chem. Soc., *42*, 1030 (1920).

88 M. Hartmann and E. Wybert, Helv. Chim. Acta, *2*, 60 (1919).

89 W. Steinkopf and A. Wolfram, Ann. Chem., *437*, 22 (1924).

90 W. Steinkopf and W. Ohse, Ann. Chem., *448*, 205 (1926).

91 V. duVigneaud, H. McKennis, Jr., S. Simmonds, K. Dittmer, and G. B. Brown, J. Biol. Chem., *159*, 385 (1945).

91a D. J. Stuehr, O. A. Fasehun, N. S. Kwon, S. S. Gross, J. A. Gonzalez, R. Levi, and C. F. Nathan, FASEB J, *5*, 98 (1991).

92 H. Erlenmeyer, H. Ueberwasser, and H. M. Weber, Helv. Chim. Acta, *11*, 709 (1938).

93 M. Jaffé and H. Levy, Chem. Ber., *21*, 3458 (1888).

94 G. Barger, J. Chem. Soc., 2100 (1938).

95 R. Dagard, Chem. Eng. News, June 11 1990, pp. 21–23.

96 E. H. Northey, The Sulfonamides and Allied Compounds. Reinhold, New York 1948.

97 H. Erlenmeyer and W. Würgler, Helv. Chim. Acta, *25*, 249 (1942).

98 A. H. Tracy and R. C. Elderfield, J. Org. Chem., *6*, 54 (1940).

99 H. Erlenmeyer and H. v. Meyenburg, Helv. Chim. Acta, *20*, 204 (1937).

100 D. W. Wolley and A. G. C. White, J. Biol. Chem., *149*, 285 (1943).

101 D. W. Wolley and A. G. C. White, J. Exptl. Med., *78*, 489 (1943).

102 W. J. Robbins, Proc. Natl. Acad. Sci. U. S., *27*, 19 (1941).

103 F. Häfliger and W. Schindler, U. S. Pat. 2554736 (1951).

104 P. A. J. Janssen, C. J. E. Niemegeers, and K. H. L. Schellekens, Arzneim.-Forsch., *15*, 104 (1965).

105 J. P. English, R. C. Clapp, Q. P. Cole, E. F. Halverstadt, I. F. Campen, and R. O. Roblin, Jr., J. Am. Chem. Soc., *67*, 295 (1945).

106 G. W. Wheland, Resonance in Organic Chemistry. Wiley, New York, pp. 695–784.

107 D. T. Witiak and R. C. Cavestri, in: Burger's Medicinal Chemistry, 4th edn., M. E. Wolff, Ed. Wiley, New York 1981. Part III, pp. 553–568.

108 A. Burger, A Guide to the Chemical Basis of Drug Design. Wiley, New York 1983, pp. 28–29, 53–54, 109–113.

109 D. G. Cooper, R. C. Young, G. J. Durant, and C. R. Ganellin, in: Comprehensive Medicinal Chemistry, C. Hansch, Ed. in chief. Vol. 3, J. C. Emmett, Ed. Pergamon, Oxford 1990, pp. 368–382.

110 R. R. Burtner and J. W. Cusic, J. Am. Chem. Soc., 65, 262 (1943).

111 R. Meier and K. Hoffmann, Helv. Chim. Acta, 7, Suppl. VI, 106 (1941).

112 H. Ramsey and A. G. Richardson, J. Pharmacol. Exptl. Therap., 89, 131 (1947).

113 A. C. Cope, P. Kovcic, and M. Burg, J. Am. Chem. Soc., 71, 3658 (1949).

114 D. L. Tabern and E. H. Volwiler, J. Am. Chem. Soc., 57, 1961 (1935).

115 E. E. Swanson and W. E. Frey, J. Am. Pharm. Ass. Sci. Ed., 29, 509 (1940).

116 C. R. Ganellin and G. J. Durant, in: Burger's Medicinal Chemistry, M. E. Wolff, Ed. 4th edn. Wiley, New York 1981. Part III, pp. 487–551.

117 R. C. Hirt, R. G. Smith, H. L. Strauss, and J. Koren, J. Chem. Eng. Data, 6, 610 (1961).

118 J. G. Bonner and J. C. Lockhardt, J. Chem. Soc., 3858 (1958).

119 O. H. Miller and L. Fischer, J. Am. Pharm. Ass. Sci. Ed., 30, 45 (1941).

120 O. Schaumann, Arch. exptl. Pathol. Pharmakol., 196, 109 (1940).

121 J. E. Hertz, J. Fried, and E. F. Sabo, J. Am. Chem. Soc., 78, 2017 (1956).

122 A. D. Ainley and H. King, Proc. Roy. Soc. Ser. B, 125, 60 (1933).

123 R. M. Pinder and A. Burger, J. Med. Chem., 11, 267 (1968).

124 E. A. Nodiff, K. Tanabe, C. Seyfried, S. Matsmera, Y. Kondo, E. H. Chen, and M. P. Tyagi, J. Med. Chem., 14, 921 (1971).

125 C. J. Ohnmacht, A. R. Patel, and R. E. Lutz, J. Med. Chem., 14, 926 (1971).

126 E. F. Rogers, H. D. Brown, I. M. Rasmussen, and R. E. Heal, J. Am. Chem. Soc., 75, 2991 (1953).

127 A. Burger and R. D. Foggio, J. Am. Chem. Soc., 78, 4419 (1956).

128 E. C. Jorgensen, in: Thyroid Hormones, C. H. Li, Ed. Academic Press, New York 1978. Chapter 3, pp. 107–204.

129 K. Chae and J. D. McKinney, J. Med. Chem., 31, 357 (1988).

130 B. C. Rudy and B. Z. Senkowski, in: Analytical Profiles of Drug Substances. Vol. 3. K. Florey, Ed. Academic Press, New York 1974, pp. 307–331.

131 H. Mitsuya, J. K. Weinhold, P. A. Furman, M. H. St. Clair, S. Nusinoff-Lehrman, R. C. Gallo, D. Bolognesi, D. W. Barry, and S. Border, Proc. Natl. Acad. Sci. U. S., 82, 7096 (1985).

132 T.-S. Lin, J.-Y. Guo, R. F. Schinazi, C. K. Chu, J.-N. Xiang, and W. H. Prusoff, J. Med. Chem., 31, 336 (1988).

133 C. L. Gemmill, J. A. Anderson, and A. Burger, J. Am. Chem. Soc., 78, 2434 (1956).

134 R. E. Cortell, J. Clin. Endocrinol., 9, 955 (1949).

135 A. G. J. Guerbet, French Pat. 828486 (1938).

136 E. J. Ariens, in: Drug Design, Vol I. E. J. Ariens, Ed., Academic Press, New York 1971.

137 A. Korolkovas, Essentials of Molecular Pharmacology: Background for Drug Design. Wiley, New York 1970.

138 C. W. Thornber, Chem. Soc. Rev., 8, 563–580 (1979).

139 C. A. Lipinski, Annu. Rept. Med. Chem., 21, Chapter 27. Academic Press, Orlando, Florida, 1986.

140 C. Mentzer, P. Gley, D. Molho, and D. Billet, Bull. soc. chim. France, 271 (146).

141 P. Gley, C. Mentzer, J. Delor, D. Molho, and J. Millon, Compt. rend. soc. biol., 140, 748 (1946).

142 P. Meunier and C. Mentzer, Bull. soc. chim. biol., 25, 80 (1943).

143   P. D. Leeson, D. Ellis, J. C. Emmett, V. P. Shah, G. A. Showell, and A. H. Underwood, J. Med. Chem., *31*, 37 (1988).
144   G. L. Grunewald, A. E. Carter, D. J. Sall, and J. A. Monn, J. Med. Chem., *31*, 60 (1988).
145   G. Petranyi, N. S. Ryder, and A. Stütz, Science, *224*, 1239 (1984).
146   P. A. Zoretic, P. Soja, and T. Shiah, Prostaglandins, *16*, 555 (1978).
147   C. J. Harris, N. Whittaker, G. A. Hicks, J. M. Armstrong, and P. M. Reed, Prostaglandins, *16*, 773 (1978).
148   J. H. Jones, W. J. Holtz, J. B. Bicking, E. J. Cragoe, L. R. Mandel, and F. A. Kuehl, J. Med. Chem., *20*, 1299 (1977).
149   J. B. Bicking, C. M. Robb, R. L. Smith, E. J. Cragoe, F. A. Kuehl, and L. R. Mandel, J. Med. Chem., *20*, 35 (1977).
150   J. H. Jones, W. J. Holtz, J. B. Bicking, E. J. Cragoe, L. R. Mandel, and F. A. Kuehl, J. Med. Chem., *20*, 44 (1977).
151   R. L. Smith, J. B. Bicking, N. P. Gould, T.-J. Lee, C. M. Robb, F. A. Kuehl, L. R. Mandel, and E. J. Cragoe, J. Med. Chem., *20*, 540 (1977).
152   T. A. Eggelte, H. deKoning, and H. O. Huisman, Rec. Trav. chim., *96*, 271 (1977).
153   P. A. Zoretic, B. Branchard, and N. D. Sirka, J. Org. Chem., *42*, 3201 (1977).
154   J. Bruin, H. deKoning, and H. O. Huisman, Tetrahedron Lett., *1975*, 4599.
155   G. Bollinger and J. M. Muchowski, Tetrahedron Lett., *1975*, 2931.
156   R. L. Smith, T.-J. Lee, N. P. Gould, E. J. Cragoe, H. G. Oien, and F. A. Kuehl, J. Med. Chem., *20*, 1292 (1977).
157   Merck, U. S. Pat. 4087435.
158   Beechams, Belg. Pat. 861956.
159   Beechams, Belg. Pat. 861957.
160   Miles, U. S. Pat. 4127612.
161   Pfizer, U. S. Pat. 4,132847.
162   J. Vlattas and L. Dellavecchia, Tetrahedron Lett., *1974*, 4455.
163   F. M. Hauser and R. C. Huffman, Tetrahedron Lett., *1974*, 905.
164   J. T. Harrison, R. J. K. Taylor, and J. H. Fried, Tetrahedron Lett., *1975*, 1165.
165   J. T. Harrison, V. R. Fletcher, and J. H. Fried, Tetrahedron Lett., *1974*, 2733.
166   E. I. duPont de Nemours, Brit. Pat. 1428431.
167   J. T. Harrison and V. R. Fletcher, Tetrahedron Lett., *1974*, 2729.
168   J. W. H. Watthey, M. Desai, R. Rutledge, and R. Dotson, J. Med. Chem., *23*, 690 (1980).
169   H. Van de Waterbeemd and B. Testa, J. Med. Chem., *26*, 203 (1983).
170   J. T. Strupczewski, R. C. Allen, B. A. Gardner, B. L. Schmidt, U. Stache, E. J. Glamkowski, M. C. Jones, D. B. Ellis, F. P. Huger, and R. W. Dunn, J. Med. Chem., *28*, 761 (1985).
171   G. M. Shutske, L. L. Seleseak, R. C. Allen, L. Davis, R. C. Effland, K. Ranbom, J. M. Kitzen, J. C. Wilker, and W. J. Novick, Jr., J. Med. Chem., *25*, 36 (1982).
172   N. B. Eddy, C. F. Touchberry, and J. E. Lieberman, J. Pharmacol. Exptl. Therap., *98*, 121 (1950).
173   M. M. Klenk, C. M. Suter, and S. Archer, J. Am. Chem. Soc., *70*, 3846 (1948).
174   J. Büchi, M. Prost, H. Eichenberger, and R. L. Leiberherr, Helv. Chim. Acta, *35*, 1527 (1952); *36*, 819 (1953).
175   E. C. Kleiderer, J. B. Rice, V. Conquest, and J. H. Williams, Dept. of Commerce PB-981, July 1945.
176   T. Y. Shen, in: Clinoril in the Treatment of Rheumatic Disorders, E. C. Huskisson and P. Franchimont, Eds. Raven Press, New York 1976, p. 1.

177 T. Y. Shen and C. A. Winter, in: Advances in Drug Research, Vol. 12. N. J. Harper and A. B. Simmonds, Eds. Academic Press, Orlando, Florida, 1978, p. 90.
178 R. L. Smith, J. B. Bicking, N. P. Gould, T.-J. Lee, C. M. Robb, F. A. Kuel, L. R. Mandel, and E. J. Cragoe, J. Med. Chem., 20, 540 (1977).
179 J. Vlattas and L. Dellavecchia, Tetrahedron Lett., 1974, 4459.
180 A. P. Bender, J. Med. Chem., 18, 1094 (1975).
181 K. A. Jensen, F. Lundquist, E. Rekling, and C. G. Wolffbrandt, Dansk. Tideskr. Farm., 17, 173 (1945).
182 R. H. K. Foster and A. J. Carman, J. Pharmacol. Exptl. Therap., 91, 195 (1947).
183 G. A. Alles and M. A. Redeman, J. Pharmacol. Exptl. Therap., 96, 338 (1949).
184 L. E. Craig, Chem. Rev., 42, 285 (1948).
185 R. Hunt and R. R. Renshaw, J. Pharmacol. Exptl. Therap., 25, 315 (1925); 29, 17 (1926).
186 W. H. Hartung, Ind. Eng. Chem., 37, 126 (1945).
187 J. Kovacs and T. Horvath, J. Org. Chem., 14, 306 (1949).
188 W. D. Avison and A. L. Morrison, J. Chem. Soc., 1469 (1950).
189 H. Kägi and K. Miescher, Helv. Chim. Acta, 32, 2489 (1949).
190 H. L. Friedman, Some Bio-Isosteric Anomalies, Abstracts, 126th Meeting, American Chemical Society, New York 1954. See also A. Burger, J. Chem. Educ., 33, 362 (1956).
191 B. S. Griffin and A. Burger, J. Am. Chem. Soc., 78, 2336 (1956).
192 C. M. Suter, Chem. Rev., 28, 269 (1941).
193 F. M. Berger, J. Pharmacol. Exptl. Therap., 93, 470 (1948).
194 T. Fusco, S. Chiavarelli, G. Palazzo, and D. Bovet, Gazz. chim. ital., 78, 951 (1948).
195 A. M. Kunkel, A. H. Oikemus, and J. H. Wills, Fed. Proc., 11, 365 (1952).
196 S. Thesloff and K. R. Unna, J. Pharmacol. Exptl. Therap., 111, 99 (1954).
197 C. R. Scholz, Ind. Eng. Chem., 37, 120 (1945).
198 D. Bovet and F. Bovet-Nitti, Structure and Pharmacological Activity of Drugs Acting on the Autonomic System. Interscience, New York 1948.
199 A. M. Lands, Symposium on Chemical-Biological Correlation, Natl. Acad. Sci. Natl. Res. Council, Publ. No. 206. Washington, D. C., 1951, p. 73.
200 D. Woods, Brit. J. Exptl. Pathol., 21, 74 (1940).
201 D. Woods and P. Fildes, Chemistry Industry, 59, 133 (1940).
202 R. Kuhn, E. F. Möller, G. Wendt, and H. Beinert, Chem. Ber., 75, 711 (1942).
203 I. M. Klotz and R. T. Morrison, J. Am. Chem. Soc., 69, 473 (1947).
204 L. D. Friedman and G. O. Doak, Chem. Rev., 57, 479 (1957).
205 J. D. Thayer, H. J. Magnuson, and M. S. Gravatt, Antibiotics Chemotherapy, 3, 256 (1953).
206 T. R. Herrin, J. S. Fairgreave, R. R. Bowen, N. L. Shipkovitz, and J. C.-h Mao, J. Med. Chem., 20, 660 (1977).
207 E.-s Huang, J. Virol., 16, 1560 (1975).
208 J. C.-h Mao, E. E. Robishaw, and L. R. Overby, J. Virol., 15, 1281 (1975).
209 J. C.-h Mao and E. E. Robishaw, Biochemistry, 14, 5475 (1975).
210 L. R. Overby, R. G. Duff, and J. C.-h Mao, Ann. N. Y, Acad, Sci., 284, 310 (1977).
211 M. H. Maguire and G. Shaw, J. Chem. Soc., 1756 (1955).
212 R. D. Bennett, A. Burger, and W. A. Volk, J. Med. Chem., 23, 940 (1958).
213 G. D. Diana, E. S. Zalay, U. J. Salvador, F. Pancic, and B. Steinberg, J. Med. Chem., 27, 691 (1984).
214 F. H. Westheimer, Science, 235, 1173 (1987).

215 G. M. Blackburn, F. Eckstein, D. E. Kent, and D. T. Perree, Nucleosides and Nucleotides, *4*, 165 (1985).

216 M. J. Camarasa, P. Fernandez-Resa, M.-T. Garcia-Lopez, F. G. De las Heras, P. P. Mendez-Castrillon, P. Alarcon, and L. Carrasco, J. Med. Chem., *23*, 481 (1980).

217 B. Wichrowski, S. Jouquey, C. Broquet, F. Heymans, J.-J. Godfroid, J. Fichelle, and M. Worcel, J. Med. Chem., *31*, 410 (1988).

218 K. Sturm, R. Muschaweck, and M. Hropot, J. Med. Chem., *26*, 1174 (1983).

219 C. A. Lipinski, Annu. Repts. Med. Chem., *21*, Chap. 27, refs. 74, 75 (1986).

220 D. H. Rich, M. Kawai, H. L. Goodman, J. Engelke, and J. W. Suttie, FEBS Lett., *152*, 79 (1983).

221 G. Sosnovsky, J. Lukszo, E. Gravela, and M. F. Zuretti, J. Med. Chem., *28*, 1350 (1985).

222 D. H. Kinder and J. A. Katzenellenbogen, J. Med. Chem., *28*, 1917 (1985).

223 J. G. Atkinson, Y. Giraud, J. Rokach, C. S. Rooney, C. S. McFarlane, A. Rackham, and N. N. Share, J. Med. Chem., *22*, 99 (1979).

224 H. von Kohler, B. Eichler, and R. Salewski, Z. anorg. Chem., *379*, 183 (1970).

225 P. Krogsgaard-Larsen and T. Rodolkov-Christiansen, Europ. J. Med. Chem., *14*, 157 (1979).

226 J. L. Kraus, Pharmacol. Res. Commun., *15*, 183 (1983).

227 J. L. Kraus, Pharmacol. Res. Commun., *15*, 119 (1983).

228 E. S. Stratford and R. W. Curley, Jr., J. Med. Chem., *26*, 1463 (1983).

229 H. W. R. Williams, E. Eichler, W. C. Randall, C. S. Rooney, E. J. Cragoe. Jr., K. B. Streeter, H. Schwan, S. R. Michelson, A. A. Patchett, and D. Taub, J. Med. Chem., *26*, 1196 (1983).

230 D. C. Schlegel, B. L. Zenitz, C. A. Fellows, S. C. Laskowski, D. C. Behn, D. K. Phillips, I. Botton, and P. T. Speight, J. Med. Chem., *27*, 1682 (1984).

231 A. F. Spatola, Annu. Repts. Med. Chem., *16*, 199 (1981).

232 A. F. Spatola, in: Chemistry and Biochemistry of Amino Acids, Peptides and Proteins, B. Weinstein, Ed. Marcel Dekker, New York 1983. Vol. 7, Chapter 5.

233 M. E. Wolff and A. McPherson, Nature (London), *345*, 365 (1990).

234 M. Goodman, Biopolymers, *24*, 137 (1987).

235 H. Erlenmeyer and H. Rey-Bellet, Helv. Chim. Acta, *37*, 234 (1954).

236 D. J. Cram, Science, *240*, 760 (1988).

237 R. T. Brittain, J. B. Farmer, D. Jack, L. E. Martin, and W. T. Simpson, Nature (London), *219*, 862 (1968).

238 D. J. Triggle and C. R. Triggle, Chemical Pharmacology of the Synapse. Academic Press, London 1976. Chapter III.

239 A. Hilditch and G. M. Drew, Trends Pharmacol. Sci., *1985*, 396.

240 P. B. W. M. Timmermans, A. T. Chin, and M. J. M. C. Thoolen, in: Comprehensive Medicinal Chemistry, C. Hansch, Ed. in chief. Vol. 3, J. C. Emmett, Ed. Pergamon, Oxford 1990, pp. 133–186, G. B. Main, ibid., pp. 187–228. A. S. Horn, ibid., pp. 229–290. F. Ince, ibid., pp. 291–322.

241 N. J. Bach, E. C. Kornfeld, N. D. Jones, M. O. Chaney, D. E. Dorman, J. W. Paschal, J. A. Clemens, and E. B. Smalstig, J. Med. Chem., *23*, 481 (1980).

242 R. I. Thrift, J. Chem. Soc., *C*, 288 (1967).

243 R. M. Pinder, D. A. Buxton, and D. M. Green, J. Pharm. Pharmacol., *23*, 995 (1971).

244 J. B. Cannon, Prog. Drug Res., E. Jucker, Ed., Birkhäuser, Basel, *29*, 303 (1985).

245 H. E. Katerinopoulos and D. I. Schuster, Drugs of the Future, *12*, 223 (1987).

246 A. J. Stoessel, E. Mak, and D. B. Calne, Lancet II, 1330 (1985).

247 C. Kaiser and T. Jain, Med. Res. Rev., *5*, 145 (1985).

248 Y. A. Chang, J. Ares, K. Anderson, B. Sahol, R. A. Wallace, T. Farooqui, N. Uretsky, and D. D. Miller, J. Med. Chem., *30*, 214 (1987).
249 R. A. Brown, R. C. Brown, J. C. Hall, J. Dixon, J. B. Farmer, R. A. Foulds, F. Ince, S. E. O'Connor, W. T. Simpson, G. W. Smith, B. Springthorpe, and A. C. Tinker, Spec. Publ. Roy. Soc. Chem., *55*, 169 (1986).
250 G. W. Smith, J. C. Hall, J. B. Farmer, and W. T. Simpson, J. Pharm. Pharmacol., *39*, 636 (1987).
251 A. Hamada, N. Chang, N. Uretzky, and D. D. Miller, J. Med. Chem., *27*, 675 (1984).
252 B. Belleau, U. Gulini, B. Goursalin, and F. R. Ahmed, Canad. J. Chem., *63*, 1268 (1985).
253 J. W. McCubbin and I. H. Page, J. Pharmacol. Exptl. Therap., *105*, 437 (1952).
254 W.-H. Chin, T. H. Klein, and M. E. Wolff, J. Med. Chem., *22*, 119 (1979).
255 D. G. Cooper, R. C. Young, G. J. Durant, and C. R. Ganellin, in: Comprehensive Medicinal Chemistry, C. Hansch, Ed. in chief. Vol. III, J. C. Emmett, Ed. Pergamon, Oxford 1990. Chapter 12.5, pp. 324–421.
256 G. J. Durant, M. E. Parsons, and J. W. Black, J. Med. Chem., *18*, 830 (1975).
257 H. Bretschneider and W. Klötzer, Monatsh. Chem., *87*, 136 (1956).
258 H. Bretschneider, W. Klötzer, and G. Spiteller, Monatsh. Chem., *92*, 128 (1961).
259 R. G. Shepherd, W. E. Taft, and H. M. Krazinski, J. Org. Chem., *26*, 2764 (1961).
260 G. Zbinden, in: Molecular Modification in Drug Design, R. F. Gould, Ed. American Chemical Society, Washington, D. C., 1964, p. 25.
261 M. Pigini, M. Gianella, F. Gualtieri, C. Melchiorne, P. Bolle, and L. Angelucci, Europ. J. Med. Chem., *10*, 29, 33 (1975).
262 R. C. Barrass, D. B. Goult, R. M. Pinder, and M. Sheels, Biochem. Pharmacol., *22*, 2891 (1973).
263 H. Erlenmeyer, J. P. Jung, and E. Sorkin, Helv. Chim. Acta, *29*, 1960 (1946).
264 J. Aeschlimann and M. Reinert, J. Pharmacol. Exptl. Therap. *43*, 413 (1931).
265 H. Casier and R. Verbeke, Arch. intern. pharmacodynamie, *83*, 452 (1950).
266 W. Robertson, J. H. Krushinski, G. D. Pollock, and J. S. Hayes, J. Med. Chem., *31*, 461 (1988).
267 K. Kato, S. Ohkawa, S. Terao, Z. Terashita, and K. Nishikawa, J. Med. Chem., *28*, 287 (1985).
268 R. Johnson, E. G. Nidy, J. W. Aiken, N. J. Crittenden, and R. R. Gorman, J. Med. Chem., *29*, 1461 (1986).
269 W. B. Wright, J. B. Press, R. S. Chan, J. W. Marsico, M. F. Haug, J. Lucas, J. Tauber, and A. S. Tomcufcik, J. Med. Chem., *29*, 523 (1986).
270 G. W. Raiziss, M. Severac, and L. W. Clemence, U. S. Pat. 2476508 (1949).
271 A. L. Tatum and G. A. Cooper, J. Pharmacol. Exptl. Therap., *50*, 198 (1934).
272 W. J. Ehlhardt, B. B. Beaulieu, Jr., and P. Goldman, J. Med. Chem., *31*, 323 (1988).
273 H. Haguchi, Mol. Pharmacol., *13*, 362 (1977).
274 S. Inoue, T. Shamura, T. Tsurvoka, Y. Ogawa, H. Wanatabe, J. Yoshidea, and T. Nuda, Chem. and Pharm. Bull. (Japan), *23*, 2669 (1975).
275 S. J. Norton and E. Sanders, J. Med. Chem., *10*, 961 (1967).
276 R. N. L. Harris and R. Teitel, Austral. J. Chem., *30*, 649 (1977).
277 R. Adams and V. V. Jones, J. Am. Chem. Soc., *69*, 1803 (1947).
278 R. C. Crounse, J. D. Maxwell, and H. Blank, Nature (London), *194*, 694 (1962).

279 J. P. Chambon, P. Feltz, M. Heaulme, S. Restle, R. Schlichter, and C. G. Wermuth, Proc. Natl. Acad. Sci. U. S., *82*, 1802 (1985).

280 H. W. R. Williams, Canad. J. Chem., *54*, 3377 (1976).

281 R. E. Bambury, D. T. Feeley, G. C. Lawton, J. M. Weaver, and J. Wemple, J. Med. Chem., *27*, 1613 (1984).

282 K. Wallenfels, K. Friedrich, J. Rieser, W. Ertle, and H. K. Thieme, Angew. Chem. Internat. Edn., *15*, 261 (1976).

283 C. H. Boehringer, Sohn, U. S. Pat. 4085216.

284 SmithKline Corp., U. S. Pat. 4117128.

285 E. M. Vaughan Williams and P. Polster, Europ. J. Pharmacol., *25*, 241 (1974).

286 N. Claeys, C. Goldenberg, R. Wanderstrick, E. Devay, M. Descamps, G. Delaunois, J. Bauthier, and R. Charlier, Chim. Ther., *9*, 377 (1972).

287 J. Bossert and M. Vater, Naturwissenschaften, *58*, 578 (1971); Drugs of Today, *11*, 154 (1975).

288 Ciba-Geigy Corp., Brit. Pat. 1464324.

289 J. P. Fournier, R. C. Moreau, G. Narcisse, and P. Choay, Europ. J. Med. Chem., *17*, 81 (1982).

290 G. R. Brown and A. J. Foubister, J. Med. Chem., *27*, 79 (1984).

291 J. R. Huff, P. S. Anderson, J. J. Baldwin, B. V. Clineschmidt, J. P. Guare, V. J. Lotti, D. J. Pettibone, W. C. Randall, and J. P. Vacca, J. Med. Chem., *28*, 1756 (1985).

292 B. R. Baker, in Medicinal Chemistry, 3rd edn. A. Burger, Ed. Wiley-Interscience, New York 1970. Chapter 12, pp. 215 ff.

293 G. B. Elion, Science, *244*, 41 (1989).

294 G. B. Elion, A. Kovensky, G. H. Hitchings, E. Metz, and R. W. Rundles, Biochem. Pharmacol., *15*, 863 (1966).

295 R. K. Robins, J. Am. Chem. Soc., *78*, 784 (1956).

296 P. Schmidt and J. Druey, Helv. Chim. Acta, *39*, 986 (1956).

297 W. H. Prusoff and C. D. Ward, Biochem. Pharmacol., *25*, 1233 (1976).

298 R. Duschinsky, E. Pleven, and C. Heidelberger, J. Am. Chem. Soc., *79*, 4559 (1957).

299 C. Heidelberger, Prog. Nucleic Acid Res., *4*, 1 (1965).

300 J. A. Montgomery, T. P. Johnston, and T. F. Shealy, in: Medicinal Chemistry, 3rd. edn. A. Burger, Ed. Wiley-Interscience, New York 1970. Chapter 28, pp. 722–725.

301 J. Sugar and H. E. Kaufman, in: Selective Inhibitors of Viral Functions, W. A. Carter, Ed. CRC Press, Cleveland 1973, p. 295.

302 R. W. Sidwell and J. T. Witkowski, in: Burger's Medicinal Chemistry, M. E. Wolff, Ed. 4th edn. Wiley, New York 1979. Part II, Chapter 23, pp. 546–547.

303 E. R. Walwick, W. K. Roberts, and C. A. Dekker, Proc. Chem. Soc., 84 (1959).

304 T. Y. Shen, H. M. Lewis, and W. C. Ruyle, J. Org. Chem., *30*, 835 (1965).

305 E. J. Hessler, J. Org. Chem., *41*, 1828 (1976).

306 E. DeClercq, J. Descamps, P. Desomer, and A. Holy, Science, *200*, 563 (1978).

307 H. J. Schaeffer, S. Gurwara, R. Vince, and S. Bittner, J. Med. Chem., *14*, 367 (1971).

308 H. J. Schaeffer, L. Beauchamp, P. deMiranda, G. B. Elion, D. J. Bauer, and P. Collins, Nature (London), *272*, 583 (1978).

309 G. B. Elion, P. A. Furman, J. A. Fyfe, P. deMiranda, L. Beauchamp, and J. H. Schaeffer, Proc. Nat. Acad. Sci. U. S., *74*, 5716 (1977).

310 J. T. Witkowski, R. K. Robins, R. W. Sidwell, and L. N. Simon, J. Med. Chem., *15*, 1150 (1972).

311 R. W. Sidwell, J. H. Huffman, G. P. Khare, L. B. Allen, J. T. Witkowski, and R. K. Robins, Science, *177*, 705 (1972).
312 P. C. Strivastava, D. G. Streeter, T. R. Matthews, L. B. Allen, R. W. Sidwell, and R. K. Robins, J. Med. Chem., *19*, 1020 (1976).
313 O. P. Babbar, J. Sci. Ind. Res., *20C*, 216 (1961).
314 O. P. Babbar and B. L. Chowdhury, J. Sci. Ind. Res., *21C*, 312 (1962).

Index Vol. 37

The references of the Subject Index are given in the language of the respective contribution.
Die Stichworte des Sachregisters sind in der jeweiligen Sprache der einzelnen Beiträge aufgeführt.
Les termes repris dans la Table des Matières sont donnés selon la langue dans laquelle l'ouvrage est écrit.

Index of titles
Verzeichnis der Titel
Index des titres
Vol. 1–37 (1959–1991)

Author and paper index
Autoren- und Artikelindex
Index des auteurs et des articles
Vol. 1–37 (1959–1991)

Biologische Oxydation und Reduktion am Stickstoff aromatischer Amino- und Nitroderivate und ihre Folgen für den Organismus *8*, 195 (1965) Stoffwechsel von Arzneimitteln als Ursache von Wirkungen, Nebenwirkungen und Toxizität *15*, 147 (1971)	H. Uehleke
Mode of death in tetanus *19*, 439 (1975)	H. Vaishnava C. Bhawal Y. P. Munjal
Comparative evaluation of amoebicidal drugs *18*, 353 (1974) Comparative efficacy of newer anthelmintics *19*, 166 (1975)	B. J. Vakil N. J. Dalal
Cephalic tetanus *19*, 443 (1975)	B. J. Vakil B. S. Singhal S. S. Pandya P. F. Irami
The effect and usefulness of early intravenous beta blockade in acute myocardial infarction *30*, 71 (1986)	Anders Vedin Claes Wilhelmsson
Methods of monitoring adverse reactions to drugs *21*, 231 (1977) Aspects of social pharmacology *22*, 9 (1978)	J. Venulet
The current status of cholera toxoid research in the United States *19*, 602 (1975)	W. F. Verwey J. C. Guckian J. Craig N. Pierce J. Peterson H. Williams, Jr.
Systemic cancer therapy: Four decades of progress and some personal perspectives *34*, 76 (1990)	Charles L. Vogel
Cell-kinetic and pharmacokinetic aspects in the use and further development of cancerostatic drugs *20*, 521 (1976)	M. von Ardenne
The problem of diphtheria as seen in Bombay *19*, 452 (1975)	M. M. Wagle R. R. Sanzgiri Y. K. Amdekar